KU-505-595

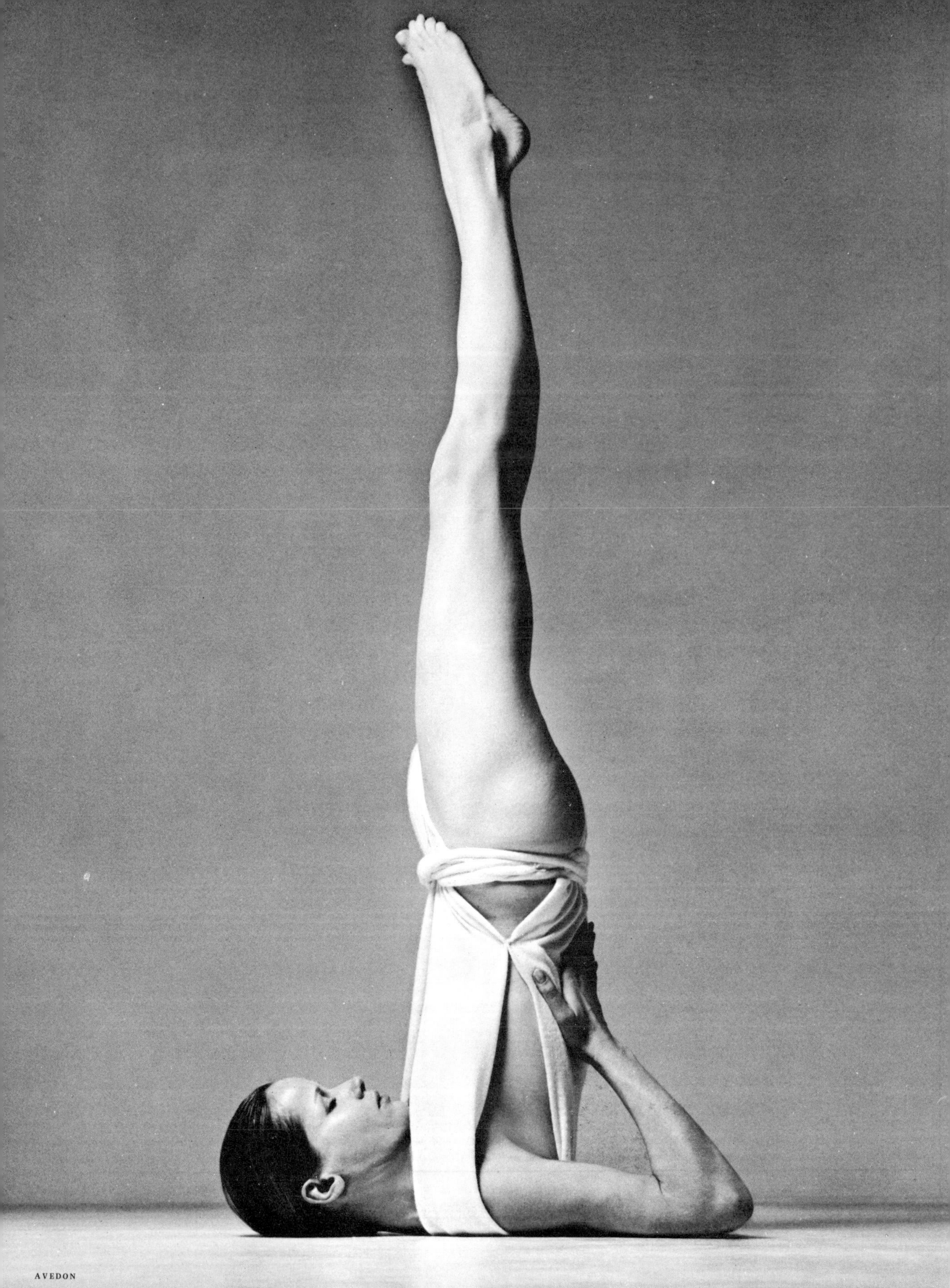

AVEDON

BRONWEN MEREDITH

VOGUE BODY AND BEAUTY BOOK

Book Club Associates, London

For Arabella

This edition published 1978 by Book Club Associates
Reprinted 1979, 1980
By arrangement with Allen Lane

Designed by Paul Bowden
Drawings by Maria Theresa Barlow
Set in Monophoto Photina by
Oliver Burridge Filmsetting Ltd
Colour separations by Newsele Litho Limited
Printed in Great Britain by Butler & Tanner Ltd
Frome and London

PART I THE BASICS

PART II THE AESTHETICS

PART III THE SCIENCES

One of the pleasures of writing this book was having at my disposal all the knowledge and expertise of all the contributors to *Vogue* since it was first published. It was like having a team of invisible collaborators and I wish to thank them all. *Vogue*, under the editorial direction of Alexander Liberman, has always been the first to introduce new ideas and to recognize the need for change in the health and beauty fields as well as in fashion. I particularly wish to express gratitude to Beatrix Miller, editor of British *Vogue*, who from the start supported my concept of the book; also to Barbara Tims who went through my original manuscript with a discerning eye and skilled pen. Alex Kroll, as editor of Condé Nast Books in London, not only kept track of everything – including me – but chose the illustrations. Maria Theresa Barlow needs special thanks for splendidly interpreting my rough sketches. I also wish to thank all the people at Allen Lane who have helped with this book, especially Eleo Gordon and the many professionals who gave precious time to explain the intricacies of their special expertise. Finally, a word of appreciation to my mother who, during the last frantic month, looked after me like a child leaving me free to worry about nothing but finishing this book.

FOREWORD

The pursuit of beauty is not narcissistic, it is an essential way to build up confidence without which there is little achievement in anything. It gives pleasure, it brings it. Beauty, today, is not a perfect face or a certain look – we have left those attitudes far behind. Beauty now is seen in the way a woman protects, reflects and projects her body power and mental energy. Beauty is individuality. It is glowing health and vitality, it is awareness and action, it is science and technology and of course marvellous looks, a perfect skin, a superb body. We are no longer interested in quick cover-up effects but in long range plans to feel and look better. Within your grasp is the accumulated knowledge of years that can provide you with your ideal health and beauty programme: a straightforward guide to the whole health and beauty spectrum bringing you the basics of body and function, of artifices and aesthetics, of scientific and medical influences . . . all adding up to complete self-awareness. Beauty is a science now. You are responsible for your body; your first move starts here. . . .

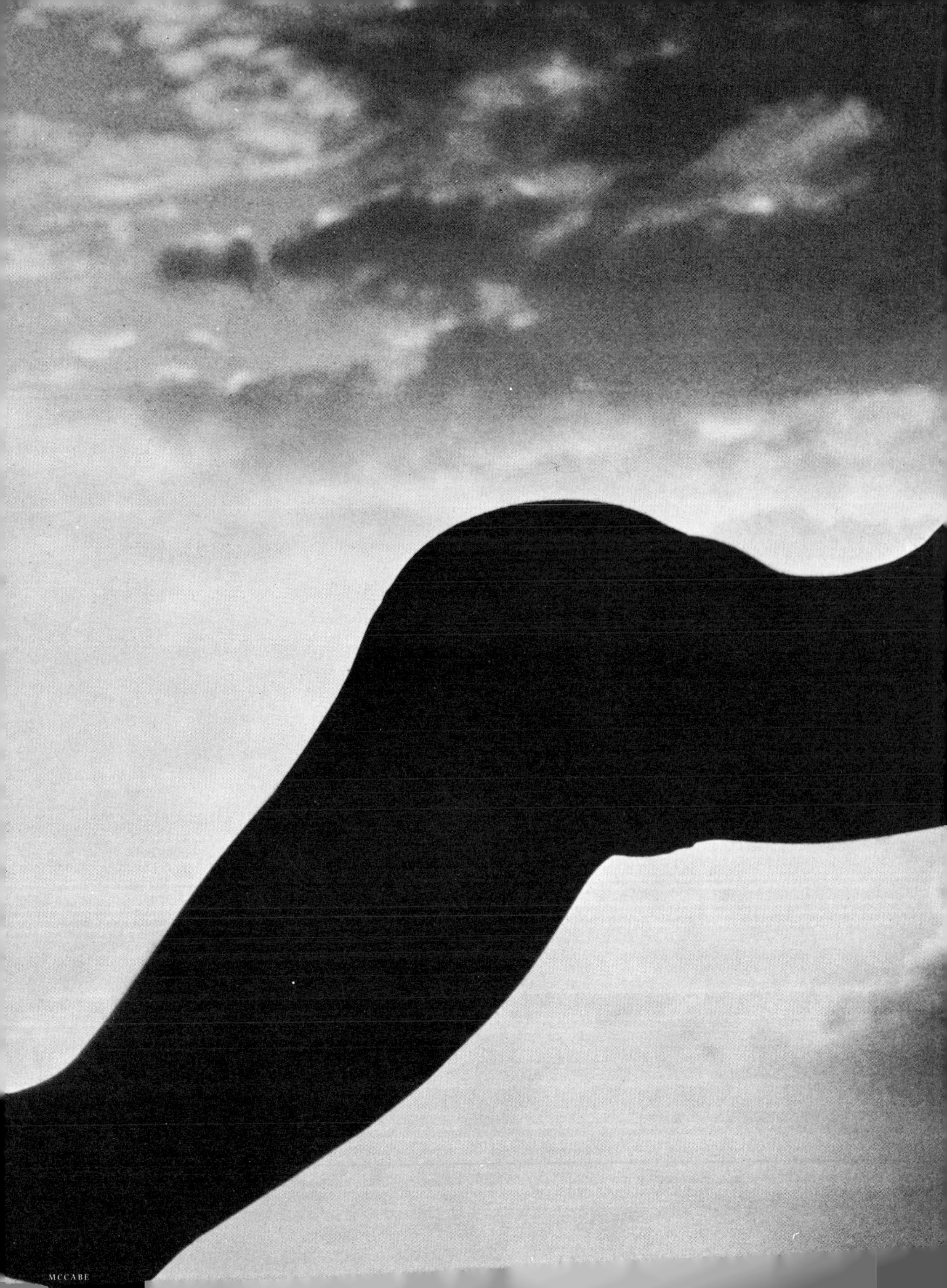

MCCABE

PART I THE BASICS

1

THE BODY

Think of the body as divided into seven systems: bones, brain, nerves, muscles, respiration, circulation, digestion, glands. All are connected and interdependent, though each has a special network of its own.

BONES

The average woman has 206 bones in her body, but not always. She, like Adam, sometimes has an extra pair of ribs. A baby is born with about 350 bones, many of which fuse during the growing years. Bone growth and final size is mostly genetic, but it can be influenced by environment and physical demands. Women usually reach their maximum height at sixteen, but that doesn't mean growth entirely ceases. The vertebral column increases from three to four millimetres between the ages of twenty and thirty. After fifty, stature often diminishes.

The function of bone is diverse. It gives shape and support, it protects certain organs and is an anchor for muscles. Although you may be able to relocate fat and influence muscles nothing can be done to alter this fundamental frame.

The word skeleton comes from a Greek word meaning 'dried bones'. Although one rarely gets an opportunity to see living bones, they are anything but dry. Bones have an outer layer of compact bone tissue that is pinky-white and crowded with tiny openings through which intertwine the network of nerves, arteries, veins and connective tissue. Inside, bones are a deep red with a mesh of spongy material containing that matter vital to life – marrow. Marrow is a combination of fat and tissue which manufactures all the red corpuscles. It also produces other constituents of blood and, most important, is a reservoir of minerals essential not only to the bone itself but to the general health of the body. Calcium and phosphorus are the two main minerals but there are also stores of magnesium, fluoride and chloride. These minerals are not stationary but constantly move on to fortify other areas and need to be replaced. Although rigid, bone is changeable and active.

The skeleton provides both firmness and also extreme flexibility. Some joints move like machinery, others remain locked. Think of what you can do with your thumb and what you can't do with your big toe.

The spinal column is the main bone structure and it supports the whole body. It is very flexible, on the average a little over 2 feet (610 cm.) long and consists of thirty-three vertebrae. These are cylindrical bones with a central canal and strung together. There is a spongy circle of cartilage between each which makes the spine elastic and shock-absorbent. Running down either side are ligaments which help to hold it together.

Attached to the spine is the framework of the chest – twelve pairs of ribs and the breastbone. The ribs are of varying lengths but they all join the spine at the back, curving round to the front where the upper ribs join the breastbone. In this manner they form a protective cage for the heart and lungs, providing ample space for expansion during breathing.

The limbs are attached to the spinal column by special structures – the arms have the shoulder blades, the legs the pelvis. The pelvis is rather like a shell, holding in its strong frame the organs of the abdomen. Freedom of limbs comes from the ball-and-socket joints. The topmost bones of all comprise the skull, where size and placement determine facial features.

BRAIN AND NERVES

The size of the brain has nothing to do with ability. One brain can be twice the size of another without showing any apparent difference in performance. The largest human brains, more than twice normal size, are those of idiots. The brain is a soft lump of 14,000,000 cells and on the surface looks like a jigsaw puzzle fitted together with extreme precision. It usually weighs about 3 pounds (1.5 k.) and is so full of water that it would flop like a jelly if not firmly supported. Anatomically it is symmetrical, but not in performance. Many of its functions are quite one sided. One half of the brain is inclined to be more active and some scientists think this may influence whether one is left- or right-handed.

The forebrain, the cerebrum, is the most important and is over five-sixths of the total. Here is where all higher functions occur – thought, memory and sensory impulses. Brain power is released when a number of factors, physical, mental and social, reinforce one another. The frontal lobe controls muscular movement through a narrow band of cortex which acts as the motor and nerve computer of the body, responding to every single action. An adjacent section receives sensations of warmth, cold and touch; another deals with sound messages. Visual reflexes go through the mid-brain.

The hypothalamus is situated below the cerebrum, mingled with general grey matter. It is an area smaller than a finger joint yet is involved in such diverse operations as balancing, water metabolism, temperature control, appetite, thirst, sleep, fatigue, emotions, weight regulation and sensual responses. Any damage, such as slight pressure from an adjacent tumour, can drastically change body health level, shape and mental attitude. In its control of temperature, the hypothalamus constantly regulates heat loss and gain. Heat is usually gained through metabolic or physical activity and sometimes from the environment, though this is normally cooler than the body. Shivering, which is simply involuntary activity of the skeletal muscles, lowers the temperature. Normal temperature is 98.4 degrees Fahrenheit (36.6 degrees Centigrade). Heat is lost through radiation, convection, conduction and by evaporation through the skin.

The nervous system is closely allied to the brain. The nerve centre of the body runs through the spinal cord. Messages travel as electrical impulses, usually following the quickest route to the spinal cord, and are transmitted from there up to the brain. There are forty-three pairs of nerves; twelve go to and from the brain itself, the rest go to and from the spinal cord. Any disturbance of the spinal cord's balance can have far reaching effects. Nerves go two ways – in and out of the brain. Those passing information to the brain are sensory nerves, those taking messages out are insensory.

MUSCLES

Muscles comprise 36% of female body weight. There are two kinds, voluntary and involuntary, and they perform as the names imply. Involuntary muscles are lighter and function without any indication of their activity. They are hidden away in the body and controlled by the involuntary nervous system. It is impossible to consciously set them in motion or stop them. Their continuous release and contraction is slow and rhythmic; through this action several functions are performed such as pushing food through the digestive channels and pumping the blood.

There are 556 muscles, each consisting of many individual fibres. The longest are 1½ inches (3–4 cm.) and some are less than a millimetre. All muscles exist at birth and grow in size without increasing in number. Strength comes after expansion of each fibre as muscles are made to work. Muscles also have connective tissue which helps to bind the fibres together and secures them to the bones. These take the form of tendons, sinews and bursae – pockets of fluid acting as pulleys at some of the joints. Most muscles are attached by a tendon at just one end, but occasionally at both.

The impulses causing a muscle fibre to twitch are electrical, mechanical or chemical. The time between the arrival of a stimulus at a fibre and the start of contraction is between two and four thousandths of a second.

RESPIRATION

Respiration is more than inhaling and exhaling, it is a very organized method of distributing oxygen around the body. All cells need oxygen to survive. A relaxed person breathes in and out some ten to fourteen times a minute drawing in between 9 and 12 pints (4.5–6 l.) of air. We carry meagre reserves of oxygen so for any physical activity there is an immediate need for more air. Strenuous exercise can require as much as 20 gallons (90 l.) of air a minute with only a second between each breath.

Breathing is controlled by the diaphragm, a large flat muscle separating the chest from the abdomen. It contracts, moving downward – ⅔ of an inch (8 mm.) in quiet breathing, almost 3 inches (7.5 cm.) in deep breathing. This movement increases the capacity of the chest, while at the same time the ribs shift from a sloping position to a more horizontal one. Air rushes in to fill the vacuum in the lungs. For exhalation, the diaphragm relaxes and is pushed upward by abdominal muscles; the ribs return to their former position.

Air is taken in through the nostrils or the mouth or both. It is cleansed by the hairs at the entrance of the nose and by the thin hairs deeper inside. The mucous cells of the nose help to humidify the air, making it less irritating to the delicate structures inside the chest. This is why it is preferable to breathe through the nose rather than the mouth. Air then enters the pharynx, a fibro-muscular passage about 5 inches (13 cm.) long; food also passes down it. Then food and air passages separate, the air going through the larynx at the front of the neck and into the windpipe (trachea), a 5-inch (13-cm.) long elastic tube. Where there's a bump on your breastbone, the windpipe divides into two main bronchi, each subdividing into much smaller bronchioles which in turn divide into many small ducts that lead into the lungs and culminate in alveoli.

The lungs are a pair of large, spongy half cones almost filling the chest area and consisting entirely of air sacs. Together they weigh about two and a half pounds, the right one usually heavier than the left. Architecturally they are rather poor as they have the same entrance as exit. This means there is usually only a partial interchange of gas and about five-sixths of the air present in the lungs is still there when the next breath is taken. Hence recommendations to breathe deeply for good health, as only in this manner is there a chance of exchanging stale air; some molecules can stay in the lungs for life.

It is at the alveoli of the lungs where gaseous diffusion most easily occurs. Each one is covered with a tracery of blood capillaries through which blood cells pass giving off carbon dioxide and taking up the oxygen just breathed in. The two ventricles of the heart are responsible for the blood flow; the right one pumps its blood into the capillary network of the lungs, the left one pumps the oxygenized blood into the capillary network of the body.

Respiration can cause some oddities. Laughter is actually deep breathing followed by spasmodic breathings out. Maybe this way of really cleaning out the lungs is responsible for the belief that if you laugh you are healthy. Yawning is a prolonged deep breath to give the body a reviving and plentiful supply of oxygen. Sighing involves extra breathing-out. Hiccups are spasmodic inhalations which end in a click due to a sudden closing of the vocal cords; either the diaphragm is at fault or the nerves controlling it.

CIRCULATION

On average there are 10 pints (5 l.) of blood in your body constantly being pumped through the circulatory system by the heart. Blood accounts for about 10% of body weight. It is a tissue consisting of red cells, white cells, platelets and plasma, with the plasma occupying a little more than half the volume.

Red corpuscles contain haemoglobin, which picks up oxygen from the lungs and delivers it to the tissues; when carrying oxygen, blood and arteries are bright red. White corpuscles are lighter and fairly transparent; they are less numerous than the red and more varied; they primarily combat infection by their mobility and ability to ingest or absorb bacteria and other foreign elements. Too many white cells, however, can be as disastrous as too few; leukaemia is an overproduction. Blood platelets are smaller than the corpuscles but much more numerous. They influence the clotting of the blood, keeping us from bleeding to death from a nick or cut. They take care of immediate needs at the site of injury. Plasma is not made up of cells; it is 90% water and the balance is proteins, salts and most of the blood cargo such as nutrients, hormones, waste-products and antibodies. Quite often an ill person needs the plasma more than the corpuscles.

Blood's most important job is transportation. During all its travels it carries water, vital to every cell; it takes oxygen from the lungs and carbon dioxide to them; it carries nutrients to the cells and waste products away; it is a distributor of hormones, a circulator of antibodies and it transports heat from the hot to the cool regions. Blood plays a part in every body function and reflects its condition; of all the substances used for testing, blood is by far the most indicative of your health.

The main pumping station, the heart, is the size of a fist and weighs less than a pound (½ k.). It doesn't lie entirely on the left side of the chest as is often supposed, but is fairly near the centre with about one-third of its bulk over on the right. It has two pumps, each having a similar output; one sends blood through the pulmonary system, the other through the rest of the body. It beats a two-fold sound, roughly seventy times a minute, or four times for each normal breath. With increased physical demand its beat quickens and it pumps blood faster.

Blood pressure is the pressure of blood in the arteries together with a measure of the tension in the arterial wall produced by the blood forced through from the heart. It depends on the output of the heart (systolic pressure) and the resistance to flow by smaller arteries (diastolic pressure). The former is always greater than the latter, and the two are always recorded in that order. An average combination in the twenties would be 120:80. It increases with age and should be frequently checked. Lack of blood pressure can be more rapidly fatal than excess of it. Fainting occurs when there is a short-lived decrease in blood flow to the brain; a stoppage, no matter how brief, would cause brain damage.

A body can lose a quarter of its blood without any apparent severe consequences. One pint (6 dl.) can be given at a transfusion and you can donate a pint (6 dl.) of blood three or four times a year without ill effects.

DIGESTION

Food provides energy and building matter for the body; digestion is the automatic process that converts it into usable units, and storage ones if necessary. The digestive system consists of the alimentary canal through which food passes; it begins at the mouth and ends at the rectum and can be anywhere from 20 to 30 feet (6 to 9 m.) long, twisting and winding to fit in the space provided. Accessory organs are the liver, kidneys, pancreas and spleen.

From the moment food is eaten, it can take from fifteen to twenty-five hours to pass through the body. It is swallowed by automatic contractions in the oesophagus (the foodpipe from mouth to stomach) that propel it onward. The wave of contraction is at the rate of an inch or so per second and is so effective that fluids will get to the stomach even if one is upside down.

On entering the stomach, the proteins, carbohydrates and fats are broken down and changed into smaller particles of protein, glucose, amino acids, fatty acids and glycerine. This is both a chemical and mechanical process; the walls secrete digestive juices and rhythmically contract, causing food units to move into the duodenum, the first part of the small intestine. The stomach's acidity is often a problem, caused by living tissue producing fairly strong hydrochloric acid; this is sometimes diluted and neutralized by food components, but the stomach walls are always protected by alkaline juices.

Practically all digestion is carried out in the small and large intestines and a great proportion of actual absorption of food takes place through the walls. The extraction of valuable food elements is done by enzymes.

LIVER: The largest single organ in the body, it weighs about 4 pounds (2 k.). One cannot live without the liver. It is made of soft, red-brown tissue divided into lobes and covered with a tough fibrous coat. A remarkable feature is that it has a double blood supply: it receives fresh arterial blood and also blood-carrying products of digestion from the intestines. At rest a quarter of the body's blood is in the liver, though a pint or two (6–12 dl.) can leave when exercise is taken. The liver is the central organ of metabolism; its functions are formidable and listed as five hundred. It is capable of replacing its own tissue and its powers of self regeneration are very high.

KIDNEYS: Each kidney is a collection of filter units that absorb virtually everything small from the blood, returning to it what is required. The kidneys eliminate waste products with the formation of urine, regulate salt and liquid intake of the body and maintain the slight alkalinity of body fluids.

PANCREAS AND SPLEEN: Pour crucial digestive juices – 1 to 1½ pints (6 to 9 dl.) daily – into the duodenum. One part of the pancreas is pure gland, secreting insulin.

GLANDS

Some glands, such as those of the skin and digestive tract, produce secretions which have an effect only where they are released; these are called exocrine glands. In contrast, the endocrine glands manufacture substances called hormones which pass directly into the blood stream and affect areas far removed from their place of origin. The secretions are fairly simple compounds many of which are now synthesized. They are effective in very small amounts and are regulators of body processes controlling growth, development, size, weight, sexual activity, reproduction and temperament.

THE PITUITARY: Situated at the base of the brain, it is the master gland. It influences the rest of the endocrine system as well as performing specific functions such as regulating growth, controlling physical and mental development, acting on the sex organs, affecting menstruation, blood pressure and sight.

THE THYROID: Found in the neck, it organizes the body's supply of oxygen. It also secretes an iodine-rich hormone, thyroxine, which works together with one from the pituitary. If the thyroid gland is defective (often due to lack of iodine) metabolism slows down often resulting in overweight and lethargy; it can lead to goitre. Excess secretion causes nervousness, irritability and protruding eyeballs.

THE PARATHYROIDS: Either side of the thyroid, they control levels of calcium and phosphorus.

THE ADRENALS: These affect the nervous system, the emotions and influence the sex glands. They are found above the kidneys. Adrenalin is one hormonal secretion; it stimulates the heart, quickens the pulse and causes a rise in blood sugar. It is released through fear and can cause anger. Cortisone is the other hormone.

THE PANCREAS: Part of the pancreas is used for digestion, the other part is a gland called the Island of Langerhans. This produces the hormone insulin which regulates the sugar level in the blood and the conversion of sugar into energy and heat. Imbalances cause diabetes or hypoglycaemia.

THE GONADS: The sex glands found in the ovaries; they produce oestrogen and progesterone which together regulate the reproductive cycle. A small quantity of male hormones are also produced; if excessive, male characteristics result.

BODY TYPE

Physique varies from person to person and any classification of figure types can only be a general guide. It is important to recognize that there are variations in frame structure, and to acknowledge that you can never change your body type. You have to learn to keep within its range, work within its possibilities. By the early twenties, the dimensions of the skeleton are settled and the appropriate muscle and fat covering is determined. Everything is a matter of proportion, judged three-dimensionally and often in truer perspective from a side view. Height has nothing to do with body type.

There are three basic shapes: ectomorph, mesomorph and endomorph and there is a degree of overlapping but no moving from one group to another. A fat ectomorph is a fat person, not an endomorph; while the slimness of a mesomorph in no way resembles the ideal of the endomorph.

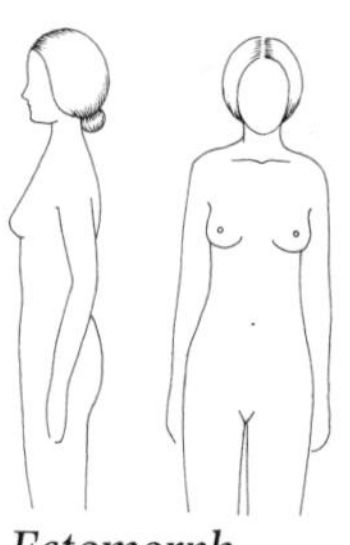

Ectomorph

ECTOMORPH: Small frame in width and depth, side view slender; narrow shoulders, often still narrower hips; ideally thin with some bust shaping, without much muscle or fat.

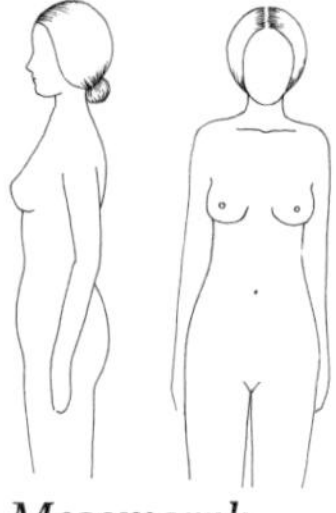

Mesomorph

MESOMORPH: Medium to large frame, ranging from athletic to rounded but always with depth and a certain degree of narrowness through ribcage, waist and hips; sometimes broad-shouldered and a forceful shape; ideally with a lot of muscle and bone, not much fat, controlled hips.

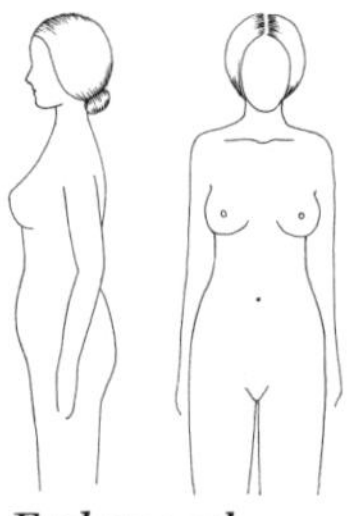

Endomorph

ENDOMORPH: A heavy build but not necessarily a large frame; rounded on all sides with a chunky middle section; shoulders often narrower than hips; ideally well-covered without excess fat and trim muscles.

BODY POSTURE

Good posture gives a better figure instantly; it is good exercise and the basis of figure beauty. The way you carry and move your body influences its shape; the effect is slow but steady, and it can work for or against you.

POSTURE EXERCISES

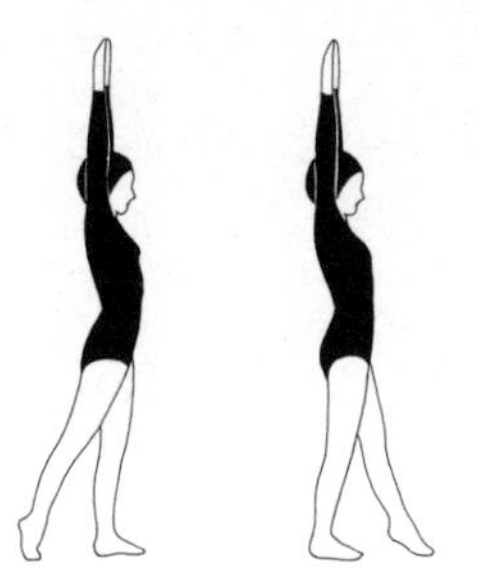

1. *Walking Stretch*

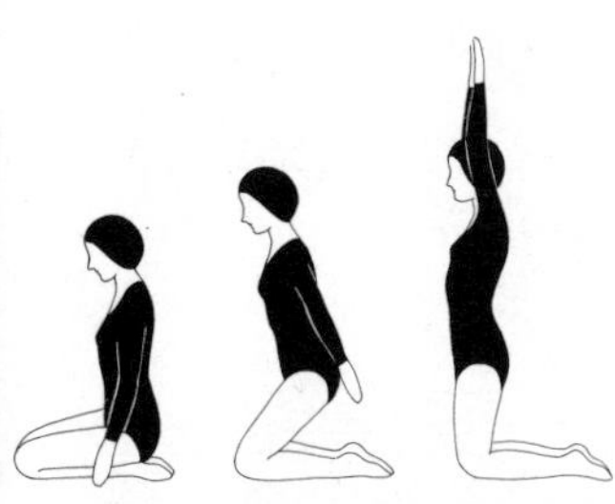

2. *Kneeling Stretch*

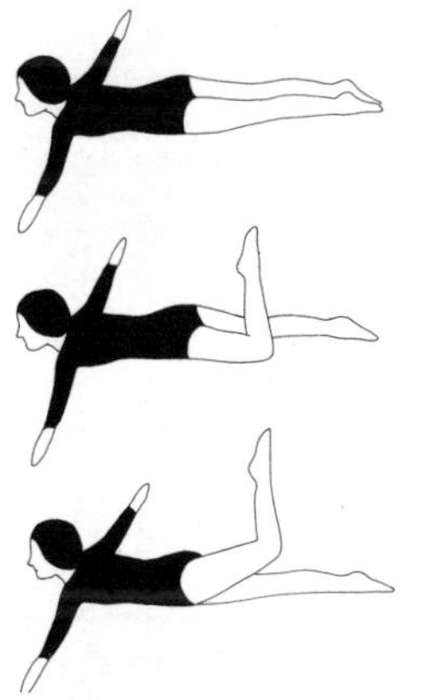

3 *Lying Stretch*

Many figure faults have their origin in faulty posture; aches and body fatigue too. When the spine is carried correctly, it has an easy alignment; when incorrectly held it gives a hollow back, squashes the vertebrae together, sets up friction and tension, and eventually can cause joint thickening and bone displacement.

The habit of good posture can mean a young-looking figure for life; it creates an impression of vitality, confidence and attractiveness.

Standing – Your spine is a long cord; imagine there is a thread running through it and it is being pulled up tautly from above your head. This lifts and stretches straight the whole body; it also makes you feel much lighter and springier. Pull in stomach, tuck buttocks under, chest high, shoulders back but relaxed and pulling the arm sockets downwards, head in alignment with chin parallel to the ground. When picking something up, bend from the knees with one foot slightly in front of the other, bottom tucked under. Good posture strengthens the supportive muscles and through habit they automatically keep firm and in place.

Walking – Check alignment before you start and be sure toes point straight ahead. Relax arms, allowing them to swing, following the body naturally and with ease. Movement should come from the thighs, not the hips; as you walk breathe deeply and slowly to the count of four in, four out. Keep the back straight, up and down hill, up and down steps, lifting and lowering yourself by using thigh muscles. Don't lean forward with buttocks stuck out at the back.

Sitting – Before sitting, be sure your back is to the chair and one leg almost touching it, the other a little in front. Keeping the back straight and head aligned, lower yourself by bending the knees. Legs look better together, straight in front or slightly to the side.

1. Align back, hold arms straight above head, thumbs hooked; pull arms back without arching spine. Walk around the room for two minutes, breathing in deeply to the count of four, out to the count of four.

2. Kneel, sitting on heels, back straight, arms at side; using thigh muscles, keeping back straight and bottom under, rise to kneeling position bringing arms up over head; return to heel sitting; never arch back. *10 times.*

3. Lie on stomach, arms stretched out, palms down, shoulders flat, head slightly raised. Bend left leg at knee to a right angle; keeping ribcage firmly on floor, move bent leg across straight one, aiming to touch the floor with the knee; at first it is impossible. *6 times with each leg.*

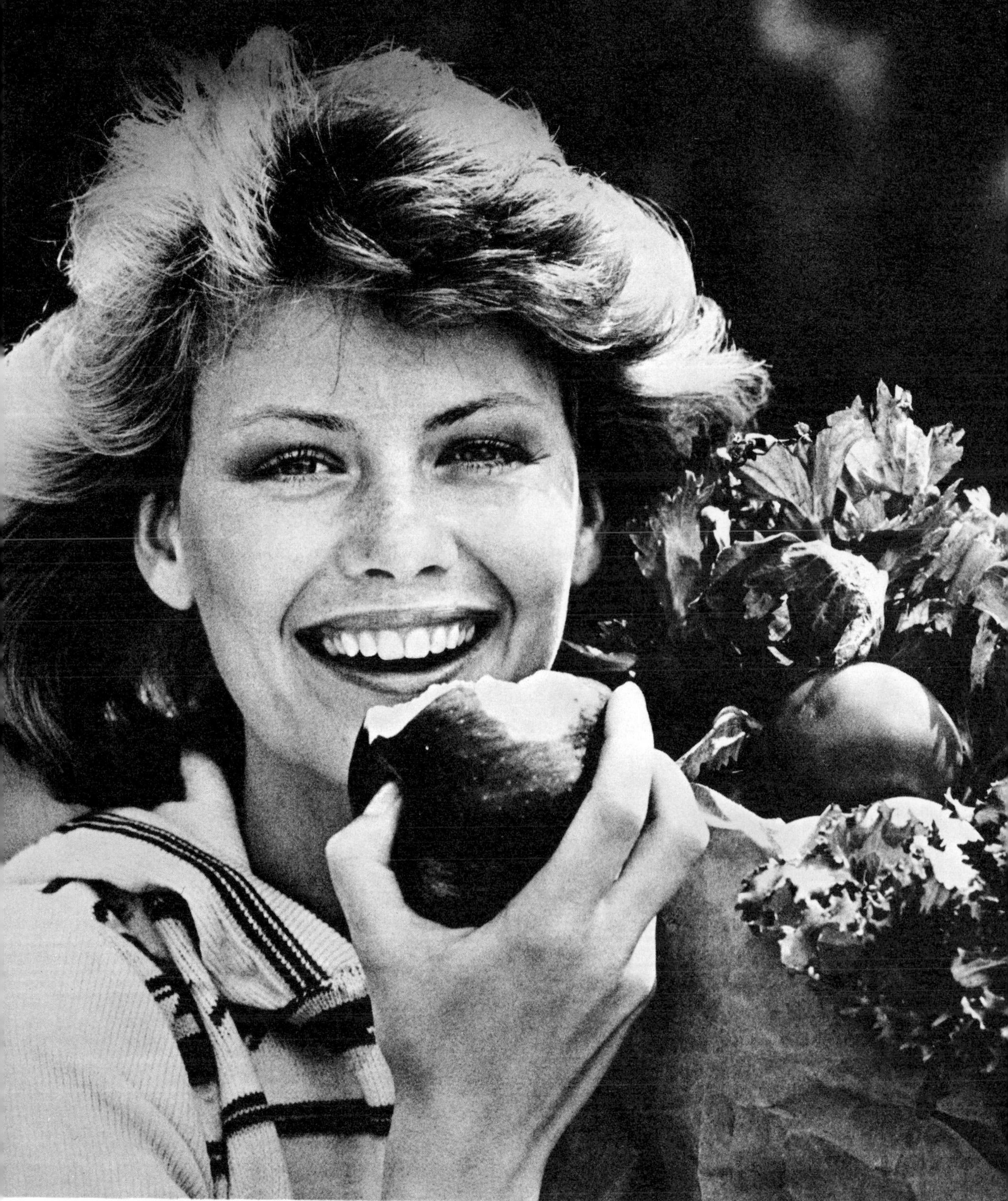

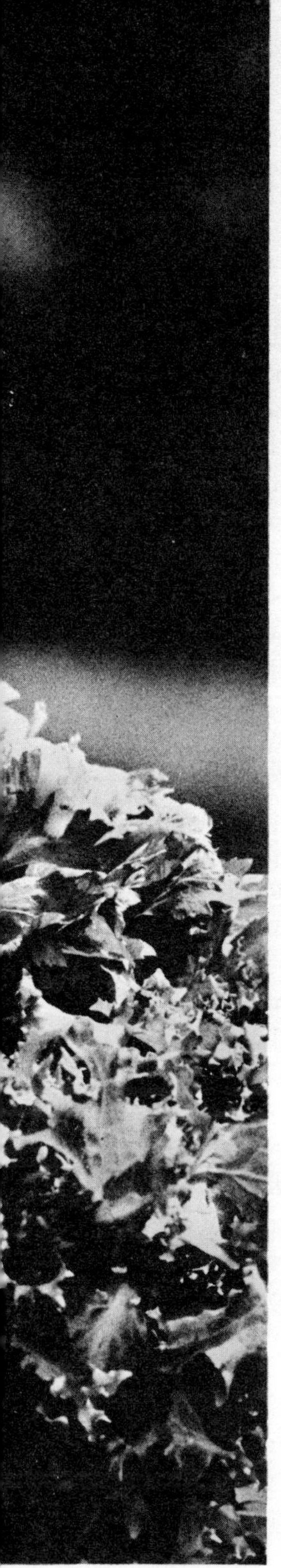

2

NUTRITION

Nutrition is a comparatively new science. We are warned constantly about the adverse effects of refining, processing, of additives and of pollution but there is disagreement on certain points, the main one being health food versus regular food. People eat health food for many reasons: because they like plain good food, because they are worried about chemical additives either in the growing or in the processing of food, or because they feel that food is directly linked to how they look and feel. But there are alternatives to the specialized health shop. There is enough fresh food around to supply all the nutrients anyone normally needs. This is the rational way to nutrition and it takes only a basic knowledge of food constituents, their preservation and utilization, to work out a conscientious diet. It is being aware of food values that matters, so that you do not unconsciously give your body worthless foods – or worse, poisonous ones. A lot is ordinary common sense:

Fresh is best.
Eat plenty of vegetables and fruit, raw when possible.
Certain manufactured, processed or refined food should be avoided.
Sugar and all its derivatives should be cut down to a minimum, preferably cut out.
Eat foods rich in fibre (formerly known as roughage).
Eat less fat.

We should eat as much wholesome, fresh, uncontaminated food as possible. It is the best way to get essential vitamins and minerals. Most of the food we eat has been tampered with in some way; the goodness taken out by refining and processing, chemicals added to prolong shelf life, stabilize, preserve, flavour, colour, sweeten, thicken – all of which may please the eye and the taste, but not the stomach and health.

Be wary of anything white – white flour, bread, pastries, rice, sugar. White means a blank, that most nourishment has been taken out and all sorts of synthetic things put in. Wholegrain cereals, flour, bread and brown rice should replace this fortified white stodge.

Sugar is the number one enemy of good nutrition and sugar supplies about 20 per cent of an average diet in the Western world.

Sugar was unknown to man until 200 years ago, so the body handles it as a foreign substance. In nature sugar is packaged with vitamins and minerals – in fruit as fructose and in vegetables as starch. The refined product is straight sucrose, which the body absorbs much faster than natural sugars, and because it is so similar to blood sugar which has already been metabolized into glucose, it escapes the body's processing action. The body is forced to use its vitamins and minerals and acids to fight the invasion, and this surge of activity can lower blood sugar and body energy levels leaving one tired, mentally slow, irritable, and susceptible to disease. The odd sweet or chocolate bar gives an initial spurt due to acceleration of metabolism, but shortly afterwards you are more depleted than ever. Substitute honey for sugar; brown sugar is next best.

Fruit and vegetables should make up the highest proportion of your diet. They can supply all necessary vitamins and minerals. Wash thoroughly but not overmuch. Eat skins whenever possible, they are often the richest part.

Eat less fat. Evidence is conflicting on this issue but it seems reasonable to keep it to a minimum. This means cutting a lot of fat off meat, restricting butter, using unsaturated fats and vegetable oils. It does not necessarily mean skimmed milk and cottage cheese – that is a personal choice.

The missing ingredient in many diets is fibre. It was once called roughage and considered essential to the proper working of the bowels. Overlooked over the last twenty years, it is now thought to be directly related to the high incidence of colon-rectal cancer, also to the increased prevalence of diabetes, gallstones, appendicitis, varicose veins, haemorrhoids and obesity. Yet fibre passes virtually unchanged through our intestines and is excreted as waste matter.

Fibre is the structural part of a plant, the connective tissue that supports the cells – leaves, stems, seeds, flowers, fruits, bulbs, roots and tubers are all sources of fibre. In itself it doesn't contain nourishment, but it is believed that its bulk is needed to provide a smooth intestinal voyage for other nutrients. What is known is that a high-fibre diet takes longer to consume and you are more likely to reach a point of satiation before you eat too much. Also it takes a lot of chewing, therefore more saliva and gastric juices are produced which aid in the digestion of other nutrients.

Again fruit and vegetables are the main suppliers of fibre, and best eaten raw with their skins, or lightly cooked. Whole grains in cereals and flours are good for fibre and for other reasons; bran, a very good source, can be taken in water, sprinkled on other foods or made into bread.

When working out a nutritious diet think in terms of vegetables, fruits, proteins, grains (the carbohydrate group) and fats in that order of importance.

PROTEINS: Primarily for building and repairing body tissue and helping to counteract daily wear and tear. Essential to life, they satisfy hunger and have so many functions it would be impossible to list them all. A few of the more important are: ability to build hormones and enzymes which aid in energy production; digestion of food and excretion from the tissues and body; the making of haemoglobin within the red corpuscles; maintaining the acid-alkaline balance of the body; assisting in clotting the blood; forming antibodies to fight infection and disease.

Proteins are found in flesh foods, dairy products (eggs and milk are the best source of all), soya beans and nuts, grains (especially wheatgerm) and some vegetables.

CARBOHYDRATES: Provide energy for physical and mental exertion by supplying immediate calories; they assist in the assimilation and digestion of other foods. A deficiency leads to low energy level, poor health and mental depression. There are three forms of carbohydrates — sugars, starches and cellulose. The sugar and starch are converted to glucose for energy; excess not spent as energy is quickly stored as fat. In an effort to burn up this excess, the body uses extra vitamin B, thus depriving other organs. The cellulose carbohydrates (a large part of fruit and vegetables) have no energy value but provide the fibre necessary to regulate the bowels. The best carbohydrates are found in vegetables, fruits, whole grain flours and cereals. Acceptable sugar carbohydrates are honey, blackstrap molasses and dried raisins. Unacceptable sugar and starch carbohydrates are the refined sugars, flours, cereals and breads.

FATS: Provide a delayed source of energy and act as carriers for fat-soluble vitamins. Fats also make calcium available to body tissues, thus promoting growth. They prevent the skin from becoming dry. It is important to have fatty deposits to protect the vital organs and a layer under the skin preserves heat and protects the body against cold. A deficiency of fats can lead to a deficiency of vitamins, and to skin disorders. Excess means obesity and indigestion. There are two types: saturated fats which are hard at room temperature and come mostly from animal sources; and unsaturated fats, usually liquid and from vegetable sources. Some nutritionists say it doesn't matter whether one has animal or vegetable fat, while others point out that hard animal fats create high cholesterol content in the blood. Play safe and limit animal fats like butter and solid unsaturated fats such as margarine and be liberal with the liquid vegetable oils – olive, corn, wheatgerm, sunflower, sesame, avocado and peanut. They all contain linoleic acid which is particularly beneficial to the skin.

There are no wonder foods but there are some foods that contain a particularly concentrated amount of vitamins and minerals. They include honey, brewers' yeast, blackstrap molasses, wheatgerm, yoghourt, powdered skimmed milk and sunflower seeds.

COOKING

A few basic rules are important: no frying in additional fat; meat, poultry and game can be cooked in its own fat or with a little oil (always vegetable oil, avoid butter) or roasted, braised or boiled. When cooking vegetables use a minimum of water and cook for the minimum of time otherwise vitamins and minerals are destroyed. Don't add chemicals such as bicarbonate of soda, use a few drops of lemon juice instead. Learn to bake with wholegrain flours and sugar substitutes.

SELECTION AND SERVINGS

Constantly vary vegetables and fruits, consulting the vitamin and mineral listings to see which are most nutritious. Balance the flesh and dairy products – eggs for breakfast, cheese for lunch, meat for dinner, for example. This is not a diet for weight loss but be sensible and keep to moderate portions. Eat raw fibre food first, it fills you up. An average meat serving should be about 20 grammes. A vegetable serving should be about a cup, the same for rice or other grains. One large baked potato or three new boiled ones. Salads and raw vegetables in any quantity but not too much fruit because of its high sugar content: one apple, orange or banana, a small bowl of berries, a slice of melon, half a grapefruit.

THE MAINTENANCE DIET

This is the blueprint for a daily eating plan that ensures that all the protein, vitamins and minerals, with the right amount of energy foods, are consumed. It concentrates on healthy, wholesome foods and is not at all meagre. It is a preventive health measure as well as one that provides a high degree of energy and helps to keep weight at a constant level. Count calories if you like but it is really not necessary if you keep to the servings suggested. A day's intake should average 2,300 calories, the number needed to balance energy output.

PROTEIN GROUP – 20% OF TOTAL

meats: beef, veal, lamb, pork, ham, bacon, liver, kidney, heart, brains, sweetbreads, tripe
poultry: chicken, turkey, duck, goose, guinea fowl
game: venison, pheasant, quail, rabbit
fish: fresh and salt water varieties, shellfish
dairy products: eggs, cheese, yoghourt, milk
nuts: almonds, Brazil nuts, peanuts, walnuts, pecans
vegetables: avocados, soya beans, lentils
grains: barley, oatmeal, rice, wheatgerm, wholegrain flours, brewers' yeast

VEGETABLE GROUP – 65% OF TOTAL, TOGETHER WITH FRUIT

leafy vegetables: asparagus, artichokes, broccoli, cabbage, cauliflower, celery, chicory, endive, kale, spinach, lettuce, watercress
root vegetables: onions, radishes, potatoes, beetroot, carrots
fruit vegetables: tomatoes, peppers, aubergines, courgettes, cucumbers, marrows, pumpkins, squashes

FRUIT GROUP

citrus: lemons, oranges, grapefruits, tangerines
orchard: apples, pears, plums, apricots, peaches, cherries, grapes
berry: raspberries, strawberries, bilberries, cranberries, gooseberries
tropical: mangoes, bananas, pineapples, papayas, cantaloups, melons

GRAIN AND CEREAL GROUP – 10% OF TOTAL

Wholegrain flours and breads, oatmeal, barley, brown rice, wheatgerm, bran.

FAT GROUP – 5% OF TOTAL

Unsaturated fats such as margarine, limited butter, all vegetable oils.

DAILY FORMULA

Breakfast:

Generally considered essential, as your blood sugar level is low in the morning and a good breakfast will get you going. Some protein must be eaten.

fresh fruit or unsweetened juice
protein – egg, cheese, fish or meat (not less than 20 grammes)
slice of wholewheat bread or toast with butter, honey or home-made preserves or wholegrain cereal such as oatmeal or muesli
coffee or tea.

Lunch:

This is the time to eat raw foods such as salads combined with some protein, but if it's more convenient to have the main meal at midday, reverse dinner menu – nutritionally it doesn't make any difference.

fresh salad or raw vegetables
protein – egg, cheese, fish or meat
wholewheat bread, toast or roll
dessert – yoghourt or fresh fruit
coffee, tea or glass of wine.

Dinner:

This is the main meal of the day, it should be leisurely and can be many courses. Start with something fresh.

salad or fresh fruit or crudités
home-made soup
protein – meat, fish, game or poultry
cooked vegetables – always include one leafy green variety
choice of potatoes, rice or pasta
dessert – fruit, yoghourt, cheese or gelatine with fruit
2 glasses wine coffee or tea.

FLAVOURINGS: All natural herbs; limited salt, preferably sea salt.
SWEETENERS: No white sugars; use honey, natural brown sugar or molasses.
DRESSINGS: For salads, oil and vinegar with added herbs and mustard, home-made mayonnaise; avoid creamy synthetic dressings.
SAUCES: Limit those containing flour or cornstarch; use no sugar.

SNACKS: Fresh fruits and vegetables or their juice; cheese and other protein titbits. No sweet biscuits or cakes.

BEVERAGES: Four glasses of water a day, and when possible sparkling mineral water. Limited wine and spirits; coffee, tea.

VITAMINS

Vitamins are not forms of energy or builders themselves but they regulate metabolism and help convert fat and carbohydrates into energy. They also help to repair tissues. Though each of the vitamins has specific functions within the body, they work as a team, which means that if one vitamin is deficient, it may well affect the efficiency of the others.

You cannot test for vitamin deficiency. Only when it is at the extreme stage do visible symptoms occur in the blood chemistry. So how much vitamin should be supplemented and on what grounds? A new branch of science called orthomolecular medicine uses large doses of vitamin supplements in the treatment of disease. This megavitamin (the name for huge doses) therapy cites success stories such as vitamin C as a barrier against some virus infections, and vitamin E as an aid in heart ailments and in retarding the ageing process. Megavitamins do not have an overall seal of approval despite reasonable evidence to support the claims. Some nutritionists point out that overdoses of certain vitamins can have bad side effects. However, there are strong indications that vitamins may be our best protection against environmental stress and pollutants.

Vitamins fall into two groups: those soluble in fat (A, D, E and K) which generally are stored in the body and do not require daily replacement, and those soluble in water (C and B complex) which must be supplied each day as excess is excreted in the urine. The fat soluble ones are measured in International Units (a tiny measurement) and the water soluble ones in milligrammes (mg) which is one thousandth of a gramme. Below are itemized the most important vitamins, indicating their best sources and their effect on the body. New vitamins are being discovered and named, e.g. P, Q, U, B-15 and B-17 (laetrile), but their properties and functions are not fully formulated, nor their claims supported (e.g. laetrile in the treatment of cancer). If you take your vitamins from fresh natural sources every day you should receive an adequate supply. It is almost impossible to get an overdose. Vitamin supplements are essential if you are without fresh foods and take care not to destroy vitamin content in processed foods by exposure to toxins, light, etc.

VITAMIN A (RETINOL)

Function: Maintains a healthy complexion and helps keep skin in good condition. Promotes good eye-sight and is essential to the formation of visual purple, a substance which adapts the eye to darkness. Protects surface tissues of the respiratory tract. Helps to repair body tissues and skeletal growth.
Good source: Alfalfa sprouts, apricots, broccoli, butter, carrots, chicken liver, cod liver oil, dandelion greens, eggs, kale, kidneys, lamb's liver, mangoes, papayas, parsley, peppers (hot red), spinach, watercress.
Deficiency results: Inflammation of the eyes and inability to adjust to darkness. Dryness and premature ageing of the skin. Aggravation of the respiratory system that leads to infections.
Overdose results: Loss of appetite, headaches, hair loss and aching bones.
Destroyed by: Exposure to sunlight can cause serious loss of vitamin A, although it is not destroyed by cooking; air pollution and watching T.V. have adverse affects; it is not well absorbed if taken in conjunction with excessive mineral oil.
Daily need: 5,000 International Units. It is stored in the liver so daily intake is not absolutely essential.

VITAMIN B COMPLEX

There are 13 separate vitamins which should be taken together in the correct proportion because a large dose of one may cause a deficiency of the others. It is impossible to work this out for oneself but in a fresh food diet nature does it for you. Synthetic vitamin supplements are accurately balanced. All these vitamins dissolve in water and any excess is excreted so it is essential to replace them daily. This is not always easy as refining flours and cereals removes almost all of them and large amounts are destroyed by light and heat during cooking. Extra B vitamins are required when under stress, by pregnant women and alcoholics. Best sources for the whole complex are: green leafy vegetables, brewers' yeast, whole grains and offal including liver and kidney.

VITAMIN B-1 (THIAMINE)

Function: Necessary for conversion of carbohydrates into glucose for energy. Important for smooth functioning of nervous system, heart, liver.
Good source: Alfalfa sprouts, asparagus, Brazil nuts, brewers' yeast, brown rice (not white), haricot beans, lamb's liver, muesli, rolled oats, sunflower seeds, wheatgerm, wholewheat bread (not white).

Deficiency results: Fatigue, forgetfulness, nerve pain, numbness and tingling. A severe restriction causes beriberi, but this is rarely found outside the tropics.
Overdose results: Has been known to cause low blood pressure and trembling, but it is very difficult to take an overdose.
Destroyed by: Soaking and cooking, alcohol and tobacco.
Daily need: 1.5 mg.

VITAMIN B-2 (RIBOFLAVIN)

Function: Helps to break down all food. Necessary for good vision and clear eyes. Needed for cell respiration.
Good source: Almonds, avocados, brewers' yeast, chicken liver, cottage cheese, kidneys, milk, mushrooms, spinach, turnip greens, wheatgerm, wild rice, yoghourt.
Deficiency results: Bloodshot and itching eyes, sensitivity to bright lights, broken blood vessels, split corners of mouth, dermatitis, dandruff, split finger-nails.
Overdose results: Tingling sensations.
Destroyed by: Light – rapidly.
Daily need: 2 mg.

VITAMIN B-3 (NIACIN)

Function: Assists in breakdown and use of proteins, fats and carbohydrates. Important to mental health. Maintains health of skin, tongue, gums and digestive system. Is most beneficial in conjunction with the other B vitamins.
Good source: Chicken, chicken's liver, halibut, kidneys, lamb's liver, mackerel, peanuts, salmon, sardines, turkey, whole grains and breads.
Deficiency results: Lethargy, bad concentration, bad balance, depression, nervousness, diarrhoea, dental decay, halitosis (bad breath).
Overdose results: Flushes, tingling sensations, activation of peptic ulcer.
Destroyed by: Not established.
Daily need: 15 mg.

VITAMIN B-5 (PANTOTHENIC ACID)

Function: Essential for balanced functioning of the adrenal gland, therefore important to the nervous system; cholesterol and fatty acids cannot be formed without it.
Good source: Bran, brewers' yeast, kidneys, lamb's liver, mushrooms, peanuts, whole grains.

Deficiency results: Malfunction of the adrenal gland which means loss of control against stress, irritability, dizziness, nervous headache, blackouts; numbness and tingling of muscles, sometimes cramps. Can lead to premature grey hair – an adequate amount may prevent it. Lack of it plays a major role in the onset of arthritis.
Overdose results: Not established.
Destroyed by: Acid such as vinegar. More stable in hot liquid (such as boiling) than in dry cooking (such as grilling or roasting).
Daily need: Estimated at 5–10 mg.

VITAMIN B-6 (PYRIDOXINE)

Function: Aids in metabolic breakdown of foods; helps form antibodies and red blood cells. Important in regulation of nervous system.
Good source: Bananas, blackstrap molasses, Brazil nuts, chicken, lamb's liver, mackerel, walnuts, wheatgerm, wholewheat grains and bread.
Deficiency results: Nervousness, irritability, depression, mouth disorders, muscular weakness, anaemia, haemorrhoids, dermatitis.
Overdose results: Not established.
Destroyed by: Oral contraceptives, so supplements may be necessary for women on the Pill. A little is taken away by soaking and cooking food.
Daily need: 2 mg.

VITAMIN B-12 (CYANOCOBALAMIN)

Function: Essential for normal functioning of body cells, particularly those of the bone marrow, nervous system and gastro-intestinal tract. Necessary for formation of red blood cells.
Good source: Cheese, eggs, herrings, kidneys, lamb's liver, milk, oysters, sardines, soya beans.
Deficiency results: Most serious is pernicious anaemia; also bronchial asthma, disturbance of central nervous system, unpleasant body odour.
Overdose results: High haemoglobin count.
Destroyed by: Foods used in conjunction with raw egg white.
Daily need: .005 mg.

BIOTIN (VITAMIN B COMPLEX)

Function: Helps form fatty acids, then burns them up together with carbohydrates for energy.
Good source: Blackcurrants, blackstrap molasses, cauliflower, dried milk, kidneys, lamb's liver, leeks, raw egg yolks (only), rolled oats (dry).

Deficiency results: Unlikely, but absorption problems can occur resulting in fatigue and depression, dermatitis and greyish skin colour.
Overdose results: Not established.
Destroyed by: Exposure to air, baking soda; raw egg white prevents absorption. Unaffected by heat.
Daily need: Very small amount, not established.

CHOLINE (VITAMIN B COMPLEX)

Function: Aids distribution of fats from the liver to the cells. Plays a role in nerve transmission.
Good source: Beans, fish, heart, lecithin granules, lentils, wheatgerm, whole grains.
Deficiency results: Cirrhosis of the liver, hardening of arteries, high blood pressure.
Overdose results: Not established.
Destroyed by: Strong alkali. Not affected by heat or storage.
Daily need: Not established.

FOLIC ACID (VITAMIN B COMPLEX)

Function: Helps form red blood cells and nucleic acids, both essential for reproduction. Carries carbon to form the iron-containing protein in haemoglobin.
Good source: Almonds, cod, comfrey, lamb's liver, oysters, raw cabbage, raw kale, walnuts, watercress.
Deficiency results: Anaemia, low white blood count, depression.
Overdose results: Not established.
Destroyed by: Not established.
Daily need: 1.5 mg – stress and the intake of excess alcohol increase needs.

INOSITOL (VITAMIN B COMPLEX)

Function: Together with choline, necessary for the formation of lecithin, which keeps the liver free of fats.
Good source: Bran, blackstrap molasses, lecithin granules, nuts, oats, sesame seeds, wheatgerm.
Deficiency results: Cirrhosis of the liver, poor appetite, hardening of arteries.
Overdose results: Not established.
Destroyed by: Not established.
Daily need: Not established.

PABA (PARA-AMINOBENZOIC ACID, VITAMIN B COMPLEX)

Function: Enables other vitamin B agents to function properly. Especially important in forming red blood cells. May help prevent onset of grey hair.
Good source: Broccoli, cabbage, kale, kidneys, lamb's liver, rice (brown).
Deficiency results: Fatigue, irritability, depression and digestive disorders.
Overdose results: Not established.
Destroyed by: Not established.
Daily need: Not established.

VITAMIN C (ASCORBIC ACID)

Function: Main use is to maintain level of collagen, a protein necessary for the formation of skin, ligaments and bones; therefore helps to mend fractures, heal wounds, form scars. Helps prevent haemorrhaging. Said to aid and prevent some types of virus and bacterial infections (the common cold, for instance).
Good source: Acerola cherries, alfalfa sprouts, blackcurrants, broccoli, Brussels sprouts, cabbage, cauliflower, grapefruit, lemon juice (diluted), orange juice (including pith and peel), papaya, paprika, parsley, peppers, pineapple, rose-hip powder, strawberries, tangerines, watercress.
Deficiency results: Tooth decay, bleeding gums, aching joints, susceptibility to infections, slow healing, tendency to bruise or bleed, bad vision, low body warmth. Prolonged deficiency can lead to scurvy.
Overdose results: Suspected as a contributing factor to kidney stones; large doses cause diarrhoea, activation of peptic ulcer.
Destroyed by: Light, heat, air, prolonged storage, excess cooking, copper and iron utensils. Most easily destroyed of all vitamins.
Daily need: 50 mg. Body's need is increased when under stress, tired, suffering an infection, injury, surgery. More also needed if you smoke, take aspirin or live in a hot climate.

VITAMIN D (CALCIFEROL)

Function: Encourages the transport of calcium and phosphorus to tissues which build bone.
Good source: Cod liver oil, eggs, halibut liver oil, herrings, mackerel, salmon, sardines, sunshine, ultra-violet light (in moderation).
Deficiency results: Weak, brittle bones, spinal curvature, muscle cramp, joint pains, hardening of the arteries, rickets.
Overdose results: Loss of appetite, headache, drowsiness; widespread calcification of non-bony tissues can occur.

Destroyed by: Air pollution inhibits its production via sunlight. Stable when exposed to heat, keeps under storage conditions. Primarily stored in the liver.
Daily need: 400 international units – more if you are on the Pill.

VITAMIN E (TOCOPHEROL)

Function: Not well understood. It unites with oxygen to protect red blood cells and keep them from rupturing. Thought to improve the circulatory system and counteract the process of ageing; used to increase fertility and treat sterility. Externally, used on burns, bruises and wounds to accelerate healing and help alleviate scars.
Good source: Apples, carrots, cabbage, celery, eggs, muesli, olive oil, rolled oats, sunflower seeds, sunflower seed oil, wheatgerm, wholemeal bread, wholemeal flour.
Deficiency results: Degeneration of reproductive tissues, sexual frigidity, early onset of old age, sluggish circulation, varicose veins, liver problems, muscle weakness.
Overdose results: Elevated blood pressure.
Destroyed by: Cooking, storage, iron utensils.
Daily need: 20 International Units – more when under stress.

VITAMIN K

Function: Prevents haemorrhaging, stimulates production of substances involved in the normal clotting process.
Good source: Broccoli, Brussels sprouts, cabbage, cauliflower, eggs, oats, potatoes, strawberries, wheatgerm, wholewheat grains.
Deficiency results: Haemorrhaging deficiencies, but very rare as this vitamin is manufactured by bacteria in intestines.
Overdose results: Fast clotting – thrombosis.
Destroyed by: Alcohol, light and rancidity. Sulphur drugs and antibiotics interfere with its absorption (eating yoghourt can restore it).
Daily need: Widely available, only supplemented in disease conditions.

MINERALS

Minerals occur in minute quantities in the human body and are essential to certain metabolic processes; they help draw chemical substances in and out of the cells; they control the amount of water necessary to the life process; they influence the secretion of glands; they affect muscle responses; and they are important in transmitting messages through the nervous system.

We obtain our minerals through food, but unlike vitamins, which plants manufacture, minerals have to be extracted from the earth by plants. Once in the body, when their work is done, they are excreted in the urine and sweat, so must be regularly replaced.

The problem is that with chemical interference in the soil and atmosphere we are getting too little of some minerals and too much of others; and because the amounts are so minuscule, even a speck of mineral matter can upset metabolism. Reading about deficiencies and their results may inspire you to take capsule supplements. Don't; the borderline between under- and over-doses is too fine. Supplement your diet with natural foods rich in minerals so that the positive and negative electrical charges that minerals carry will be neutrally balanced for proper absorption.

CALCIUM

Functions: To build and maintain bones and teeth; also important in regulation of heart muscles and nerve transmission.
Good source: Almonds, blackstrap molasses, broccoli, cheese (hard varieties such as Parmesan, Swiss, Cheddar), clams, haricot beans, kelp and other seaweeds, milk, powdered milk, olives, sardines, sesame seeds, shrimps, yoghourt.
Deficiency results: Deterioration of bones; weakened tooth structure; muscle cramps, numbness and tingling in arms and legs; blood clotting.
Overdose results: Excess calcium is normally excreted by the body; if not there is a chance of widespread calcification.
Daily need: 600 mg.

CHLORINE

Function: Important in cell metabolism; helps regulate the balance of acid and alkali in the blood.
Good source: Celery, kelp, lettuce, salt (and other sodium-containing foods), spinach, tomatoes.
Deficiency results: Weak water retention, atherosclerosis.
Overdose results: Not established; excess chlorine is usually excreted.
Daily need: Joined to sodium, so provided that intake is sufficient, level is usually correct.

CHROMIUM

Function: Helps regulate blood-sugar levels and improves body's utilization of glucose. Thought to be instrumental in keeping cholesterol low.
Good source: Blackstrap molasses, bran, brewers' yeast, chicken, condiments, fruits, green vegetables, honey, nuts, shellfish, wholegrain cereals.
Deficiency results: Affects tolerance of glucose; hardening of the arteries.
Overdose results: Not established.
Daily need: A trace.

COBALT

Function: Necessary for the proper functioning of vitamin B-12 and for red blood cells.
Good source: Fruits, green vegetables, meat, wholegrain cereals.
Deficiency results: Pernicious anaemia; dry, scaly skin.
Overdose results: Could cause enlargement of thyroid gland but unlikely; toxic in large quantities.
Daily need: A trace.

COPPER

Function: Associated with iron in production of red blood cells; aids in forming hair pigment; a catalyst for body-building enzymes connected with muscle and nerve fibres.
Good source: Almonds, bran, Brazil nuts, chicken's liver, lamb's liver, shellfish, wheatgerm, wholegrain cereals.
Deficiency results: Very rare, but can lead to anaemia, greying or loss of hair, heart troubles and nervousness. Women need more copper during menstruation and pregnancy.
Overdose results: Toxic in large quantities, but body usually discards excess. Schizophrenics have been shown to have a high level of copper.
Daily need: 2.5 mg.

FLUORINE

Function: Improves tooth development and strengthens bones by helping to deposit calcium. Hinders tooth decay by fighting acid-forming bacteria.
Good source: Seafood, tea, fluorinated water.
Deficiency results: Poor bone and teeth formation; tooth decay.
Overdose results: Discoloured and brittle teeth, muscle stiffness, arthritis; toxic reactions.
Daily need: 1 mg.

IODINE

Function: Necessary for the production of the thyroid hormone.
Good source: Kelp, seafood, sea salt, seaweeds, shellfish.
Deficiency results: Abnormal swelling in the throat leading to a goitre; thyroid disturbances that lead to weight gain, nervous tension and lethargy; drying of skin, loss of hair.
Overdose results: Interferes with the thyroid's synthesis of hormones, reducing them to an unsatisfactorily low level.
Daily need: A trace.

IRON

Function: The most important mineral involved in the transportation of oxygen to the cells and in the formation of haemoglobin. Most beneficial when taken in conjunction with vitamin C.
Good source: Blackstrap molasses, bran, dried apricots, egg yolks, haricot beans, kidneys, lamb's liver, shellfish, soya flour, sunflower seeds, watercress, wheatgerm.
Deficiency results: Anaemia, pallid skin, loss of energy, general listlessness and restlessness; brittle nails, premature grey hair; palpitations and breathlessness. Menstruation and pregnancy use up the iron supply and it needs to be replenished.
Overdose results: Usually excreted, but poor performance of the liver or pancreas can result in excessive deposits which are toxic; skin can become pigmented.
Daily need: 15 mg.

MAGNESIUM

Function: Important in cell metabolism; it actuates more enzymes in the body than any other mineral acting as an agent in the utilization of other minerals and vitamins – calcium needs it, vitamin C useless without it. Necessary for nerve and muscle function.
Good source: Almonds, avocado, bananas, barley, blackstrap molasses, Brazil nuts, haricot beans, honey, muesli, peanuts, seafood, whole grains.
Deficiency results: Muscular weakness, heart and circulatory diseases, nervousness and depression, dizziness, diarrhoea, liability to convulsions. Alcoholics and diabetics are often short of magnesium.
Overdose results: Not likely, but could lead to sleepiness and general weakness.
Daily need: 300 mg.

MANGANESE

Function: Activates enzymes; closely related to blood-sugar levels and helps maintain reproductive processes.
Good source: Almonds, apricots, bran, kidneys, lentils, parsley, walnuts, watercress, wheatgerm.
Deficiency results: Poor equilibrium and bad co-ordination; sterility, reduction of sexual drive, abnormal body growth, still births. Deficiency extremely unlikely.
Overdose results: Not established.
Daily need: A trace.

PHOSPHORUS

Function: Found in every cell in the body and the busiest of all minerals; important for growth, maintenance and repair of cells; significant in energy and nerve transmissions; passes on genetic hereditary patterns.
Good source: Brewers' yeast, cheese, chicken, eggs, fish, liver, skimmed milk, wheatgerm.
Deficiency results: Disturbances in cell regulation; poor quality of teeth and bones; stunted growth. Older people need more phosphorus because their systems don't absorb it well.
Overdose results: The body stores phosphorus well with no known toxic results.
Daily need: 1 gramme.

POTASSIUM

Function: Often in partnership with sodium. An important mineral in muscle control including that of the heart and in the stimulation of nerve impulses; helps regulate osmosis and water balance.
Good source: Bananas, butter beans, dried apricots, figs, haricot beans, jacket potatoes, lentils, peanuts, seafood, soya beans, spinach.
Deficiency results: Muscular weakness, irritability, disturbances of the heart; deficiency unlikely.
Overdose results: Affects heart beat, slowing it down and eventually arresting action; weakness and numbness of limbs.
Daily need: 4 grammes.

SELIUM

Function: Not specifically known, but appears to be an anti-oxidant; closely related to vitamin E and may prevent certain types of cancer.

Present in the retina of the eye in fairly high concentration, indicating that it may be important in vision.
Good source: Kidney, lamb's liver, nuts, seafood, wholegrain cereals.
Deficiency results: Difficulty in absorbing and utilizing vitamin E.
Overdose results: Toxicity; brittle bones and tooth decay.
Daily need: A trace.

SODIUM

Function: Important in cellular metabolism; protects the body against excess fluid loss, balances acid-alkali levels, influences muscular activity.
Good source: Chicken, green vegetables, kelp, salt, seafood, water and wheatgerm.
Deficiency results: Rare, but in hot climates excessive perspiration may deplete the body's salt, resulting in headaches, nausea, diarrhoea and muscular cramps of legs and abdomen.
Overdose results: Swelling of body tissues (oedema); unduly aggravates high blood pressure.
Daily need: 2–5 grammes, but for those with high blood pressure, 1 gramme is the limit.

SULPHUR

Function: Present in cells to help in formation of body tissues; necessary for proper function of vitamins thiamine and biotin; acts as a detoxant.
Good source: Cheese, chicken, eggs, fish, haricot beans, meats, milk, nuts, soya beans.
Deficiency results: Rare, but associated with protein lack and its effects.
Overdose results: Toxicity, if excess comes from synthetic supplements.
Daily need: No exact amount, but widely available through protein.

ZINC

Function: Helps in the formation of enzymes and proteins, in digestion, in elimination of carbon dioxide.
Good source: Bran, eggs, lamb's liver, nuts, onions, shellfish, sunflower seeds, wheatgerm, wholewheat flour.
Deficiency results: Retarded growth, delayed sexual maturity. Pregnant women, those on the Pill and older women frequently need extra.
Overdose results: Loss of iron and copper, particularly in the liver.
Daily need: A trace.

VEGETARIANISM

This means eating no meat or fish products. Some vegetarians will eat animal by-products such as butter, cheese and eggs provided the animal isn't killed for them. Others, known as lacto-vegetarians, cut out eggs as well as meat because they are potentially living creatures. The most extreme, the vegans, eat nothing of animal origin.

Vegetarians have a reputation for being slim, healthy and energetic but their claim that their diet provides a healthier and longer life cannot be medically substantiated. Undoubtedly they are more conscious of what they eat. They are well able to get adequate protein, vitamins and minerals from meatless sources though the diet requires some variety. In cooking there is never a question of using harmful animal fats.

A vegetarian regime follows this general scheme:

Breakfast: Choice of: fruit or fruit juice, muesli, oats, wholegrain cereal, dried fruits, honey, wholewheat bread, eggs, tomatoes.
Lunch/Dinner: Salad always, protein ingredient such as nuts, cheese, egg, lentils, haricot beans, avocado, soya beans; carbohydrate ingredient such as potato, brown rice, wholegrain bread; fruit or a dessert made from it.

LIQUIDS

A daily intake of water is essential, a pint if possible, and when on a slimming diet much more. There are basically four kinds of drinking water:
hard water – contains calcium, magnesium and other salts
soft water – contains sodium (which replaces the calcium and magnesium), often some copper, iron and zinc
distilled water – has had all the minerals removed by a steam process
mineral water – natural, untreated water, bottled with nothing added, nothing removed. There are many varieties with reputations for uniform quality and stability of beneficial mineral content. They are still or sparkling and have combinations of minerals that are both good to taste and reputedly good for health. Bottled still waters have considerably less sodium content, which affects water retention, than tap water.

Most community water has been fortified with chlorine for purification and fluorine to help prevent tooth decay but evidence of the toxic effect of sodium fluoride is causing concern.

SOFT DRINKS: Many have chemicals, colourings and flavourings added. It is more nutritious to make your own juices and add sparkling water, soda or tonic mixers. The high sugar content in most soft drinks provides the body with an unnecessary overload of sugar carbohydrates.

WINES, SPIRITS AND LIQUEURS: Very pleasant in moderation; a drink or two before dinner is relaxing, wine complements food, while an after-dinner drink is often a digestive. Most doctors agree that a controlled amount of alcohol won't harm; excess does and can get to the point of being beyond the bounds of self limitation. External signs of puffiness, blotchiness, impeded speech and actions, only indicate what's going on inside. Alcohol is speedily assimilated and quickly dilates the blood vessels which explains why it is sometimes prescribed in moderate amounts for people with circulatory troubles. Within a very few minutes about 50 per cent will have passed into the blood stream and on to the liver. The liver can absorb about one-third of an ounce of alcohol an hour. Feeling 'high' starts the minute you are drinking more than that amount during that time. If you take more than the liver can handle, the surplus is pumped around the body waiting its turn to get into the liver. It literally goes to the head, acting as a sort of anaesthetic. It affects the highest centre of the brain first, the part that controls amongst other things the inhibitions. As a rule effects are quicker and more drastic in a person who doesn't drink much. Regular drinkers develop a medically unexplained slow-down in the rate at which alcohol is absorbed.

Some days one can stand more alcohol than on others. Fatigue, stress, emotional upset, depression or anger can all accelerate alcohol's anaesthetizing action, although in small doses it relieves tension. One's resistance to alcohol is roughly in direct proportion to the fullness of the stomach. This has led to the practice of drinking something creamy (even milk) or oily before setting off on a drinking evening. This doesn't absorb the alcohol but it does reduce the rate at which it is absorbed.

Wine is the most inoffensive of alcoholic beverages and said to be beneficial to the digestion as it contains enzymes active in the metabolization of food. It provides vitamins B-2, B-6, niacin, pantothenic acid and small quantities of B-1, B-12 and folic acid. Minerals are present, too, and dry red wine is a good source of iron. Wines are carbohydrates, and the sweeter or heavier the wine, the more sugar elements it contains.

Spirits and liqueurs are more concentrated alcohol and can take vitamins from the body because like any sugary carbohydrate they need the vitamin B complex. Dry spirits such as whisky, white rum, vodka, gin have less sugar content than sherry, port, vermouths and the sweet liqueurs.

THE BASIC KITCHEN

Three basic grain recipes, plus one for a soup that is all vegetables and full of vitamins. These four items constantly crop up in health cures.

Basic Muesli

2 tablespoons oats old fashioned
juice of ½ lemon
a little milk, fresh or skimmed
2 tablespoons wheatgerm
4 tablespoons water
2 tablespoons honey

Soak oats overnight in water; in the morning add lemon juice, milk, honey and wheatgerm; mix well. Then add as you wish: any fresh fruit (traditionally shredded apple), raisins, dried apricots, nuts, natural yoghourt.

Basic Wholegrain Bread

1 oz. (30 g.) dry yeast
1½ pints (9 dl.) potato water, or warm milk
1 tablespoon honey
3 lbs (1.5 k.) wholewheat flour
pinch of salt

Into a warm bowl, put the yeast with a little of the potato water (or milk), mix and add honey. Leave for twenty minutes. Into another bowl mix flour and salt, then gradually add the yeast mixture and the remainder of the potato water; blend well and knead. Put into well-oiled tins, only filling half-way. When dough has doubled, bake at 350 for 50 minutes or until the bread sounds hollow.

Basic Potato Cereal

4 cups boiling water
1½ tablespoon wholewheat flour
1½ tablespoon bran
2 raw potatoes
wheatgerm, milk, honey

Into the pan of boiling water (4 cups) add flour and bran, stir and simmer for about 3 minutes; shred raw potatoes into mixture, stir until blended, then take from heat, cover and let stand a few minutes before serving. Add the wheatgerm, milk and honey to taste.

Basic Vegetable Broth

1 cup chopped onions
3 stalks celery, chopped
3 pints (1.5 l.) water
2 large potatoes, chopped small
4 carrots, chopped
pepper and sea salt
1 cup root vegetable
1 cup any leafy vegetable

Put a little vegetable oil into a large stainless steel or ceramic pot, braise onions and celery a little, add the water and then the other vegetables except the leafy one. Season; simmer for 30 mins. and then add the leafy vegetable; cook for 3–5 mins., otherwise vitamins are destroyed.

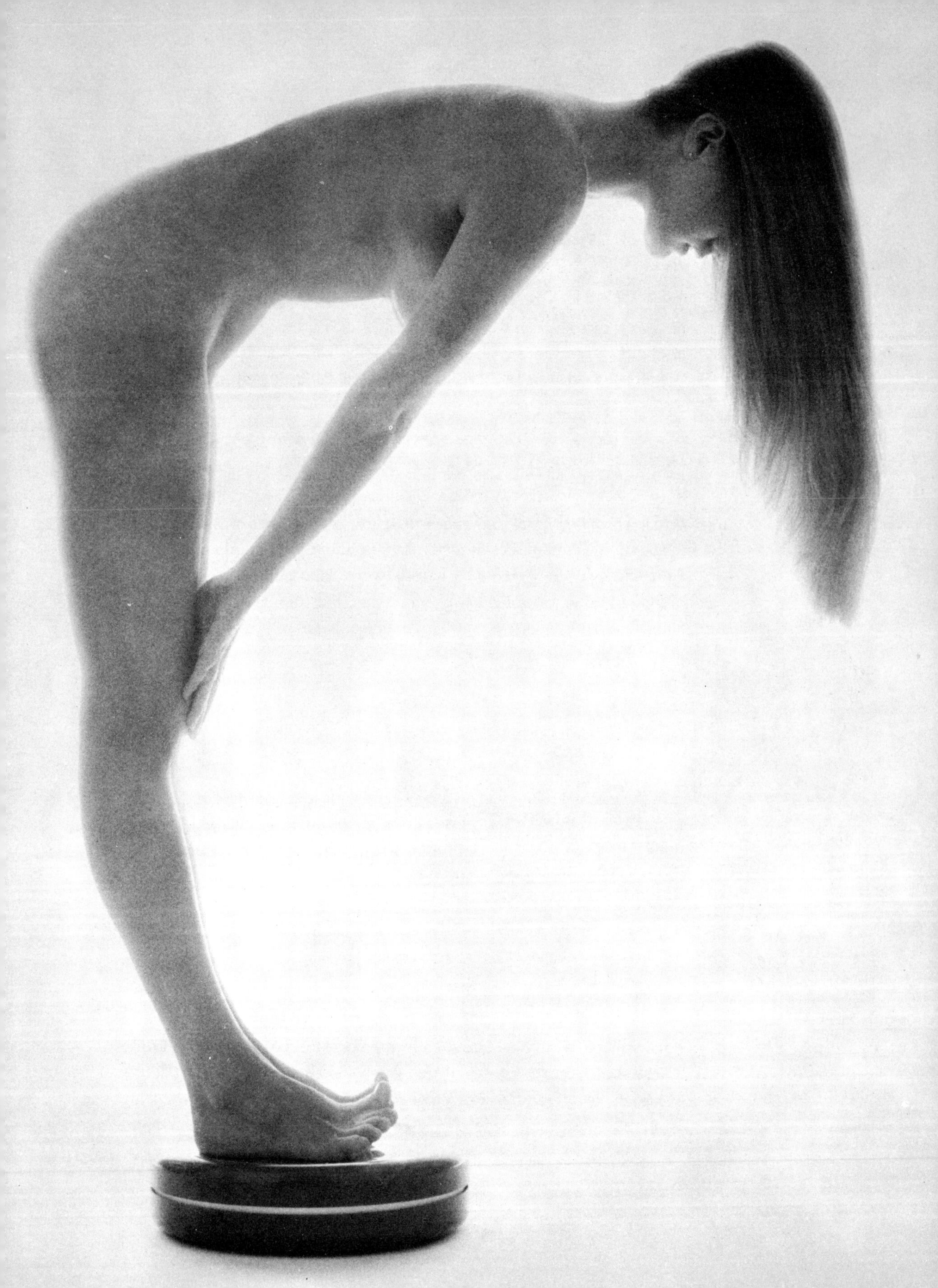

3

SLIMMING

Gradual weight loss is best. To take off pounds is one thing, to do it in a minimum time through drastic means is another. You are probably harming your own health even while you're losing weight. Ideally weight reduction should be planned on a gradual, steady basis resulting in permanent loss and a stabilized weight. For example, by steadfastly following the Maintenance Diet (Nutrition – page 25) in time the body would probably attain and sustain its ideal weight. But that time could be six months or more. Not many have that sort of patience; it is more common for an overweight person to think in terms of taking off x number of pounds for a special purpose (fashion, love, holiday) or initially to lose substantially as an inducement to get going on the long-term haul.

There are ways to quick weight loss, but the question is – which way? There are so many varieties of diet plans that it is easy to be thoroughly confused and it doesn't help to discover that even doctors do not agree about which method is the most satisfactory. Many have their pet theories and so-called recommended diets which appear contradictory.

Dieting is a very individual matter – and reaction to any specific regime varies considerably, be it psychological or chemical. There is no perfect diet that is good for everyone; nor is there any wonder food or formula that will do the trick – despite all the credit given to lemons and grapefruit. But there are several approaches to dieting that work, and it is up to you to decide which suits you best. Here is all the information: the diets summarized into categories to make it clear what theories are behind the various methods together with an assessment of their weight-loss possibilities. However, they all have one thing in common: to be successful they need will power and determined effort. Statistics reveal

LATEGAN

that out of one hundred who slim only twelve lose any substantial amount of weight, and ten are likely to gain back their loss.

What is overweight? What is normal? What is ideal? Apart from measuring in pounds and inches, there have been many ways devised to assess if you are fat or not. Most are a waste of time – can you scoop up thick folds of skin? When you pinch various spots on your body, do you hold more than an inch in your fingers? If you lie on your back can you place a ruler on your side so that it touches both your ribs and hip-bone? Do all this if you like, but the real test is to give yourself an honest look in the mirror. You know if you're carrying around too much fat. You can see it, feel it. Let your eye be the best judge.

Actual weight is not always a true indicator. Weight charts scaled to height should be used as a guide, not as a rule – ten pounds variation up or down could still mean you are at your ideal weight. Most charts record average weights tabulated by insurance companies, and these are usually quite a bit higher than the ideal. Our weight table is worked out from several independent studies and represents a guide to ideal weight for women over twenty. No adding is permitted for additional years; although metabolism and activity slow down as one ages, intake of food should be cut and balanced accordingly to keep weight steady. You usually hit your ideal weight in the mid-twenties. Most women gain roughly a pound a year after the age of thirty, which can add up to an uncomfortable lot over a number of years. Don't allow it to happen. Check the chart to give you a realistic ideal. To determine whether you are small, medium or large frame, refer to figure-type explanation (page 18). Big or small bones don't make as much difference as we would like to think. Bones roughly weigh one-sixth of your weight. They can give you an alibi for about seven pounds at the most.

Weight can fluctuate each day. To keep track of your weight weigh yourself at the same time and under the same conditions each day; weight varies not only daily but during the day as well. It also changes according to the menstrual cycle; most women are heavier and inclined to be bloated just before they menstruate. Weight can also move up and down in a seemingly alarming way – I can gain five pounds overnight after an indulgent dinner but thankfully can lose it just as fast too. Normally one swings within a three to five pound range, and it is only when you find yourself constantly returning to a lower figure that you can be sure you are losing weight on a permanent basis.

IDEAL WEIGHT FOR WOMEN OVER TWENTY

This is to be used as a guide not a rigid rule. To gauge ideal weight accurately you would have to consult a specialist. For a girl from sixteen to twenty, subtract a pound for each year under twenty.

HEIGHT (BAREFOOT)		SMALL FRAME		MEDIUM FRAME		LARGE FRAME	
		kgs.	*lbs.*	*kgs.*	*lbs.*	*kgs.*	*lbs.*
1.42 m	4′8″	39–42	86–92	41–46	90–101	44–51	98–113
1.45 m	4′9″	40–43	88–95	42–47	92–104	45–53	100–116
1.47 m	4′10″	41–44	91–98	44–49	96–107	47–54	104–120
1.50 m	4′11″	43–46	95–102	44–50	98–111	49–56	107–123
1.52 m	5′0″	44–47	96–104	46–52	102–114	50–57	110–126
1.55 m	5′1″	45–49	99–107	48–53	105–117	51–59	113–129
1.57 m	5′2″	46–50	102–110	49–55	108–121	53–60	116–133
1.60 m	5′3″	48–51	105–113	50–57	111–125	54–62	120–137
1.62 m	5′4″	49–53	108–116	52–57	114–128	56–64	123–140
1.65 m	5′5″	50–54	111–119	53–60	116–131	57–65	126–143
1.68 m	5′6″	52–56	114–123	54–62	120–136	59–67	130–147
1.70 m	5′7″	54–58	118–127	57–64	125–140	61–69	134–151
1.73 m	5′8″	56–60	122–131	59–65	129–144	63–70	138–155
1.76 m	5′9″	57–61	126–135	60–68	133–149	65–73	143–160
1.78 m	5′10″	59–64	130–140	62–69	137–152	67–75	147–165
1.81 m	5′11″	61–65	134–144	64–71	141–156	68–77	150–169
1.83 m	6′0″	63–67	138–148	66–73	145–160	70–79	154–174

Excess food is stored as fat. If you are overweight it is because at some time or other you have eaten more food than you need or the wrong food. If your body takes in more than it burns up in energy, the extra becomes a fat reserve. Today to be between twenty and thirty pounds overweight is the norm, though hardly desirable. More than that and you are on the way to obesity, which can easily get out of control. At this stage it is no longer an aesthetic problem, but a serious medical matter and no diet should be undertaken unless supervised by a doctor. It is possible that you are one of those individuals whose bodies for reasons not yet fully understood do not deal in the usual way with food. The advice for everyone who wants to diet is to check with a doctor. Few do. A normal healthy person can embark on limited sensible dieting, but should any adverse effects arise, seek medical advice immediately.

One of the oldest clichés in the diet game is that some people get fat easily no matter how little they eat, while others who constantly overeat stay thin. It's quite true that these two distinct groups exist. Recent research shows that in the case of the constant-weight types, excess food stimulates the body to increase its metabolism, and the food used up for this job exactly balances the additional intake. People who put on fat easily show no increase in metabolism when given extra food, but simply become fatter. This difference is rarely taken into consideration.

Why? No one really knows all the answers. It is impossible to distinguish the two types biologically – those who can very accurately control output and those who are not so good at it. It is a very delicate and sensitive balance; the reason may be metabolic, psychological, glandular or a complex combination of any or all. Scientists have been looking for clues in the fat cells of the body and have found that when fat people lose weight, the cause is shrinkage in the size of the fat cells, while the number of cells is unchanged.

This would seem to indicate that at maturity you have a certain number of fat cells, so that although fatness is difficult to cure, it probably is easier to prevent. It has been suggested that overfeeding in early life may account for the severe weight problem many people have as adults. Heredity may be a factor, not least because a child follows the pattern of over-eating that runs in the family. Each individual acquires an underlying cellular pattern – a sort of blue-print that is established in the early years and carries on. Each person's body has an optimum weight level that it strives to maintain. If weight is lost or gained slowly there is a force returning one to the original weight. With normal people this works in their favour, but with the fat-prone it's yet another battle, as there's a strong tendency for the overload to return. With fat gained over a long period, you must have the will-power to eat smaller quantities and better foods.

Fat cells are all over the body and they behave as an organ, which means they have a rich blood supply which enables them to metabolize. The fat organ is very large indeed, making up from 10% to 25% of body weight in an average person and half the body mass in an obese one. Some fat protects vital organs and for health reasons this fat should never fall below a certain level nor rise too high. However, the majority of cells lie in the layer of adipose tissue just beneath the skin. This layer does many useful things like cushion the body, act as an insulator, conserve heat, metabolize food and burn fat – but above all it stores fat. Here is the main reservoir of fat in the body, and it's usually too ample.

If this fat deposit becomes quite dense – which means there's rather a lot of it – the skin over the fat becomes quite puckered, rather like an orange peel, and this is called cellulite. The French invented the word, implying it was a special sort of fat and had to be treated in a special way but it is ordinary fat that is water-logged, and the best way to get rid of it is through diet accompanied by exercise, and by controlling fluid retention.

Although eating is a neural and muscular activity, it is mostly a brain function. There are certain control centres, primarily – it is thought – in the hypothalamus, from which decisions go out whether to eat, how much, when to stop. Researchers have hopes about a hormone produced by the pituitary, which seems to mobilize fat. It has been isolated but is not yet at the stage of being used. Interestingly enough it is produced by people fasting and those on a mainly fat and protein diet. People on the normal mixed diet don't produce it at all, nor do those on a low calorie intake consisting mainly of carbohydrates. And those with poor pituitary function don't make it either.

What about the glandular system and its effect on weight control? Glands are often unjustly blamed for excess fatty deposits. Glands secrete hormones into the bloodstream, which carries them around the body to act as regulators of various functions. Among other things they control the balance of food metabolism. Take the famous thyroid gland; it can produce too much hormone, thus causing cells to metabolize so fast that food is burnt up speedily as fast as it goes in. Accordingly, high thyroid persons are thin and usually nervous. Too little thyroid production results in slow cell metabolism; the cell cannot keep up with the intake of food, has no time to use it as energy, so stores it as fat. Food requirement for people with a low thyroid production is consequently less, but they frequently exceed the limit and put on weight.

Observations of these effects have led to the use of thyroid hormone for the treatment of overweight but medical opinion is very divided. Some doctors are against it, arguing that when thyroid tablets are given to a person with a normal thyroid, the gland gets lazy and stops making its own hormone. Thyroid extract is useful when there is medical evidence of low thyroid activity. Small doses will speed up metabolism and assist in weight loss, provided effective diet is being taken at the same time.

The pituitary gland has considerable influence on weight control but because it turns out dozens of hormones which stimulate or inhibit other glands, it is not easy to find out how. Under certain circumstances it produces the fat-mobilizing hormone mentioned above; this is under further experimentation. The adrenal gland, together with the reproductive system, produces a special hormone during pregnancy, which is the basis of a controversial weight shifting method used by a number of doctors (see page 65).

Some overweight people retain more water than they need. When on a diet it is necessary to differentiate between loss of weight and loss of water. Usually the latter goes first, and it can mean a magical loss of pounds overnight. In most cases this water loss is frequently recovered. There is a lot of water in the body, some in blood, some in cells, some in connecting tissue. The proportions are very carefully regulated, and one of the chief things that controls the balance is salt. You need an exact amount – no more, no less. If too much salt is taken, water accumulates with it, the tissues swell up and you weigh too much. We need about one gramme of salt a day to keep a healthy water supply. Most people consume ten to twenty times that, which means carrying an extra four pints of water. Most fresh foods naturally contain salt. It is very rare for anyone to take too little salt, and only in very hot climates is it sometimes necessary to supplement it.

If you drink a lot of water it doesn't mean you are going to retain it, in fact quite the reverse. One should have at least three pints a day when on a diet. It is good for the kidneys, and scientific approval is now being given to the old wives' tale that water can also wash off weight. Water is an important part of many slimming regimes. Many thin people drink a great deal of water with meals – something that was considered bad a few years ago – while fat people often drink less and choose more concentrated foods.

Weight loss is directly connected with energy output no matter what the metabolic speed of assimilating food. Each of us has a unique body, but one fact remains the same: if you take in more than you burn off, you will put on weight. Nutritionists calculate the amount of heat or energy released by burning food as a calorie. It is a very small unit, and when we refer to a Calorie, it is a thousand times as big as the original unit. Protein has a caloric value of approximately 4 Calories per gramme, carbohydrate 4 Calories per gramme and fat 9 Calories per gramme. An average woman uses about 2,300 Calories a day.

The principle of all diets is based on the balance of food intake with energy output. But it is not always a strict equation. New thinking is along the lines that it is not only the number of calories you take in, but also the type that helps to balance the energy output. The three groups of food – protein, carbohydrates and fat – react differently. Excess fat, not burned off, is stored as fat. Excess carbohydrate is also stored as fat, while protein has the peculiar ability of making the body burn its fuel more quickly – sometimes to such an extent that it is essential to turn some of the body fat into energy to cope with the breaking down of the protein. This is why many diets are very high in protein. Strange as it may seem, fat – though not healthy in large quantities – is inclined to metabolize quicker than carbohydrates. It is the sugar and starch that are likely to end up as stored fat.

There are certain foods to be stopped no matter what system you follow, some you can take with caution, and others you can eat without a care. Check the tables and use this as a basis for any diet menu. You will notice that it hardly varies from our Maintenance Diet and is a sound plan for healthy eating as well as for slimming.

STOP:

SUGAR CARBOHYDRATES

sugars: all types, glucose, sweets, chocolate, spreads, sweet sauces, confectionery decorations
pastries: biscuits, cakes, pies, tarts
preserves: jams, marmalade, jellies
fruit: tinned, candied or preserved in any way

STARCH CARBOHYDRATES

breads: all white breads, rolls, buns, breadcrumbs
cereals: white flour, refined grains and cereals (wheat, oats, barley, rye), packaged cereals, rice, pasta, flour, puddings, blancmange, flour sauces
vegetables: dried peas, beans and lentils, tinned root and pod vegetables, cream soups

FATS

sauces: all cream ones like mayonnaise, unless freshly made with oil, bottled sauces and relishes
nuts: peanuts, walnuts
delicatessen foods: processed meats, pâtés, sausages
no fat for frying

CAUTION:

STARCH CARBOHYDRATES

bread: wholewheat varieties, any made from unrefined grains
cereals: natural oats, unprocessed rice, wholegrain flour

CELLULOSE CARBOHYDRATES

root vegetables: potatoes, carrots, parsnips, turnips, white onions, beetroot
pod vegetables: peas, beans
fruits: some tropical varieties – bananas, water melons, avocado pears

FATS

dairy produce: butter, margarine, milk, cream

PROTEIN

dairy produce: cheese made from cows' milk, eggs
poultry: goose, duck

GO AHEAD:

PROTEINS

fish: fresh and salt water, shell varieties
meat: beef, veal, lamb, pork, ham, bacon, liver, kidney, heart, brains, sweetbreads, tripe
poultry: chicken, turkey
game: venison, pheasant, quail, guinea fowl, rabbit
cheese: made from goats' milk, mozzarella, feta, cottage cheese

CELLULOSE CARBOHYDRATES

leaf vegetables: artichokes, asparagus, broccoli, cabbage, cauliflower, celery, chicory, endive, kale, lettuce, all salad greens, spinach, watercress
root vegetables: spring onions, radishes
fruit vegetables: tomatoes, peppers, aubergines, courgettes, cucumbers, marrows
fruits: citrus – lemons, oranges, grapefruit, tangerines; berry – raspberries, strawberries, bilberries, cranberries, gooseberries; orchard – apples, pears, plums, apricots, peaches, cherries, grapes; tropical – mangoes, papaya, pineapples, cantaloupes, figs

FATS

vegetable oils: olive, soya, unsaturated fats

Herbs and seasoning are allowed, but use little salt. Never, never, fry in fat. Meat and game can be braised in a non-stick pan, on an iron griddle or on a barbecue rack. Otherwise roast, grill or boil. Fish should be roasted, steamed or grilled. Vegetables and fruit should be eaten raw whenever possible, but when cooked boil in a minimum amount of water or braise in the oven with a little oil. Sugar is forbidden in all diets; if absolutely necessary use a minimum amount of honey to sweeten a beverage.

I've already mentioned the value of water – three pints a day minimum. Coffee and tea are allowed in any quantity – without sugar and in most diets preferably without milk. Some diets permit a lot of milk, others a little, some only skimmed milk, some not at all. I'm inclined to go for skimmed milk with cautious use of whole milk and cream.

Commercial soft drinks are definitely not allowed, and that includes all tonics, sodas, and ginger ales. Some of the diet varieties can be taken in moderation, but it is best to make your own lemon drink from fresh lemons and a sparkling mineral water. This helps to take away excess fluid in the body and is a recognized regenerator of the liver.

The rule concerning alcohol is not as strict as might be supposed. It does not necessarily put on fat. If you normally drink a fair amount you should probably carry on but to a much lesser degree as the tension derived from being without may make you eat more food – with a worse result.

For the purpose of dieting think of alcohol as being equivalent to carbohydrate (roughly 1 gramme of alcohol equals 1¾ grammes of carbohydrate). Alcohol carbohydrate burns at a rather slow rate. Quite a number of alcoholic drinks contain sugar and consequently have to be avoided: beers, ales, ciders, liqueurs, sherries, ports, sweet and heavy wines. Light red and white wines are all right; so are dry spirits such as gin, vodka, rum and whisky.

Again doctors are not in agreement over alcohol. Some say that it checks the combustion of fat, others that it dilates the blood vessels and makes the body work harder, stepping up metabolism to an extent which may more than compensate for the extra calories.

Vitamins as such have no influence on weight, nor can one live on vitamins alone. Even when fasting only supplements of vitamin B and C should be taken; other additions could be dangerous. On a sensible reducing diet extra vitamins should not be required. However there are doctors who recommend taking multi-vitamin capsules, stepping up the intake of vitamin E, C and particularly the full spectrum of the vitamin B complex. This is fine but it is most important to remember that one cannot safely exceed the normal daily requirements of either vitamin A or vitamin D. As for the other vitamins, overdoses are simply washed away by the kidneys if you are drinking adequate water.

Everyone looks for a short-cut to dieting. It would seem logical that one way to eat less would be to curb the appetite. Appetite suppressants, such as the amphetamines, act on the central nervous system, and apart from getting to the centres of appetite control, they also stimulate mental and physical activity – thus increasing energy output. There are snags: some doctors consider them appetite postponers not suppressants and people have sometimes found that they quickly put on weight after stopping the drug. Amphetamines are effective for only a few weeks and can be addictive which causes a withdrawal problem. Because of this the prescription of many has been stopped.

If you look carefully at the formulae for slimming pills you will find that their active ingredient is nearly always a laxative (such as phenolphtalein). Laxatives are one of the oldest ways to lose weight, the most common being Epsom Salts (magnesium sulphate). They will get weight off temporarily due to loss of water and malabsorption of food, but the ensuing thirst usually puts back weight in the form of water desperately needed by the dehydrated body. In any case, you are not losing fat. Constant use of diuretics and purgatives can seriously harm the body.

The 'magic' foods – biscuits, package meals – are low calorie but contain a large amount of stomach filler such as methyl cellulose. This is harmless but it expands and fills up the stomach, so that you feel you have had a reasonable meal. Manufacturers put in protein and vitamins so that undernourishment is unlikely but these foods often lack essential nutrients. They are also expensive and a most monotonous way to diet.

The best and only way to go on a diet is to choose one you can stick to. Yo-yo dieting is hopeless and not worth the effort of the dieting days. The best bodies have worked out a plan of eating that is really a diet for life. They have learned to eat thin without starving and without discomfort. Plan a diet around the way you eat, one that fits into your life-style and temperament. Sometimes dieting is a matter of forcing yourself out of certain bad habits. Judge the pros and cons of each diet, balancing them against your preferences, your schedule, your finances. Then stick to what you have chosen.

There are two main schools of thought on diet. Those who believe that the clue to losing weight is simply to control the quantity you eat. These are the calorie counters who believe that food-in must always be less than energy-out when measured in calories. This is the PORTION CONTROL theory.

Then there are those who argue that it is the type of food you eat that matters and the restriction of food from certain groups. Some are all-protein diets, others contain no fat, others a lot of fat, others a few carbohydrates. These are the PROPORTION CONTROL theories and are deliberately unbalanced.

There are convincing arguments for both sides. Individual metabolism is the deciding factor.

PROPORTION CONTROL DIETS

All these restrict one or two of the food groups. It is claimed that such methods shift fat more quickly than a calorie control system and without the feeling of hunger. They can cause quite dramatic weight loss, though it is preferable to take it off slowly. Because these diets allow more food, often unlimited eating of certain things, they are more appealing to people who don't have the patience to keep track of calories or quantities.

All Protein

meat
poultry
fish
eggs
cottage cheese
3 pints water
no alcohol

FORMULA: No carbohydrates, no fats, 100% protein. Only these foods, but quantity unlimited: lean beef, veal, lamb, chicken, turkey, fatless fish and shellfish, eggs – preferably hard-boiled – cottage cheese. All fat must be cut off meat. No fat for cooking. Food must be boiled, baked, grilled or roasted. Drink at least 3 pints of water daily. As much coffee and tea as you like. Salt, pepper, herbs. Non-caloric beverages allowed. No alcohol. Supplementary vitamin tablets if necessary.

THEORY: Protein makes the body burn its fuel quickly and since in this diet there is lack of immediate fat and carbohydrate it is essential for the body to turn some of its stored fat into energy to break down the protein. Thus fatty deposits are slowly depleted. It is generally accepted that fat cannot be completely broken down in the body unless carbohydrates are present (in this case they are not). This means that during metabolism chemical compounds called ketones accumulate in the blood; they are present in the urine and also cause bad breath. The condition is called ketosis, but healthy people who chose this diet are unlikely to stick to it long enough for ketosis to reach an unsafe level. Long-termers should be under medical supervision; it can be harmful for pregnant women, as well as those with kidney problems.

Low Carbohydrate

meat
poultry
game
fish
eggs
cheese
oil
butter
salad
leaf vegetables
fruit vegetables
citrus fruit
berries
3 pints water
dry wines
dry spirits

FORMULA: Unlimited protein, caution for fats, carbohydrate limited to 250 Calories per day (about 60 grammes).

No quantity control on –

Meat: beef, lamb, veal, pork, ham, bacon, liver, kidney
Poultry: chicken, turkey, duck
Game: venison, pheasant, rabbit
Fish: all varieties
Cheese: hard varieties, cottage cheese, mozzarella and goat cheeses
Beverages: tea, coffee, a lot of water, non-calorific drinks

Limited amounts –

Eggs: any way
Fats: butter, margarine, oils, cream, milk

Control to under 250 Carbohydrate Calories (60 grammes) – total from the following:

Salads: green varieties
Vegetables: confine to leaf and fruit vegetables
Fruit: citrus fruit and berries only
Alcohol: dry wines – white or red, dry spirits – gin, vodka, whisky
Breads: wholewheat – never more than a slice a day

THEORY: This is the compromise between the Proportion and Portion theories. It is not counting calories for everything, but because it acknowledges carbohydrates in any form as a cause of weight gain, it cuts them down, though not out.

It is a slower way of losing weight than the all-protein or the protein-fat regimes. A fair amount of water is lost first and you stay on a plateau before getting really under way. The joy is that there is more to eat and something to drink, so it is considerably easier to live with over a longer period of time. At this 60 gramme a day level of carbohydrate intake there is usually no trace of ketosis. If you are not losing weight, you may cut down further on the carbohydrates. Alcohol is allowed because it is treated as a carbohydrate and comes within the controlled proportion. This diet also comes very close to our general diet rules and is not far off from the Maintenance Diet. When desired weight has been reached, it is relatively easy to make the transition to normal healthy eating, thus avoiding an immediate weight gain which happens after most diets. This low-carbohydrate scheme is not a new principle. It was originally prescribed for a rotund Victorian English gentleman, William Banting, who became famous after he published his 'Letter on Corpulence' showing how he lost 50 pounds in one year and was still going down.

Low Carbohydrate – The Grapefruit Diet

The Grapefruit Diet is based on the low-carbohydrate principle. There is no magic in the grapefruit but this fruit is used because it is very low in carbohydrates and provides necessary vitamins. It becomes most effective after five days.

Breakfast:
Half grapefruit or 4 oz. (120 g.) unsweetened grapefruit juice
2 eggs – any way
2 slices bacon
Coffee or tea

Lunch and Dinner:
Half grapefruit
Moderate portion of meat, poultry or fish
Salad with lemon juice/or portion of leafy green vegetables
Coffee or tea

Protein and Fat

meat
poultry
fish
game
eggs
cheese – hard
oil
butter
cream
salad
lemon
3 pints water
no alcohol

FORMULA: Primarily a protein and fat diet, with a small salad allowed with meals – if you must – providing such an infinitesimal amount of carbohydrate that it hardly counts. No quantity control; eat what you like at any meal.

Meat: beef, lamb, veal, pork, ham, bacon, liver, kidney
Poultry: chicken, turkey, duck
Game: venison, pheasant, rabbit
Fish: all varieties including fatty kinds like tuna and salmon
Eggs: any way, no limitations
Cheese: hard varieties, no processed ones, cottage cheese, mozzarella
Fats: butter, margarine, oils, cream (no milk)
Salads: green salad, limited to a small one each meal
Fruit: juice of one lemon a day

Food can be boiled, baked, grilled, roasted and can be cooked in a pan on the stove in its own fat – in the case of eggs, with a little fat. Drink the usual 3 pints of water daily; as much tea and coffee as desired. Salt, pepper, seasonings. Non-caloric drinks, no alcohol. Supplementary vitamin tablets if you like.

THEORY: This is basically the same principle as the all-protein diet in that, in the absence of carbohydrate, the body is forced into using stored fat for energy. Tests have shown that obese patients lose weight on comparatively high caloric diets so long as food consists mainly of protein and fat with carbohydrates kept to a minimum. Dieting is certainly made more palatable with the addition of fat, though weight loss is usually less rapid. Some people who take little or no fat find they are irritable, tired and inclined to lack concentration. Fat goes through the stomach quite slowly, so you do not feel hungry quickly after a meal and are able to stay on this diet for quite a while. We are constantly reminded about the dangers to health of too much saturated fat so although fat is permitted, it is hardly sensible to consume huge portions, nor is there usually the inclination. Again there is the problem of ketosis, but as explained above, there is no need to worry unduly about a low degree of this.

PORTION CONTROL DIETS

This is the mathematical approach to dieting, where the calorie equation rules: energy out must exceed food in, otherwise it is fat on. There's nothing wrong with it if healthily balanced.

For calorie counting you need a strong will. It is a slow, steady way of reducing weight. In theory it is simple: proteins give 4 Calories of energy per gramme, carbohydrates 4 Calories and fat 9 Calories.

The average woman needs about 2,300 Calories a day to balance energy output. For weight loss, calorie intake should be a maximum of 1,400 Calories a day. 1 pound of body fat represents 3,500 Calories. Therefore, in practice, calorie-counting diets amount to, on the average, 2 pounds loss a week on the basis of a long-term 1,200–1,400 Calories a day diet. This requires will-power.

In theory it doesn't matter how you take your calories, but it does matter nutritionally. If you follow the basic diet charts (page 57) you are on a good nutritional level.

Crash diets follow the calorie principle though they are reduced to survival level and therefore diets cannot be followed for more than a limited period. Crash diets are either for those who are only a few pounds beyond ideal and want to lose it fast, or for those who need encouragement to continue on a permanent weight-loss plan. The minimum is 800

Calories a day, less is a potential danger to health – unless completely fasting which has a different effect on metabolism.

Once ideal weight has been achieved, the calorie principle can be continued within the 2,300 Calorie limit to balance energy output. Choose foods from the 'Go-Ahead' and 'Caution' tables and you will see it is easy to keep within the caloric limit – and within the Maintenance Diet too.

CALORIE CONTROL / *1,400 a day / loss: 2 lbs (1 k.) weekly*

Breakfast: 1 glass unsweetened juice or half grapefruit
1 egg, any way but fried
1 slice wholewheat bread
1 pat butter or margarine
Coffee or tea, no sugar

Lunch: 3 oz. (90 g.) lean meat, poultry or fish
1 portion fresh vegetable or salad
1 slice wholewheat bread
1 portion fresh fruit
Coffee or tea, no sugar

Dinner: 3 oz. (90 g.) lean meat, poultry or fish
1 portion green salad
1 portion vegetable
1 slice cheese – no more than 2 oz. (60 g.)
1 portion fresh fruit
Coffee or tea, no sugar

CALORIE CONTROL / *1,200 a day / loss: 2–3 lbs (1–1.5 k.) weekly*

Breakfast: 1 glass unsweetened grapefruit juice
1 egg, any way but fried
1 slice wholewheat bread
Coffee or tea, no sugar

Lunch: 2 oz. (60 g.) lean meat, poultry or fish
1 portion green vegetable or salad
1 slice wholewheat bread
1 portion fresh fruit – not banana
Coffee or tea, no sugar

Dinner: 2 oz. (60 g.) lean meat, poultry or fish
1 portion green vegetable
1 portion salad
1 oz. (30 g.) cheese
Coffee or tea, no sugar

WEIGHT WATCHERS' PLAN / *very long term / loss: 2 lbs (1 k.) weekly*

A group therapy programme that involves a weekly meeting plus rigid adherence to a very detailed diet regime. It is portion control but through weight not calories – food is weighed on a postage scale. You must eat three meals a day, a minimum of five fish dishes a week, four to seven eggs a week, liver once, beef not more than three times. Many vegetables are unlimited. Off the list completely are the sugar carbohydrates. There are some strange rules – like eggs only for breakfast and lunch, limited vegetables for dinner only. They have no dietary or nutritional purpose, they're supposed to discipline the dieter. A typical day's menu:

Breakfast:	1 egg or 1 oz. (30 g.) hard cheese or 2 oz. (60 g.) fish 1 slice wholewheat bread Coffee or tea, no sugar
Lunch:	4 oz. (120 g.) fish, beef or poultry or 2 oz. (60 g.) hard cheese Unlimited vegetables (from a long list, mostly leafy green) 1 slice wholewheat bread
Dinner:	6 oz. (180 g.) fish, meat or poultry ½ cup limited vegetables (tomato, carrots, egg plant, peas) Unlimited vegetables in any quantity
Include each day:	three fruits – one must be a grapefruit or orange; two cups skimmed milk

CRASH DIETS

These are the drastic reducing regimes that most women resort to as an emergency measure. Over the years many fad diets have gone the rounds; here the most effective are summarized. It is important to limit diet days as indicated because of minimum nutritional value. Diets are of course monotonous, but it is this very repetition of certain foods that has proved easier to follow. Weight loss varies from one person to another, usually related to the amount you are overweight – the greater the excess the greater the loss. Average weight losses are indicated, but you could shed more or less. Do not extend the number of days; it could impair your health and also it is not always worth it as the speed of loss usually diminishes after the initial period. A crash diet can be used as an encouraging preliminary course before a long term dietary plan.

MILK AND BANANA / *5 days / loss: 5 lbs (2.5 k.)*

6 bananas
3 glasses of skimmed milk

This is the entire consumption for the day – eat at intervals when you feel like it. If necessary, add 2 cups of black unsweetened coffee.

COTTAGE CHEESE AND BANANA / *4 days / loss: 6 lbs (3 k.)*

First Day

Breakfast: 4 oz. (120 g.) cottage cheese
1 grapefruit
Black coffee or lemon tea

Lunch: 4 oz. (120 g.) cottage cheese
1 slice melon
Black coffee or lemon tea

Dinner: 4 oz. (120 g.) cottage cheese
1 grapefruit
Black coffee or lemon tea

Second Day

Breakfast: 1 banana
1 cup skimmed milk, black coffee or lemon tea

Lunch: 1 banana
1 boiled egg
Black coffee or lemon tea

Dinner: 6 oz. (180 g.) steak, grilled
2 bananas – grilled with steak if preferred
Black coffee or lemon tea

One cup of coffee or tea is allowed between meals. Repeat the routine of the two days.

BANANA DRINK / *2 days / loss: 6 lbs (3 k.)*

Recipe for drink: Juice of 2 large oranges
1 teaspoon liquid honey
Juice of 1 lemon
Mix these together well, add 1 banana very finely sliced
Mix well together

Take the drink four times a day in place of regular meals – add one cup of coffee or tea.

HONEY AND EGGS / *2 days / loss: 3 lbs (1.5 k.)*

First Day

Breakfast: Honey and egg cup: 2 egg yolks, 1 teaspoon honey and a dash of ground black pepper; beat until thoroughly blended
Black coffee or lemon tea

Lunch: Honey and egg cup
3 oz. (90 g.) hard cheese
Black coffee or lemon tea

Dinner: 1 cup clear soup
1 slice wholewheat bread
Honey and egg cup
1 portion fresh fruit
Black coffee or lemon tea

Second day

Breakfast: Honey and egg cup
1 slice wholewheat bread, bit of butter
Black coffee or lemon tea

Lunch: Honey and egg cup
5 oz. (150 g.) fish, poultry or meat
3 tablespoons boiled cabbage, spinach or courgettes
Black coffee or lemon tea

Dinner: Honey and egg cup
3 oz. (90 g.) hard cheese
1 slice wholewheat bread, bit of butter
Black coffee or lemon tea

WINE AND EGGS / *3 days / loss: 5 lbs (2.5 k.)*

Breakfast: 1 egg, hard-boiled
1 glass white wine (dry, preferably Chablis)
Black coffee

Lunch: 2 eggs, hard-boiled is best, but poached if necessary
2 glasses white wine
Black coffee

Dinner: 5 oz. (150 g.) steak, grilled with black pepper, lemon juice
Remainder of white wine (one bottle allowed per day)
Black coffee

Opposite: Benito, 1926
Overleaf left: Benito, 1926
Overleaf right: Benito, 1927

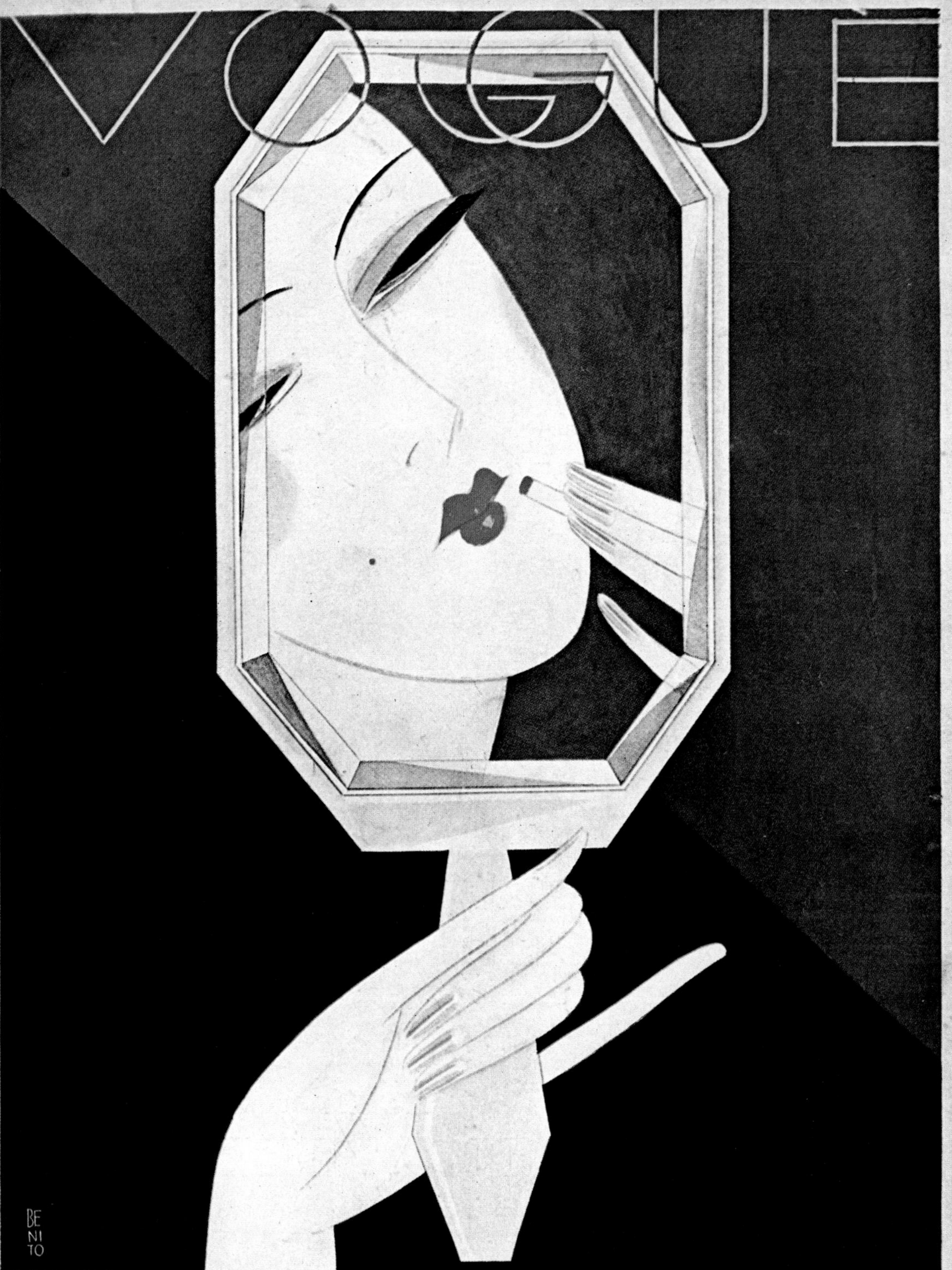

VOGUE

VOGUE

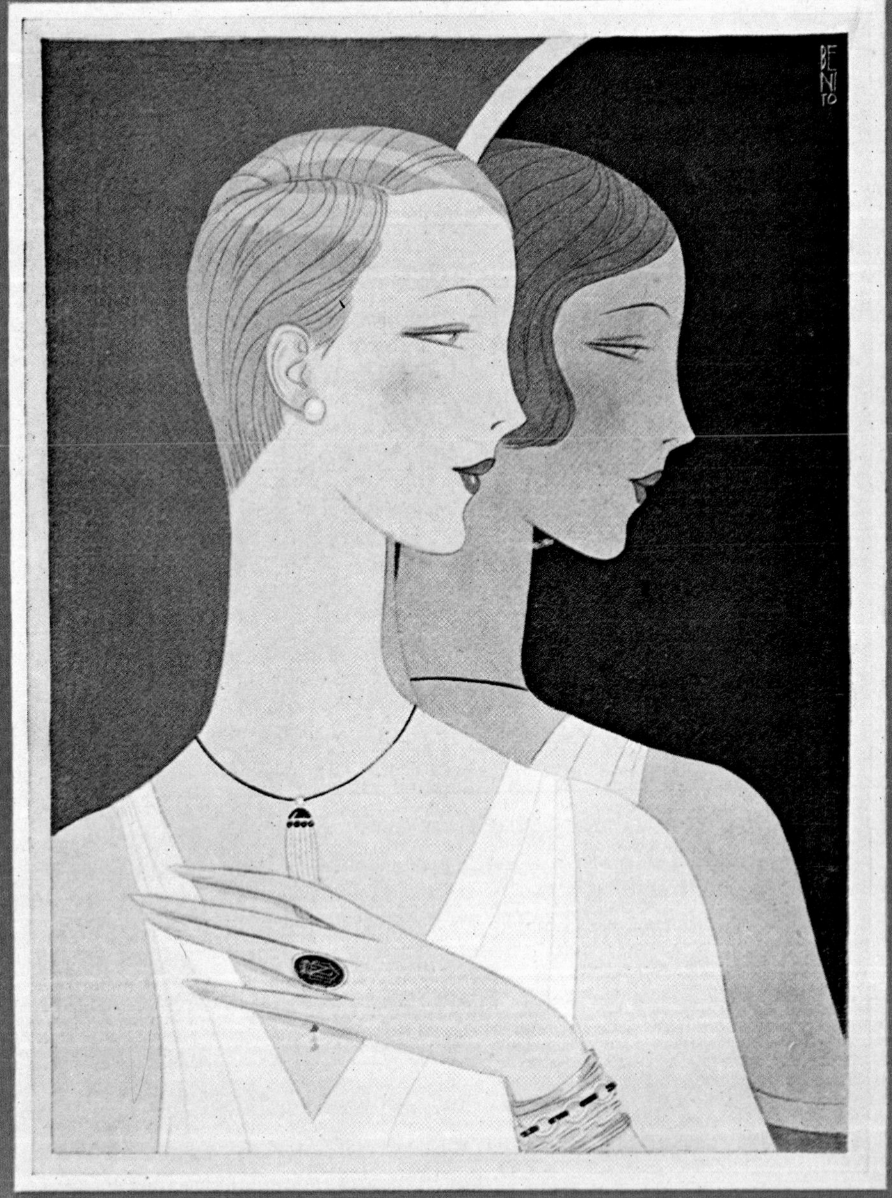

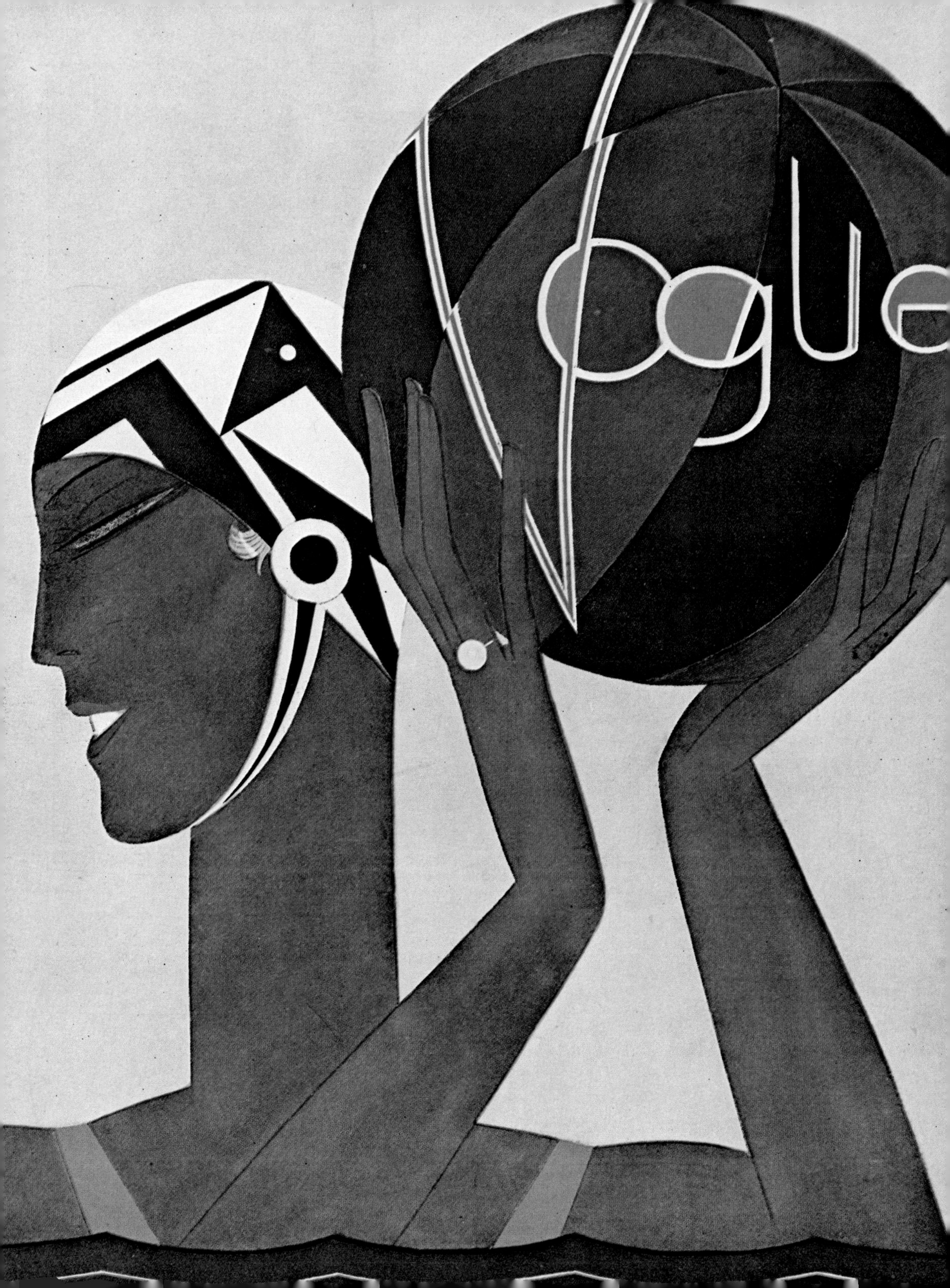
Vogue

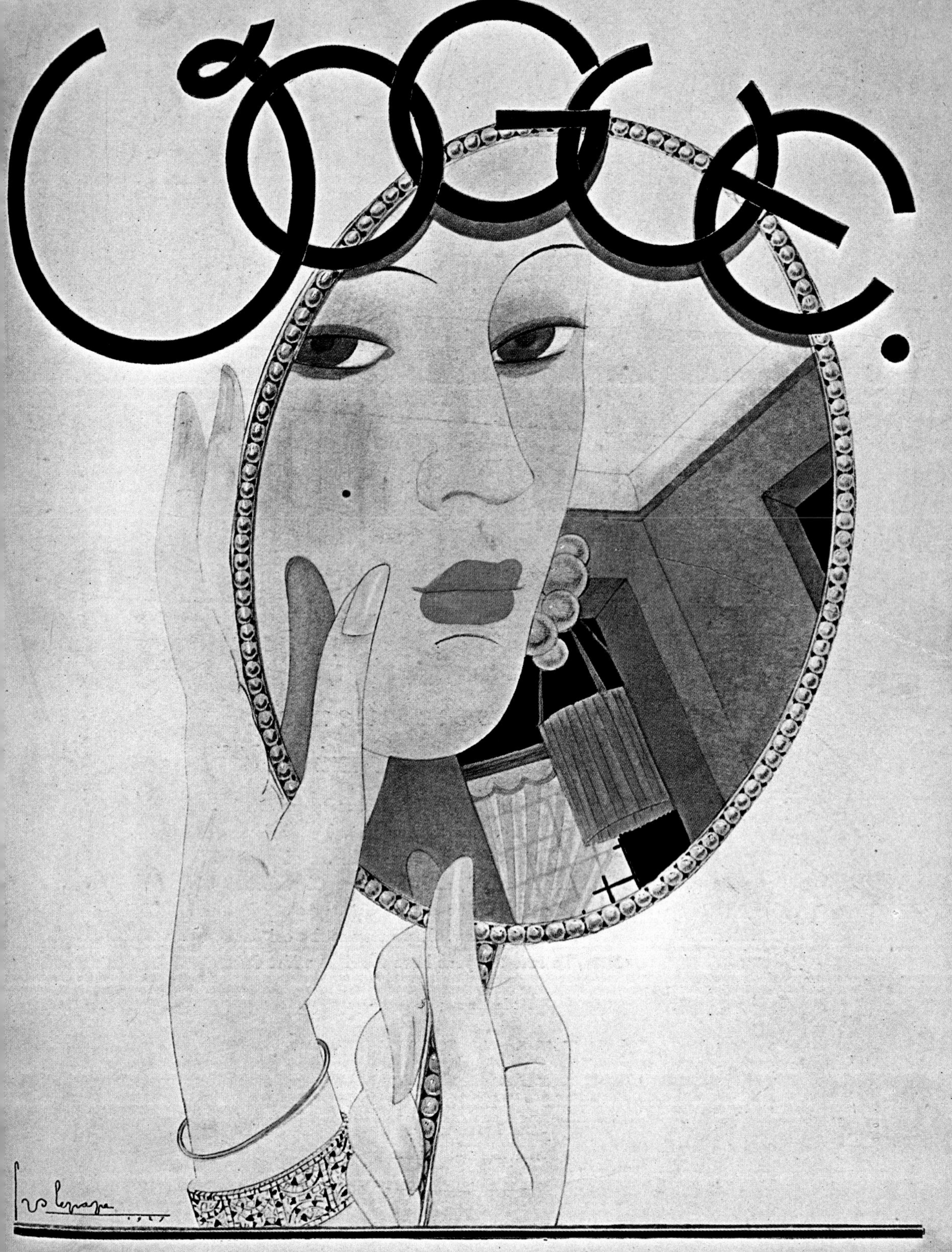
VOGUE.

WINE AND STEAK *5 days / loss: 5 lbs (2.5 k.)*

Breakfast: 2 hard-boiled eggs or 4 oz. (120 g.) grilled steak

Lunch: 4 oz. (120 g.) grilled steak
1 glass red wine

Dinner: 4 oz. (120 g.) grilled steak
1 glass red wine

Black coffee or lemon tea allowed as you like, no sugar though. Seasonings and herbs for steak, but no salt.

WINE AND CHEESE / *3 days / loss: 4 lbs (2 k.)*

Breakfast: 4 oz. (120 g.) hard cheese
1 slice wholewheat bread, toasted

Lunch/Dinner: 4 oz. (120 g.) cheese – any kind
2 slices wholewheat bread
1 glass white wine
Black coffee or lemon tea as you like

EGG AND TOMATO / *4 days / loss: 3 lbs (1.5 k.)*

Breakfast: 1 glass tomato juice
1 egg, poached or boiled
3 grilled tomatoes
1 slice wholewheat bread

Lunch: 2-egg tomato omelette or tomato and egg salad using hard-boiled egg, 2 tomatoes and adding a small sliced onion with chopped parsley

Dinner: Tomato omelette or tomato and egg salad or 2 scrambled eggs and parsley
Black coffee or lemon tea

EGG AND GRAPEFRUIT / *3 days / loss: 3 lbs (1.5 k.)*

Breakfast: ½ grapefruit
1 hard-boiled egg
1 slice wholewheat bread
Black coffee or lemon tea

Lunch: ½ grapefruit
2 eggs, any way but not fried, best if hard-boiled
Black coffee or lemon tea

Dinner: ½ grapefruit
2 eggs any way but not fried
Black coffee or lemon tea

Opposite: Lepape, 1927

EGG AND POTATO / *4 days / loss: 3 lbs (1.5 k.)*

Breakfast: 1 glass grapefruit juice
1 boiled egg
Black coffee or lemon tea

Lunch: 1 medium sized potato – baked, boiled or mashed with a little milk
1 apple
Black coffee or lemon tea

Dinner: 1 glass tomato juice
½ grapefruit
1 boiled egg
Black coffee or lemon tea

EGG AND HAMBURGER / *7 days / loss: 5 lbs (2.5 k.)*

Breakfast: 1 glass grapefruit juice
1 hard-boiled egg
Black coffee or lemon tea

Lunch: 3 oz. (90 g.) grilled hamburger, rare
1 apple
Black coffee or lemon tea

Dinner: 3 oz. (90 g.) hamburger, rare
Small green salad
Black coffee or lemon tea

AVOCADO / *3 days / loss: 3 lbs (1.5 k.)*

Breakfast: ½ avocado filled with cottage cheese
Black coffee or lemon tea

Lunch: ½ avocado sliced and mixed with sliced hard-boiled egg, 6 slices cucumber and onion to taste
Black coffee or lemon tea

Dinner: 3 oz. (90 g.) beef steak or hamburger, rare
½ avocado with cottage cheese
Black coffee or lemon tea

VEGETABLE AND FRUIT / *7 days / loss: 6 lbs (3k.)*

Vegetable Day

Breakfast: 1 glass vegetable juice
4 grilled tomatoes
Black coffee or lemon tea

Lunch: Green salad – lettuce, cucumber, celery, watercress, green peppers and onion to taste
Black coffee or lemon tea

Dinner: 1 hot green vegetable – cabbage, spinach, cauliflower, broccoli – boil and flavour with garlic and a little lemon juice
Black coffee or lemon tea

Fruit Day

Breakfast: Small fruit salad – grapefruit, orange, lemon and apple
Black coffee or lemon tea

Lunch: ½ melon
Small fruit salad as for breakfast
Black coffee or lemon tea

Dinner: Same as lunch

Alternate vegetable and fruit days, beginning and ending with a vegetable day.

RICE / *7 days / loss: 6 lbs (3 k.)*

Breakfast: 1 hard-boiled egg
2 oz. (60 g.) boiled rice (preferably brown and weigh after cooking not before)
Black coffee or lemon tea

Lunch: 3 oz. (90 g.) boiled rice (weigh after cooking not before)
3 oz. (90 g.) white fish or chicken
1 raw tomato
Black coffee or lemon tea

Dinner: Same as lunch

ONE MEAL AND LEMON / *5 days / loss: 5 lbs (2.5 k.)*

Lunch or Dinner: 8 oz. (240 g.) beef, veal or chicken grilled or roasted with no additional fat
1 portion fresh green vegetable or salad
1 orange or apple or ½ grapefruit

During the day: Juice of a fresh lemon in a wine glass of hot water – maximum of 6 times
Black coffee or lemon tea

VEGETABLE JUICES / *1 day / loss: 2 lbs (1 k.)*

Breakfast: Glass of tomato juice mixed with one raw egg and a little lemon juice
Black coffee or lemon tea

Lunch: Glass of vegetable juice – any mixture
1 slice wholewheat toast
Black coffee or lemon tea

Dinner: Glass of tomato juice with a raw egg
Black coffee or lemon tea

FRUIT ONLY / *5 days / loss: 5 lbs (2.5 k.)*

Breakfast: 1 orange or ½ grapefruit
Black coffee or lemon tea

Lunch: Fruit salad – orange, lemon, grapefruit, apple and melon
Black coffee or lemon tea

Dinner: Same as lunch – add a little cinnamon to liven the taste

STEAK TARTARE / *3 days / loss: 5 lbs (2.5 k.)*

Breakfast: Steak tartare made from 3 oz. (90 g.) fresh ground beef, 1 egg, peppers and capers
1 slice wholewheat toast
Black coffee or lemon tea

Lunch: Small green salad (eat first)
3 oz. (90 g.) steak tartare
Black coffee or lemon tea

Dinner: Same as lunch

DRINKER'S DIET / *7 days / loss 5 lbs (2.5 k.)*

Breakfast: 1 hard-boiled egg
1 portion of cottage cheese
Black coffee or lemon tea

Lunch: Up to 5 oz. (150 g.) white fish – not fried
1 small green salad or 1 portion green vegetable
2 drinks – whisky, gin or vodka or white wine

Dinner: Up to 5 oz. (150 g.) lean beef or chicken
1 small green salad
1 oz. (30 g.) hard cheese
2 drinks – whisky, gin or vodka or white wine
Black coffee or lemon tea

DIET BOOSTER:
LECITHIN, VITAMIN B-6, CIDER VINEGAR, KELP

The addition of these four to any type of diet is claimed to give it a spurt and provide a higher energy level. Tests are not conclusive on this point but personal recommendations from those who've done it, indicate that it is worth a try. The formula is: 2 tablespoons of lecithin a day, a fifty-milligramme tablet of B-6 vitamin a day, 1 teaspoon of cider vinegar after each meal and 3 tablets of kelp after each meal. The theory is that lecithin helps mobilize fat, the vitamin B-6 helps metabolize it, the cider vinegar contains potassium which helps to keep nerves on an even keel, while the kelp is rich in iodine which speeds up metabolism.

HCG DIET PLAN

This is based on daily injections of HCG (Human Chorionic Gonadotropin, a compound obtained from pregnant women's urine) together with strict adherence to a fat-free 500 Calorie a day diet; a number of medical authorities do not approve it, but many women say it is one of the few ways to not only lose weight but to shift it from the most stubborn places – such as thighs and legs – that other diets do not achieve. Treatment is for a minimum of 21 days and a maximum of 40 under the daily supervision of a doctor; weight loss is usually fairly consistent between half a pound to a pound a day. Never are you allowed to lose more than 34 pounds at a time. It is argued that the same amount of weight can be lost by forgetting the injections and just existing on the miserly diet; maybe, but the injections mobilize the fat and once in the bloodstream make you feel as though you have eaten so there are no hunger pangs. Also, the fat is encouraged into more even distribution. No cosmetics containing grease can be used during treatment.

Breakfast:	Tea or coffee in any quantity without sugar – only 1 tablespoonful of milk allowed in 24 hours
Lunch or Dinner:	3½ oz. (105 g.) of veal, beef, chicken breast (skinned raw), fresh white fish, shrimp, lobster or crab 4 oz. (120 g.) of only one of the following vegetables: cabbage, onions, beet greens, spinach, Brussels sprouts, chicory, tomatoes, celery, cucumber, fennel, lettuce, watercress, radishes 1 breadstick or 1 piece of Melba toast 1 apple or orange, or ten cherries, 2 oz. (60 g.) strawberries or half a grapefruit Black coffee or tea with lemon is allowed

FASTING

The ultimate diet. If you wish to lose between 2–10 pounds (1–5 k.) over a period of two to four days, there is a very good chance you can do it this way. It is possible to lose up to 4 or 5 pounds (2–2½ k.) on a one-day fast, up to 10 pounds (5 k.) on a weekend regime and up to 20 pounds (10 k.) on a week-long abstinence. If you are in general good health, fasting within limits is not dangerous; in fact the contrary for it gives body metabolism a much needed rest and revitalizes the digestive system. Fasting on one's own should have a limit of four days, but under medical supervision and preferably in a clinic, most women can safely fast for several weeks.

A fast means eating absolutely nothing. You can drink, indeed you have to, the medical recommendation of a minimum of 2 quarts (2 l.) of water a day. Some fasts suggest drinking natural vegetable or fruit juices, others allow black coffee or lemon tea, but it is generally accepted that when fasting for weight loss rather than health, it is best to drink only water – mineral water, if possible, but not distilled water. There is no limit to the amount of water you may drink, nor is there any reason for concern if you don't seem to be eliminating as much as you take in; much of it evaporates through the pores.

Hunger amazingly disappears during a fast. After eighteen hours of no solid food, one usually loses hunger pangs and the desperate desire to eat. There is no need to take any vitamin supplements, but if you must, only take vitamin B and C as the others could cause complications.

The rate at which you lose weight is generally in proportion to the degree you are overweight – the more, the faster. It is also said that after fasting, chances are much better for permanent weight control than after other diets. A few pounds may come back at the beginning; this doesn't mean you are eating too much but that the sodium content in food causes the body once again to retain a certain amount of fluid. After an initial fast and weight loss, you should be able to lose an additional two pounds a week on a daily diet of not more than 1,400 Calories (see page 57).

You can fast for one or two days a week, but the total in any one month should not be more than 10 days. A fast should be gradually broken. At first add orange juice to the water, then take some yoghourt, later melba toast and honey. Eat a little every three hours until your body gets back again into the rhythm of regular meals. You will probably find that after a fast, it takes less food to satisfy you, also frequently the taste for sweet and fatty foods is less.

SLIMMING DISEASE

Anorexia nervosa is a psychiatric illness usually caused by compulsive dieting. There is such a thing as too much dieting. It doesn't happen often and it is a relatively small problem compared with troubles caused by overweight. Even the keenest slimmers find that hunger eventually overcomes intentions and any target weight is reached with relief. Not so for a small proportion of women who find that once started they are unable to stop slimming even when they are thinner than is normal. It becomes an obsession. Only prolonged medical attention can reverse it and unless checked this diet mania can lead to starvation.

The prevalence of the disease is on the increase. It usually starts with a desire to be extremely thin or alternatively with a morbid fear of fatness. In the early stages it looks like crash dieting of an extreme kind, but there the similarity ends. Any degree of thinness is not thin enough, and the next step is a refusal to eat almost any solid food and to take a minimum amount of fluids. It is a vicious circle for as the anorexia victim eats less and less she develops an aversion to food. At this point she really cannot eat and cannot be persuaded to try. If she does indulge in a bout of eating she will force herself to be sick. By this time she is usually rather pleased with her emaciated state.

One of the first metabolic symptoms is a specific endocrine disorder that causes periods to stop; other signs are dry skin and often swollen ankles. Medical attention should be sought right away, for it has gone far beyond the point of being a 'diet mad' matter – and beyond self control. Serious cases are immediately hospitalized and treatment starts with several weeks in bed using drugs to overcome resistance to eating and to stimulate the appetite. Psychiatric help is used and in some cases sleep therapy. Most patients leave within two to three months, but often the patient goes back to the old starvation habits, sometimes triggered by an emotional crisis. It can take years to cure and repeated relapses are not unusual. It mostly affects teenage girls. There are many theories as to the cause, but little is specific. Sometimes when a girl is fat and teased about it during childhood she develops an obsession to be thin in puberty. Others are said to wish to retain the shape of a child in order to avoid the sexual implications of growing to womanhood. In a mature woman a hypothalamic dysfunction is cited, or desire to get attention by subconsciously gambling with death.

SLIMMING AIDS:

Most salons use electrical machines that provide passive exercise. They are based on a system of electrical impulses invented 150 years ago by Faraday. Two pads – one negatively charged, the other positive – force body muscles to expand and contract between thirty-five to forty times a minute, thus exercising them. When the available energy these muscles need for exercise is used up, fatty deposits are converted into additional energy. The art lies in the correct placement of the pads so they tighten the appropriate muscles to reshape the figure. Another electrically induced way of slimming employs glass vacuum cups for massage; these stimulate the muscles by suction.

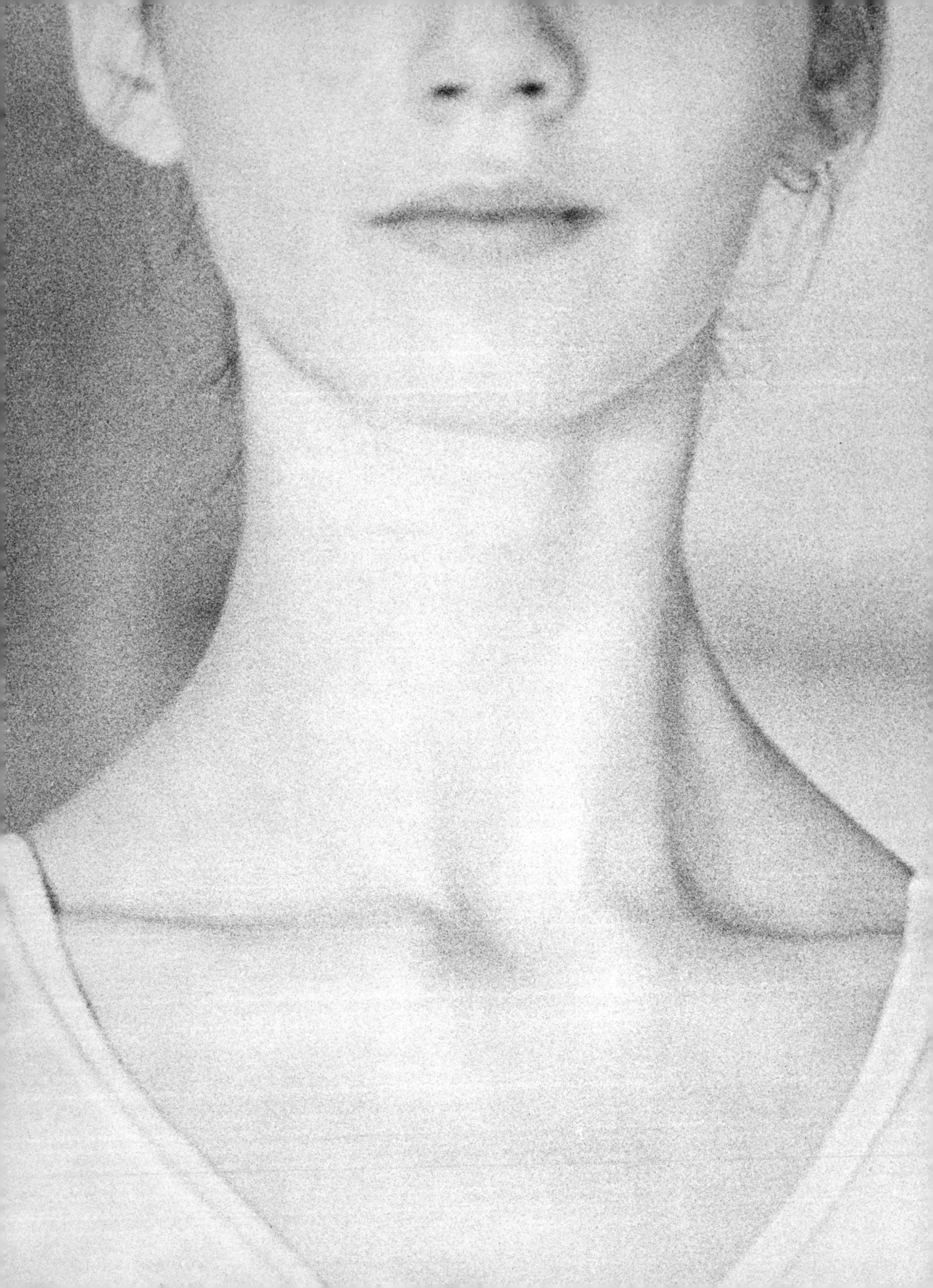

4

EXERCISES

Exercise is vital to overall health. It promotes good circulation and increases oxygen intake and flow. It firms muscles, moves joints, gives flexibility and suppleness; it can help to dispel nervous tension and delay some ageing symptoms. The reason we do not devote more time to it is because of laziness and boredom.

Most physical jerks are thoroughly boring, and it is essential to find the kind of exercise that fits your figure, age, temperament, skills and preferences. There are dozens of systems to choose from; all good ways of getting you into shape and building up energy reserves. One of the surprises for the beginner is the enjoyment that exercise brings. There is pleasure in motion and once you discover this you will find exercise indispensable.

To be effective, exercise must be part of your daily schedule. A burst of activity followed by a few days off just doesn't work. And there is no point in torturing your body with a crash programme: you might jeopardize your health, particularly if you are used to a sedentary life. Slow but sure is the only way. Gradually the body will respond and become capable of doing every movement at its own steady pace.

Exercise cannot alter your weight to any appreciable degree, but it can alter your figure by toning and tightening the body's outer layer of muscles thus helping to restore firmness. It can take inches off upper arms, midriff, waist, hips, thighs and buttocks – but it takes them off slowly.

Exercises are individual and on the following pages are the blueprints for the most effective systems. Each group incorporates a series of eight movements which together exercise the entire body. They are paced so that you can gear them to your own rhythm and timing. They can be

HEUMANN

done in 15 minutes a day – though there's no restriction if you want to do more. Each system has a different approach, different techniques of balance, movement and muscle control. The end result is the same: better health, energy, vitality. You don't have to stick to one routine; change weekly or do two different ones in a day if you wish – variety will retain your interest and keep you exercising.

Before you start, a little preparation and attention to basics:

Decide where and when; make a definite time and be firm and punctual.

If there's no convenient carpet area, get an exercise mat, large towel or blanket for the floor.

Wear leotards, bathing suit, underwear or nothing.

Exercise barefoot if possible.

Move to music, it keeps you at a certain pace, maintains interest.

Each exercise is a series of integrated movements, go from one to the other with smooth, controlled motions.

Body movements should be balanced by deep rhythmic breathing; exhale when body is bent and chest compressed, inhale as you stretch or straighten.

Work gradually into schedule; five minutes at first.

INFORMAL EXERCISE AND SPORTS

Some sort of exercise each day is so important – walking, jogging, swimming, tennis, bicycling. Informal activities and sports, done regularly and in easy stages, contribute to your general health, fitness and all over firmness. Every activity raises your pulse rate above normal and keeps it there while a fresh supply of oxygen pumps through your system. Each breath revitalizes the heart-lung complex and noticeably improves well-being. An under-exercised heart results in lack of energy. Walking should be a daily constitutional of not less than a mile.

Two of the most effective forms of exercise are swimming and jogging. Almost everyone can do one or the other. In swimming the buoyancy of the water makes movement easier, while the pressure makes it more effective. It uses almost every muscle in the body and physical strength is not necessary.

Take a warm shower first, finishing up with body-temperature water. Then a few arm circles to limber up. Breast stroke helps to firm and shape arms and legs, upper chest muscles. Back crawl is good for the shoulders, shaping the bosom and firming upper thighs. Front crawl uses the muscles of upper and lower arms, upper chest, while the leg action tightens the buttocks and the front of the thighs. In swimming you can measure endurance and progress: if you swim regularly you will be amazed at the degree of improvement in a relatively short time. Try to swim three or four times weekly, for forty-five-minute periods.

Jogging is the simplest form of exercise and uses most muscles in the body, especially those in the legs. The lungs are forced to bring in more oxygen, the heart has to beat faster to supply this to the muscles, so the entire circulatory system is put in peak motion. Begin jogging by combining it with walking for periods of fifteen minutes. It is better to do a few warm-up exercises beforehand, then break into a slow trot for about a quarter of a mile. When you are tired walk until you have recovered your breath, then trot again. Do not over exert yourself at first, but try to build up a steady rhythm, keeping that as your beat and speeding it up as you get fitter.

MASSAGE:

Massage relaxes you, relieves tension through touch and, most important, makes you conscious of your own body and its potential. In massage you are not so much toning muscles as trying to achieve a recovery from muscle fatigue; the blood flow is stimulated, the body becomes supple and energy is restored.

A false assumption is that rubbing and manipulation of tissues break up unwanted fat deposits and wash them away in the bloodstream. Women with cellulite problems who explore the possibilities of massage find that although the fat is broken up to some extent it simply moves from one place to another.

Massage helps exercise and diet take effect sooner and makes you feel slimmer and better. It is best to have massage after exercise or late in the afternoon when tension is at its height. It is the great tranquillizer – far superior to a pill – acting on the autonomic nervous system and nerve endings all over the body.

There are several ways of giving a massage and masseurs normally work out their own techniques which are as individual as handwriting. Stroking and kneading may vary from light to heavy depending on the area, but all movements should be gentle, slow, and rhythmic. Most masseurs use a bland oil or emollient, but you can choose what you want. Certain aromatic oils have particularly beneficial effects.

CLASSIC BEGINNER

These formal movements are an introduction to motion, and prove that simple easy rhythms if done every day can quickly bring about a new suppleness and make you more relaxed. When mastered, go on to the intermediate exercises.

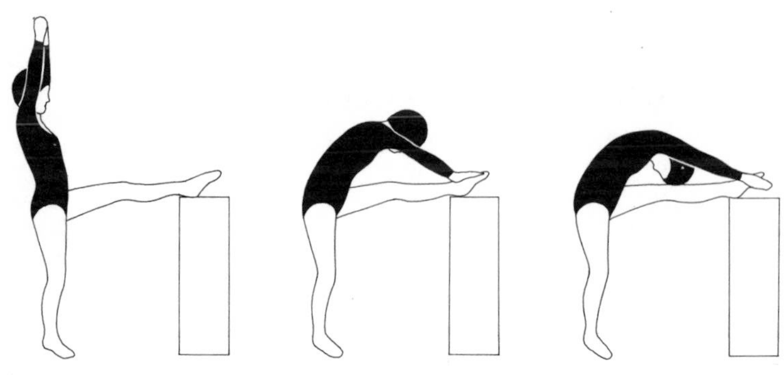

Raised Leg Stretch – Stand a leg's distance away from a support a fraction higher than your leg. Lift leg, rest it there. Stretch hands over head. Bend forward, try to touch feet, head on knee. Keep supporting leg straight. *3 times.* Reverse legs.

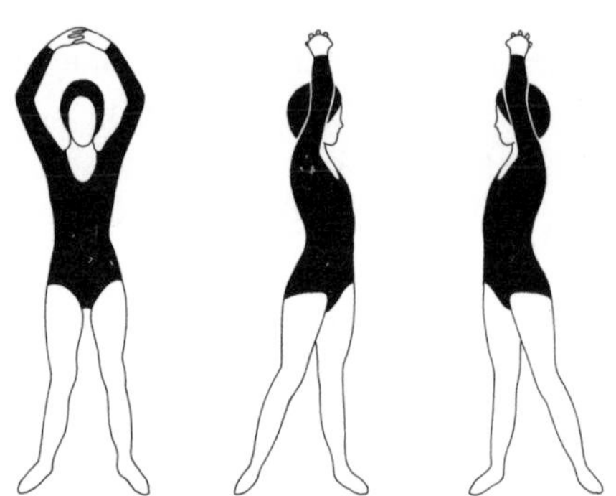

Torso Twist – Stand feet apart, hands over head, fingers linked. Slowly twist the body to left, then right. Move only the torso. *10 times, working up to 20.*

Hip Swing – Lie on back, arms slightly from sides, knees bent. Swing legs down to left, then to right. *20 times.*

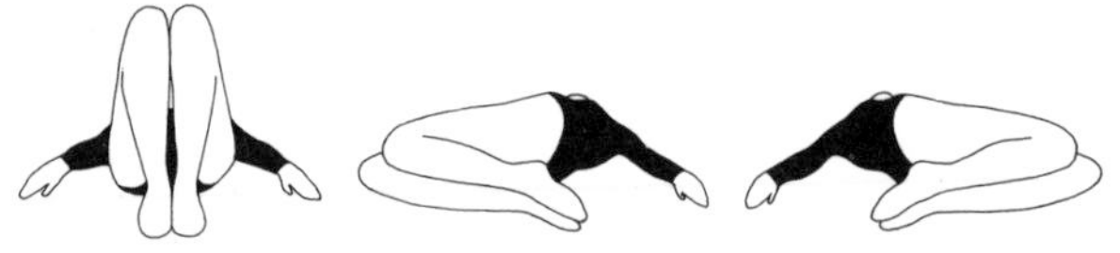

Stomach Control – Lie on back, head and shoulders on floor. Bend legs, raise knees to chest, slowly extend legs, lower and hold at 45°. Count 3. Bend legs back to chest. *6 times, work up to 10.*

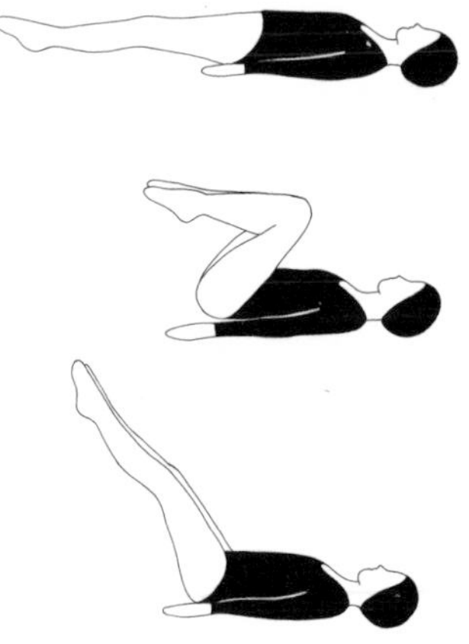

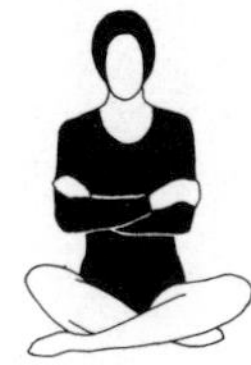
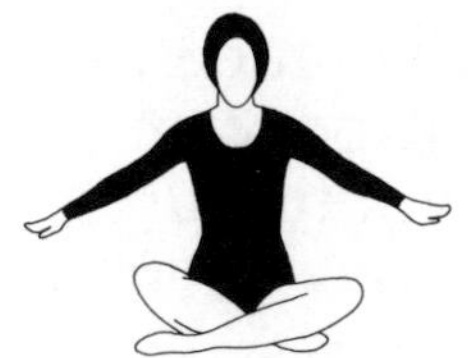
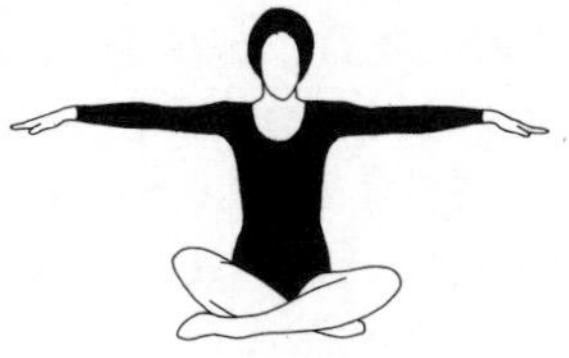

Chest Brace – Sit cross-legged, arms folded. Open arms, gently stretch out and push back. Count 3. Relax. *10 times.*

Stretch and Relax – Stand, legs a little apart, arms high. Stand on toes, stretch high. Curve back, relax knees, arms down. Relax completely, unfurl. *6 times.*

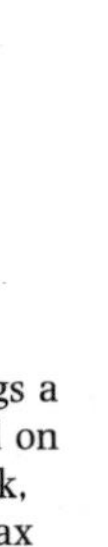
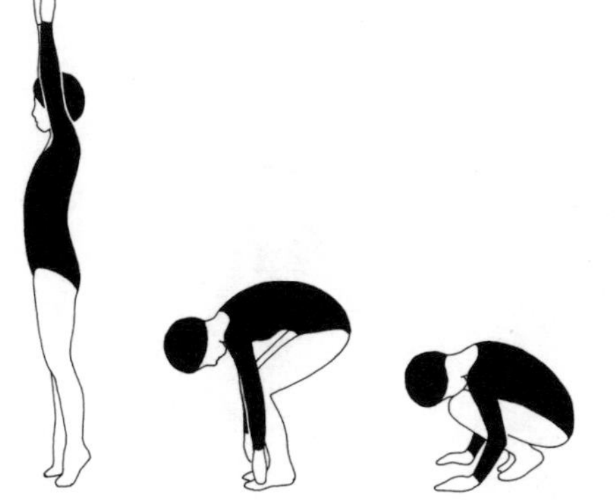

Leg Swing – Stand holding a support. Swing outside leg high in front, then way back leaning forward. *20 times.* Reverse legs.

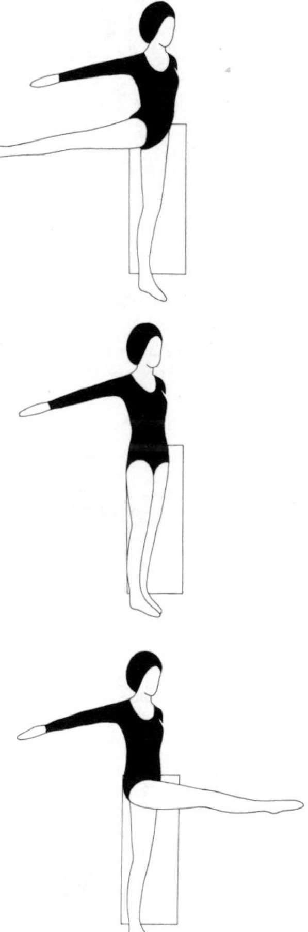

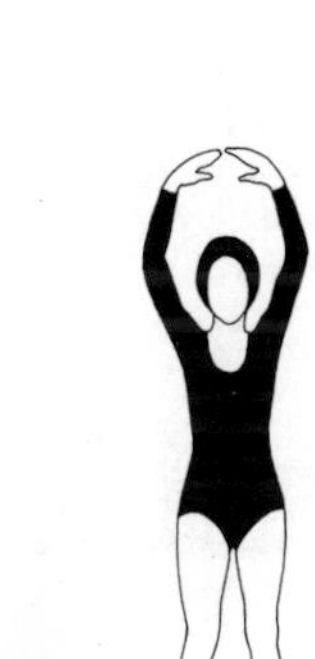
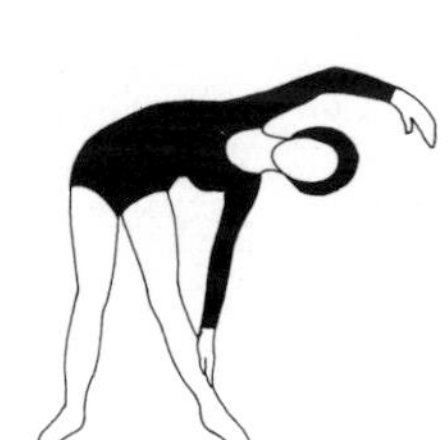
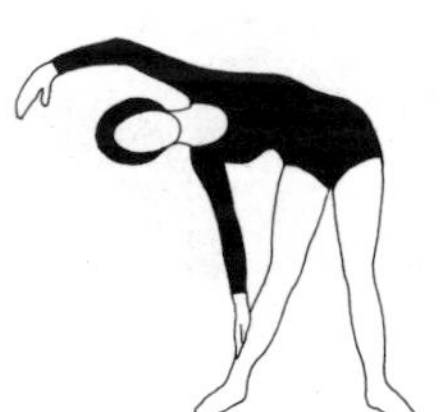

Waist Stretch – Stand feet apart, hands over head. From the waist, bend far to left, then to right. *10 times, working up to 20.*

CLASSIC INTERMEDIATE

For bodies used to a little movement but not really limber, more advanced forms of basic actions already introduced. Now you can be aware of control as well as rhythm. Pay attention to correct breathing. On exertion take deep breaths to fill the lungs; on relaxation, exhale very slowly.

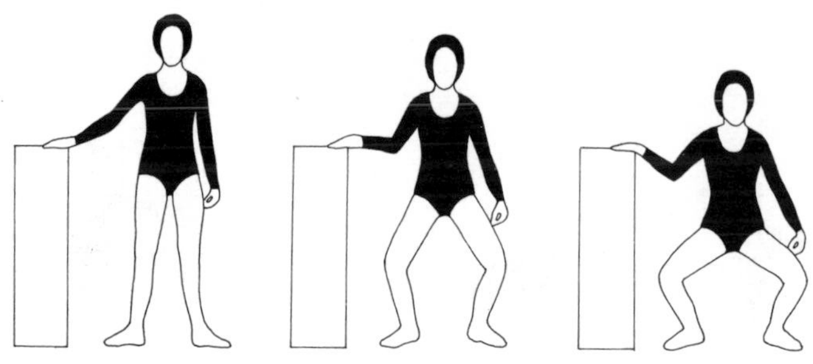

Knee Bends – Stand feet apart, holding on to support if necessary. Keeping back straight, bend both knees outward and down, keeping pelvis forward. *5 times, work up to 10 then 20.*

Kneeling Posture – Kneel, bend keeping back straight, hands clasped behind back. Stretch and curve forward until head is on floor. Return. *10 times, working up to 20.*

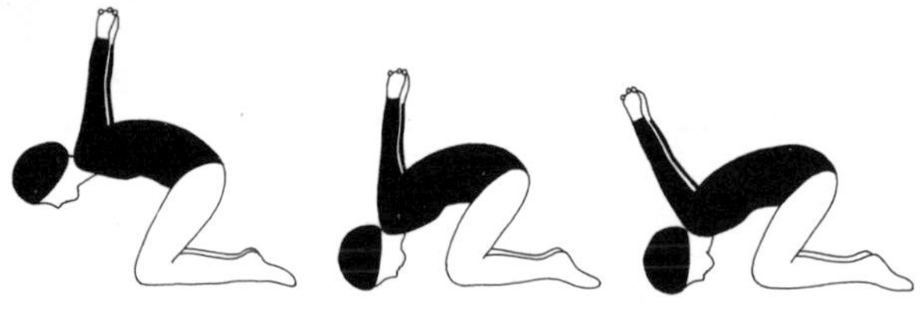

Knee-Tapping – Lie on back with legs well apart, knees bent. Clasp ankles. Bring left knee inwards and down to tap on floor, then right knee. *10 times each knee, working up to 20.*

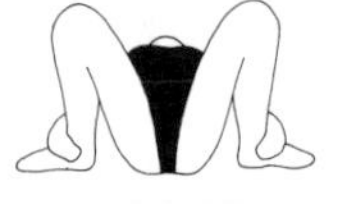

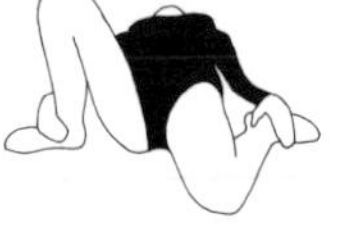

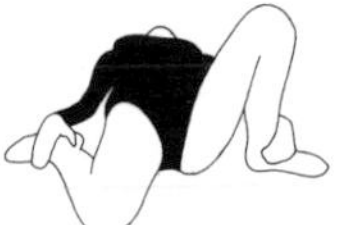

Scissor Raise – Lie on side, head on hand, other hand on floor in front. Keeping torso firm, slowly raise leg high. Lower slowly. *10 times.* Reverse legs.

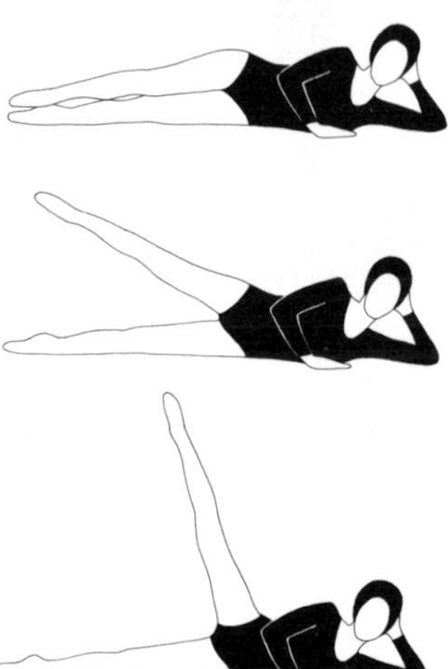

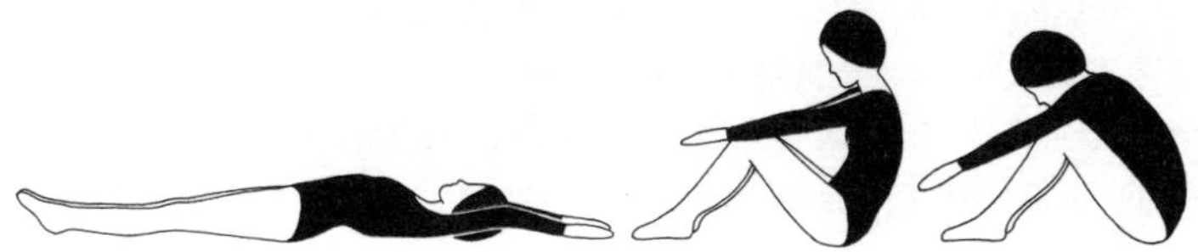

Stomach Control – Lie flat on back, arms over head. Breathe out, pulling up and stretching forward. Breathe in and return. *6 times, working up to 12 and increasing speed.*

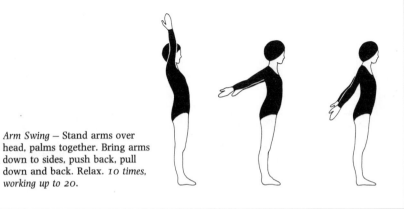

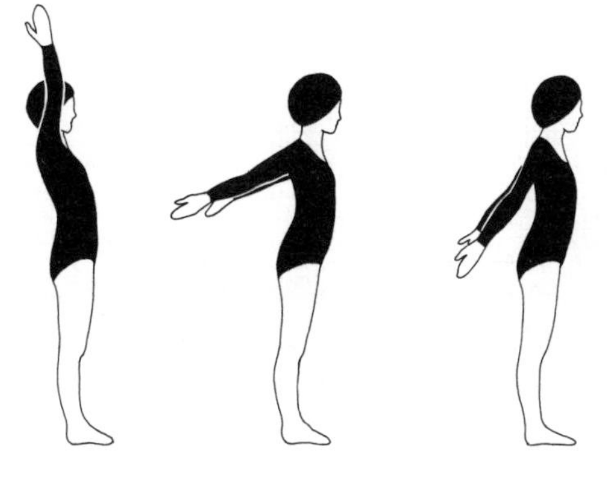

Arm Swing – Stand arms over head, palms together. Bring arms down to sides, push back, pull down and back. Relax. *10 times, working up to 20.*

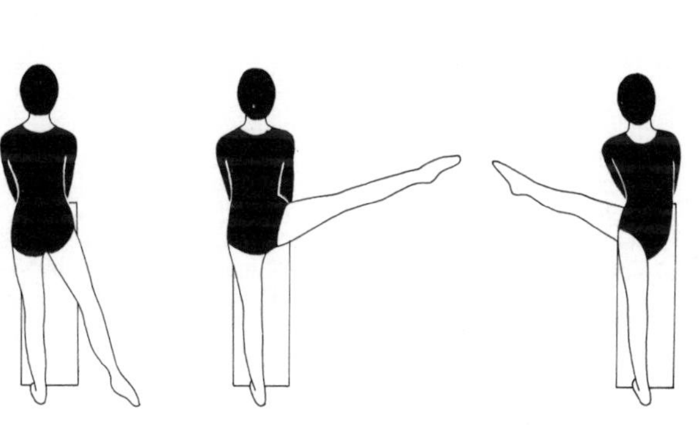

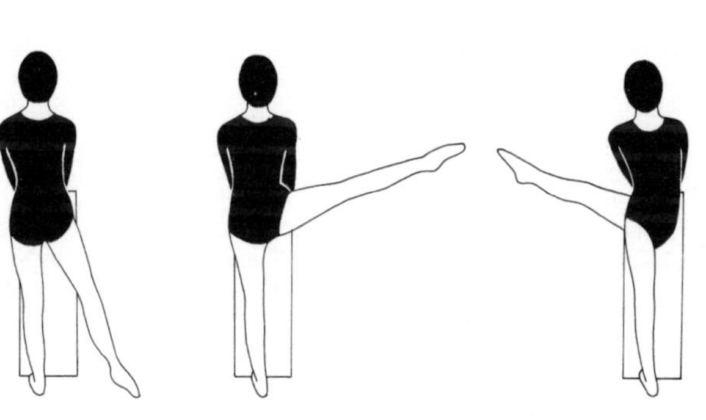

Crossover Swing – Stand about 2 feet away from a support. Keeping legs straight, stretch and lift one leg, swing across body. *20 times.* Reverse legs.

Waist Bend – Stand feet well apart, link hands over head. Keeping arms and body straight, bend slowly to right, push to the limit. Count 3. Reverse sides. *10 times, working up to 20.*

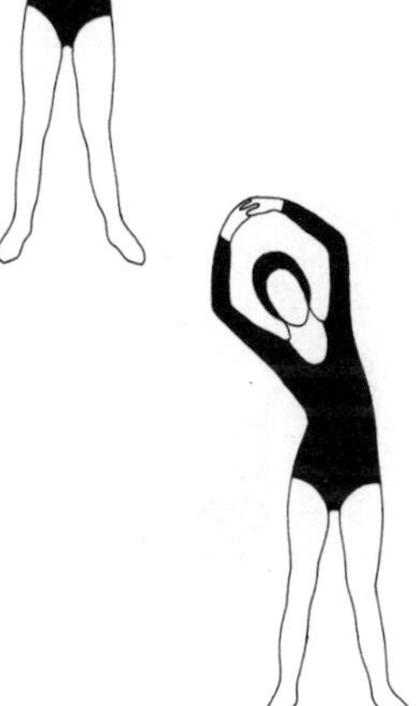

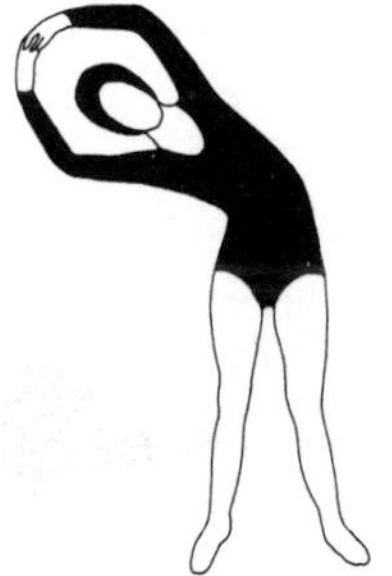

CLASSIC ADVANCED

For these exercises the muscles require more subtle control and should be able to sustain positions longer. Endurance should come with ease. Smooth and clockwork precision is expected. Do beginner series to warm up, activate muscles.

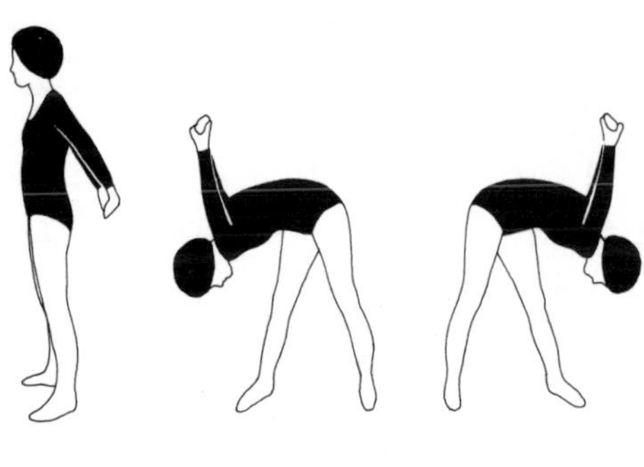

Body Bend – Stand legs apart, hands linked behind hips. Drop upper body forward, with head near knees, move head to right and left. *10 times each side.*

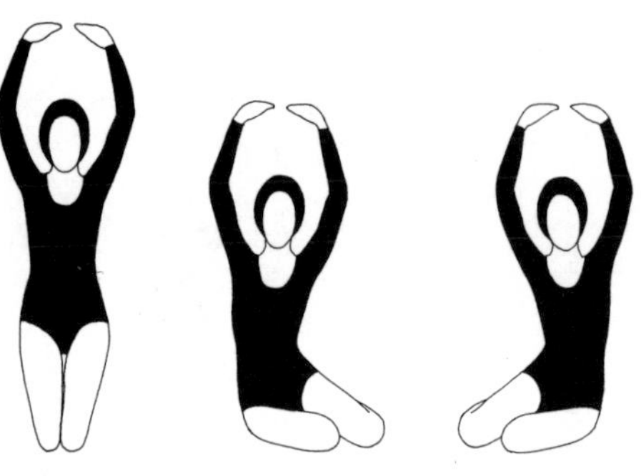

Bottom Bounce – Kneel with hands over head, fingers touching. Keeping body facing forwards, lower buttocks to touch floor on right, then swing to left and down. *5 times each side, working up to 10.*

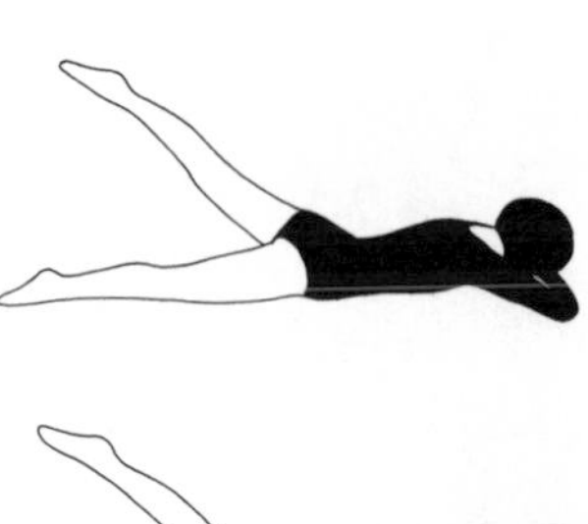

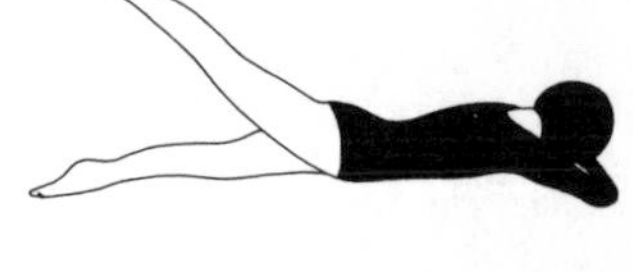

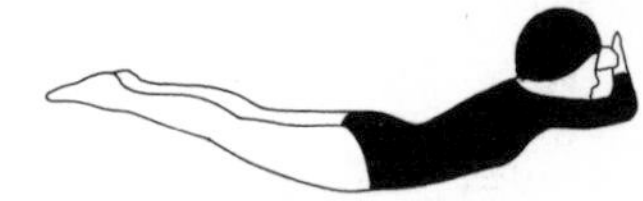

Leg and Head Lift – Lie on front. Raise left leg high. Count 2, lower. Reverse legs. Raise both legs simultaneously, lift shoulders and head with hands on forehead; count 2. *5 times, working up to 10.*

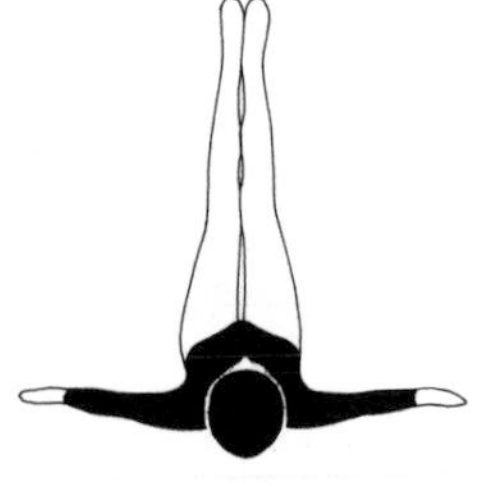

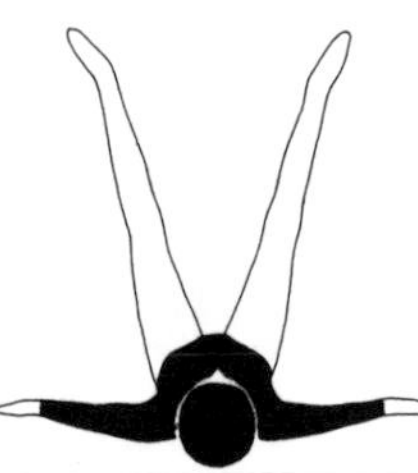

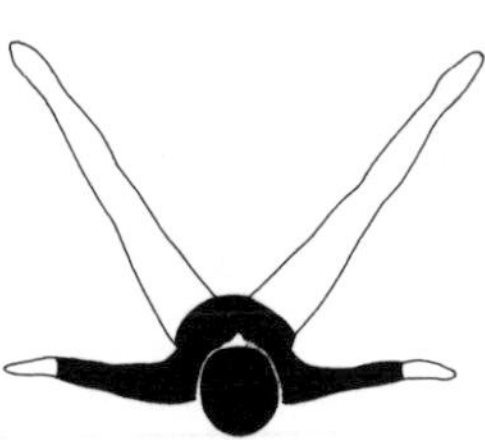

Thigh Control – Lie, arms out at sides, legs at right angles to torso. Spread legs wide, bring together. *Non-stop 20 times.*

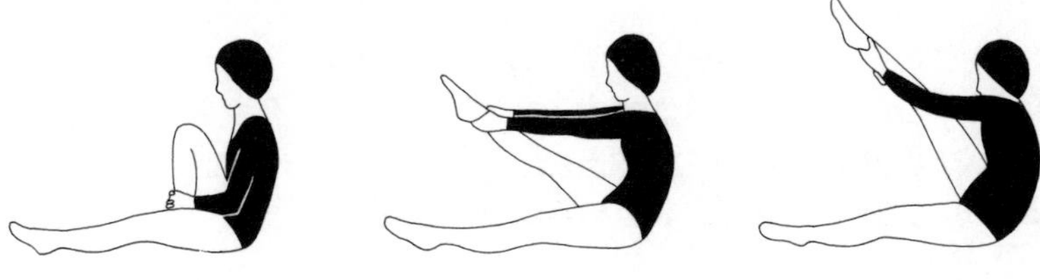

Complete Leg Stretch – Sit, left leg straight, right leg bent. Clasp ankle, bringing heel right against buttocks. Holding firm, straighten leg pulling up high. Count 3, lower leg. *3 times each leg.*

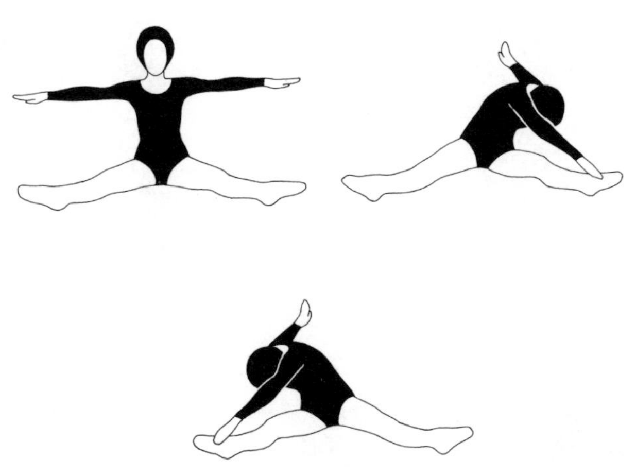

Sitting Stretch – Sit upright, legs wide apart, arms outstretched. Swing forward to touch left foot with right hand, then vice versa. *20 times in rhythm.*

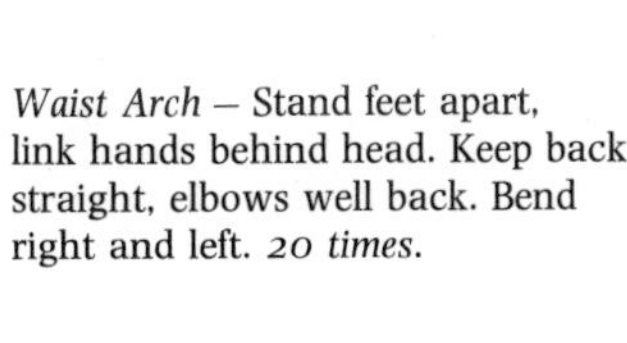

Waist Arch – Stand feet apart, link hands behind head. Keep back straight, elbows well back. Bend right and left. *20 times.*

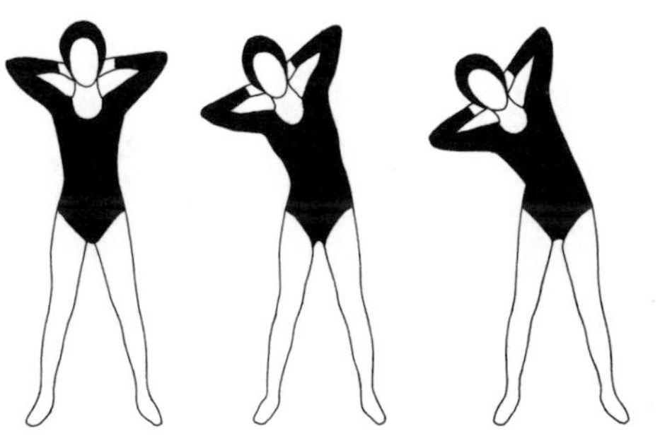

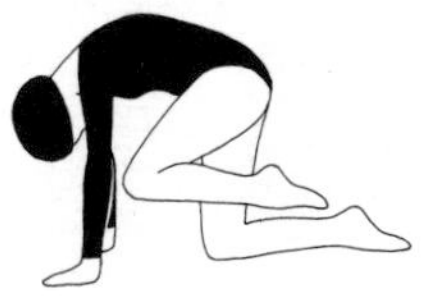

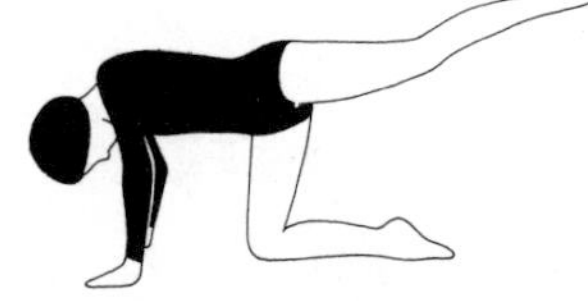

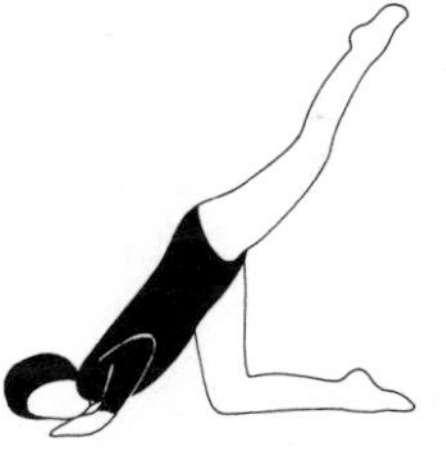

Kneel and Stretch – Kneel, arms straight, head down. Bend left knee to chest, push straight back and up. Count 2. Bend elbows allowing head to rest on floor, holding body in diagonal line from toe to shoulder. Count 2. Relax. Reverse legs. *5 times each leg.*

STICK

These are straightforward classic exercises with a prop to give movements a systematic form. Suggested for women who need some sense of direction for hands; in addition stick controls arm movements, paces distance and provides good balance. Use long pole, broom handle or curtain rod.

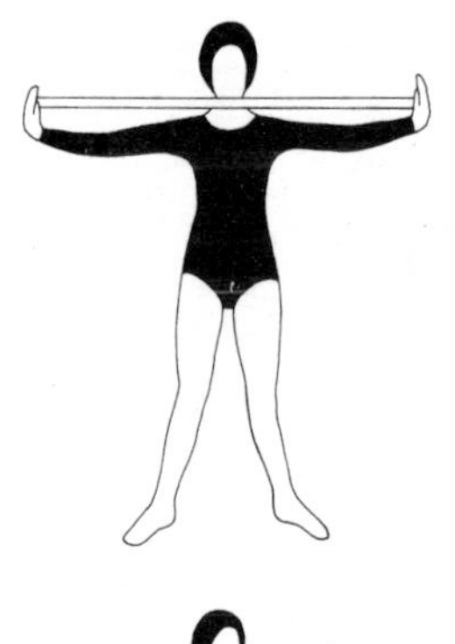

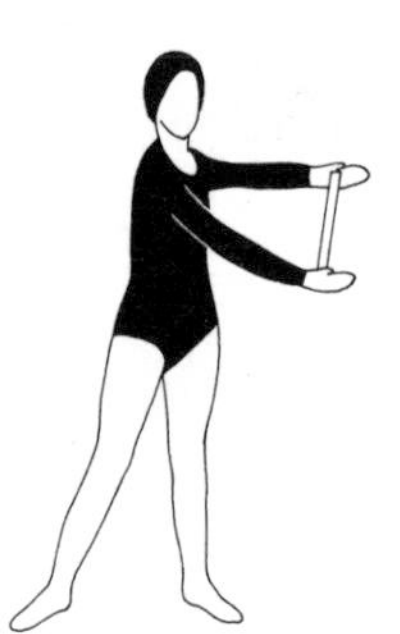

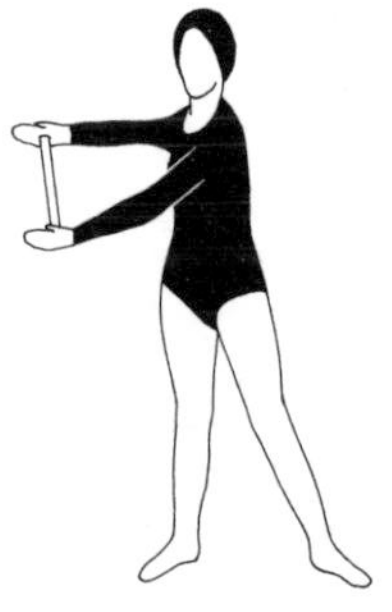

Fore-arm Reach – Feet apart, stick ends held between palms, arms stretched really wide. Swing arms from side to side, holding stick firmly. *20 times.*

Shoulder Brace – Feet together, body balanced on balls of feet. Hold stick in hands behind body, arms straight. Swing wide to each side, back and forth working shoulder muscles. *20 times.*

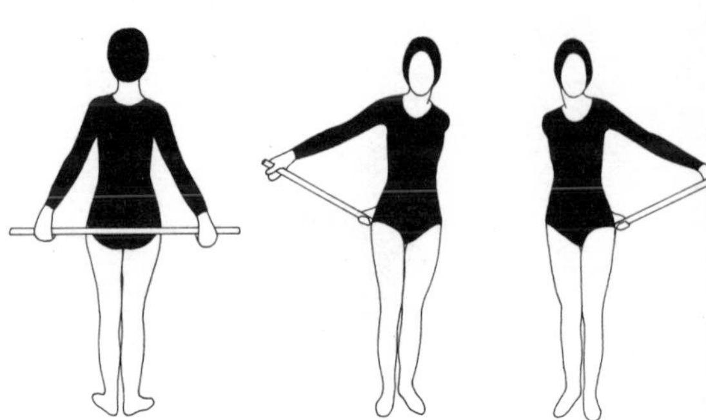

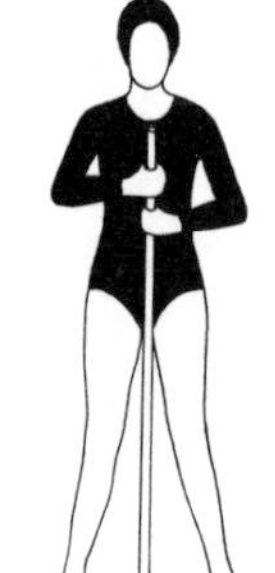

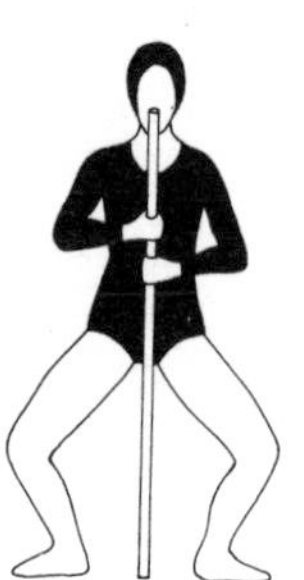

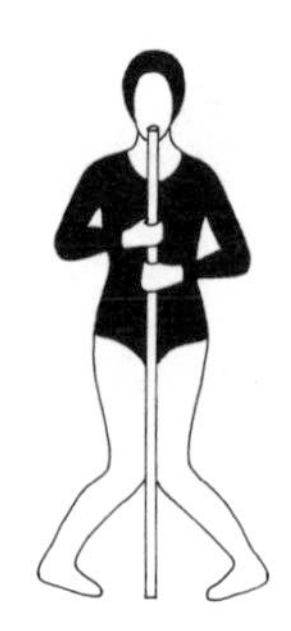

Foot Switch – Stand feet a few inches apart, stick held vertically. Bend knees, turn toes out, straighten up. Bend knees, turn toes in, straighten up. *In-out quickly 20 times.*

Leg Swing – Stand upright, stick vertical. Hold with both hands, balance it. Swing one leg forward and back as far as possible, holding stick firm. *30 times each leg.*

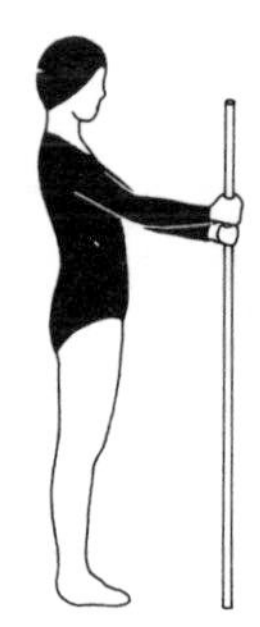

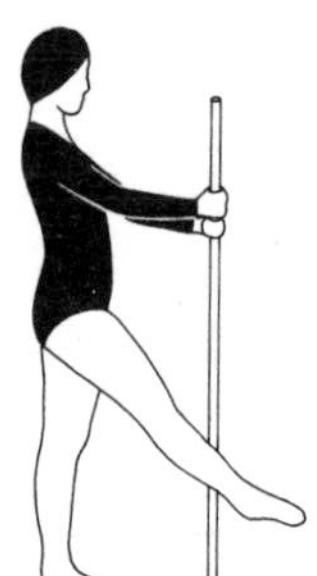

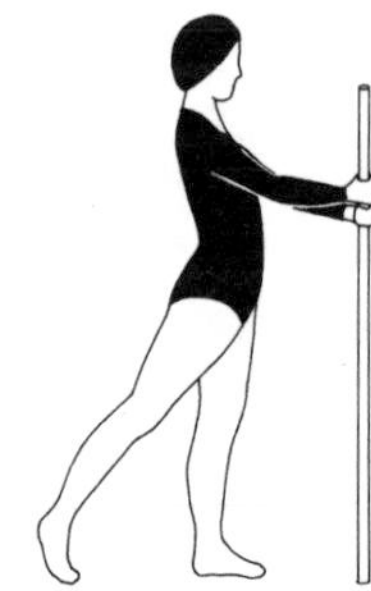

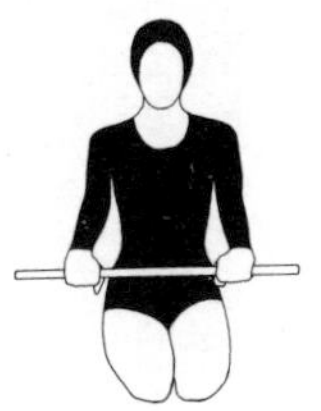

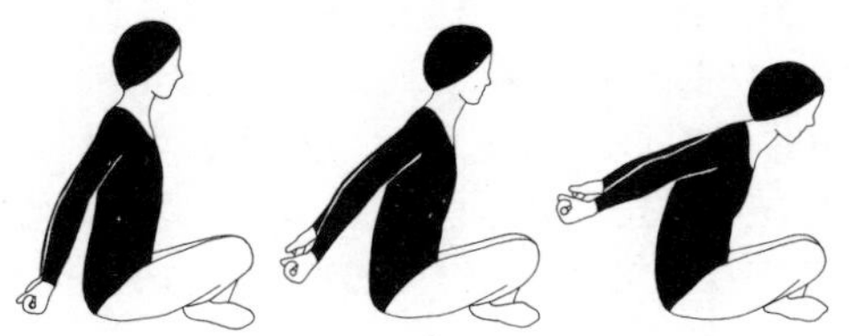

Behind the Back – Sit cross-legged, hold stick behind back, palms upward. Push stick up and down very slowly, keeping arms straight. *30 times.*

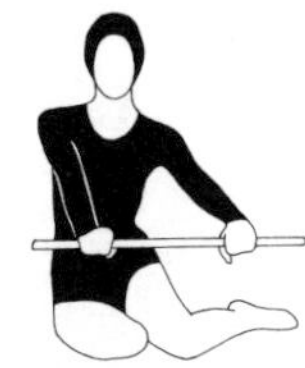

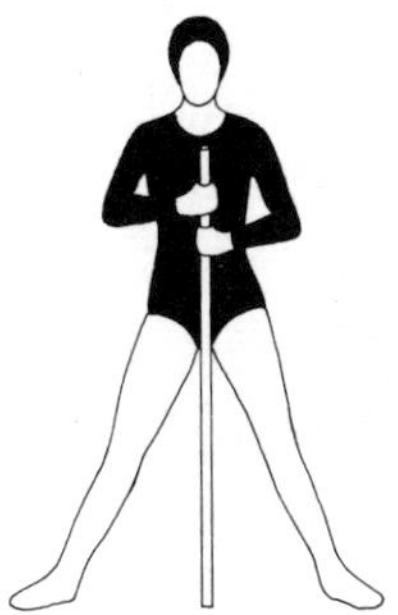

Side Dip – Stand legs apart, holding stick with both hands. Keeping back straight and buttocks tucked under, dip left then right knee in rhythm. *20 times.*

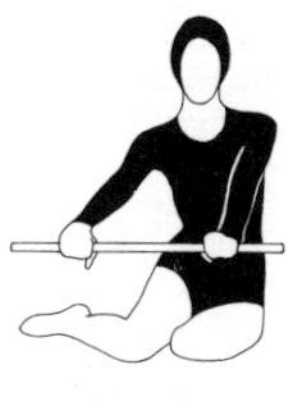

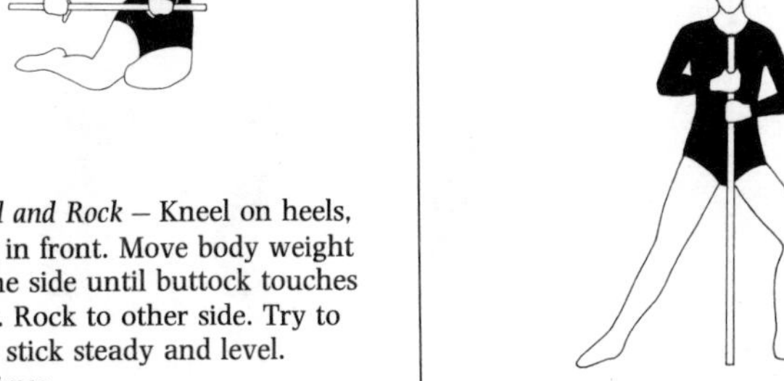

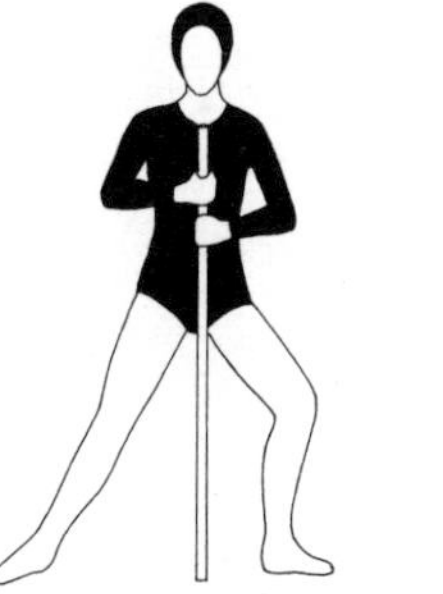

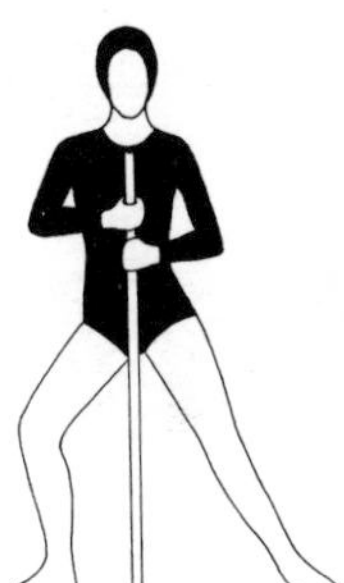

Kneel and Rock – Kneel on heels, stick in front. Move body weight to one side until buttock touches floor. Rock to other side. Try to keep stick steady and level. *20 times.*

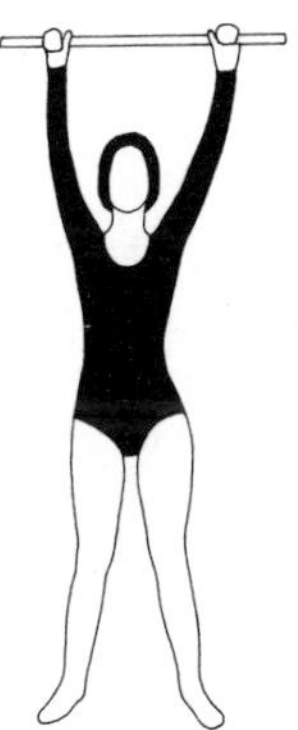

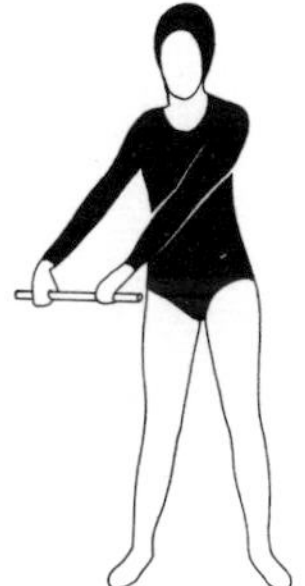

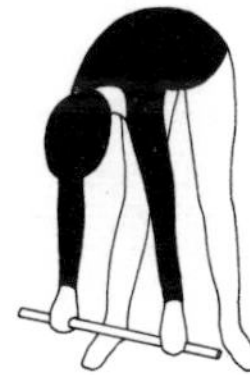

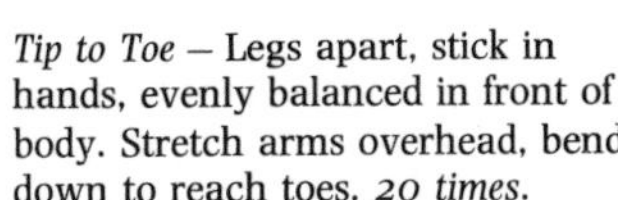

Tip to Toe – Legs apart, stick in hands, evenly balanced in front of body. Stretch arms overhead, bend down to reach toes. *20 times.*

WEIGHTS

Excellent for those with stamina and anxious for quick reshaping. Extra pounds make muscles work harder. Start with 3 pounds (1.5 k.), work up to 5 (2.5 k.), finally to 10 (5 k.). There are weights to hold, tie or slip on. Or make your own sacks. Warning: too much for too long can develop ugly muscles.

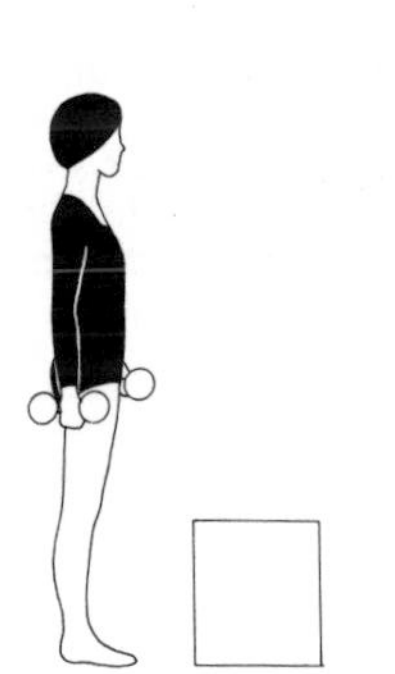
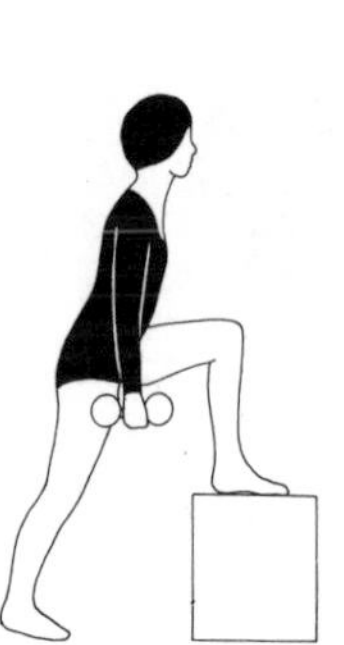
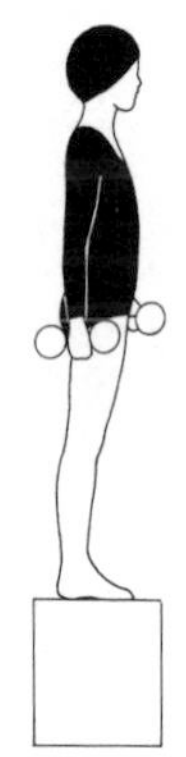

Step-Up – Stand in front of chair, or high step, weight in each hand. Put one foot on chair, draw other leg up to it. Step down same way. *10 times each leg.*

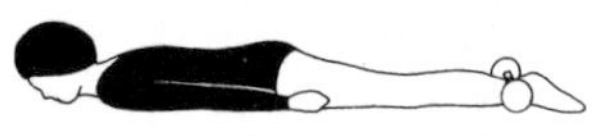
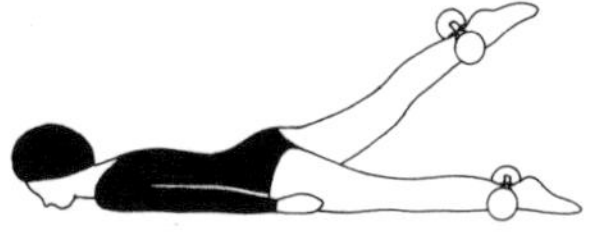
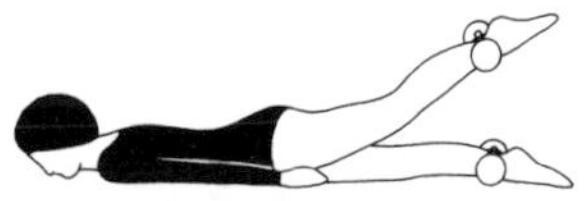

Horizontal Lift – Lie on floor, weights tied on each ankle. Raise one leg as high as possible, count 6, lower slowly. Reverse legs. *6 times each leg.*

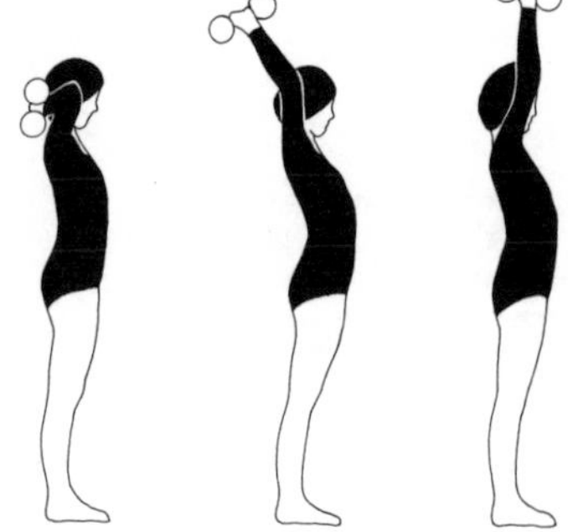

Arm Raising – Feet together, weight in each hand behind head, elbows close to ears. Raise and lower 3 times quickly. Relax. *10 times.* Rest 3 minutes.

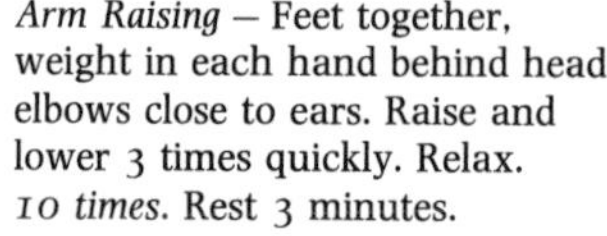

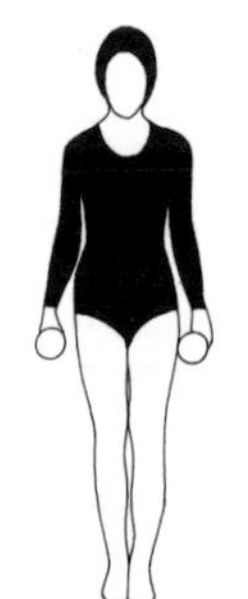
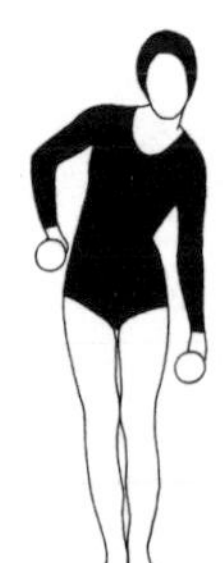
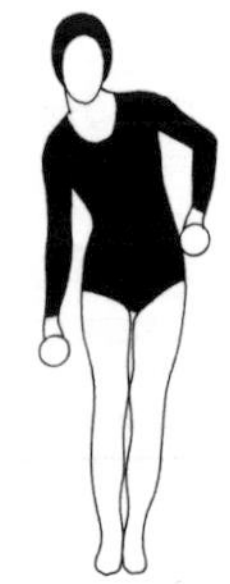

Body Bend – Stand feet together, knees slightly flexed, weight in each hand. Pull right arm up, bend body to left, then vice versa. *10 times.* Rest 3 minutes.

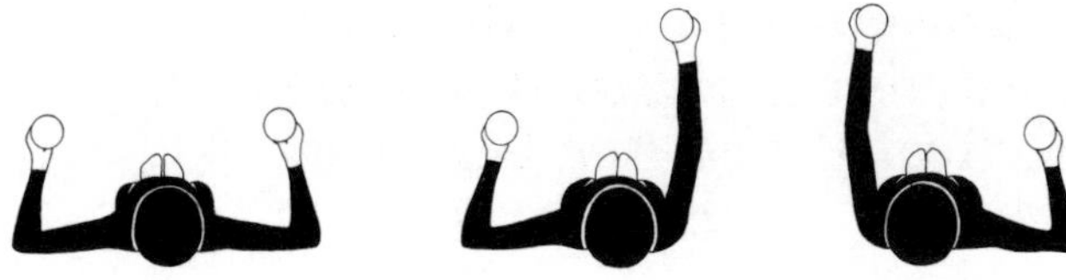

Arm Push – Lie on back, weight in each hand. Elbows bent, upper arms flat on floor. Push alternate arms towards ceiling. *6 times each arm.*

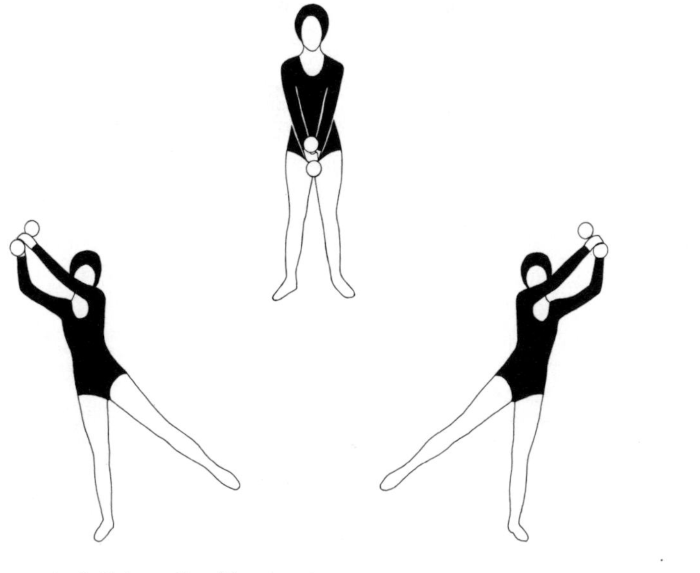

Angle Swing – Stand legs apart, holding one weight in both hands. Swing arms up and out way over to the right. At height of swing, lift left foot for balance. *10 times each side.*

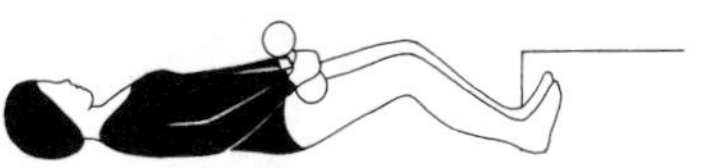

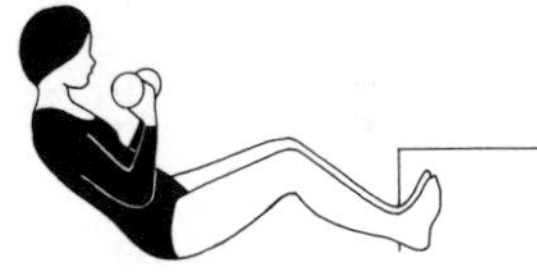

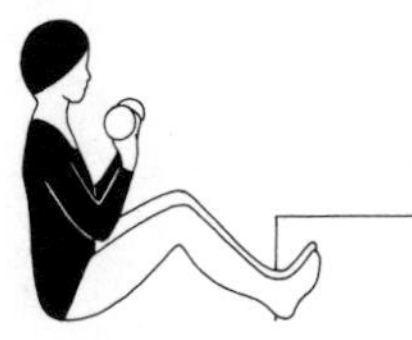

Stomach Pull – Lie on floor with feet on underside of couch, one weight in both hands. Slowly raise body up and down 3 times, knees and feet firm. Relax. *6 times.*

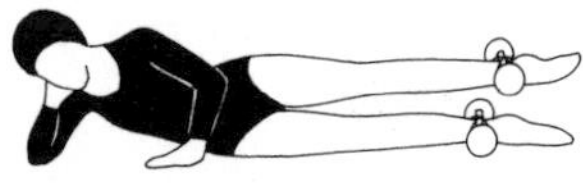

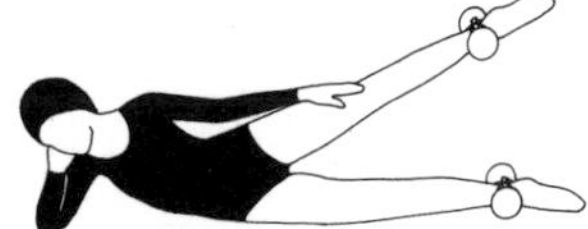

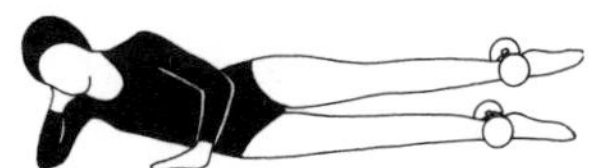

Side Lift – Weights on each ankle, lie on side, supported by one elbow and hand. Lift leg, help with hand near knee, lower slowly. *6 times each leg.*

WATER

Callisthenics in the water is one of the most pleasant and easiest ways to exercise. The buoyant nature of the body gives the illusion of little effort, yet it's the pressure of water that makes movements so effective. Perfect for beginners and older women. Water at shoulder height; best in pool.

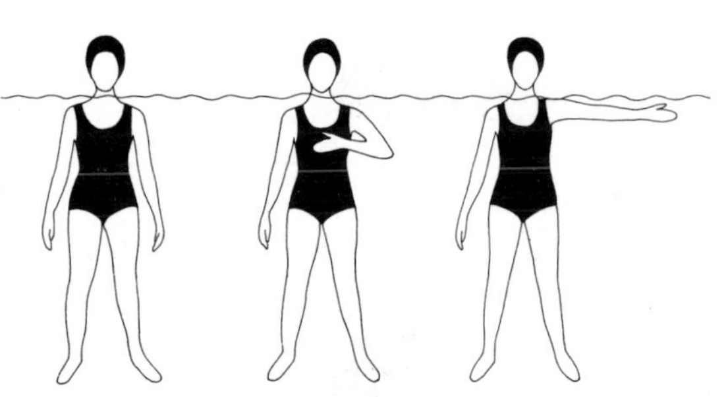

Arm Push – Stand feet apart, arms at sides. Bend arm across in front of bosom, palm facing body. Straighten elbow then push arm back hard against water. Relax to side. *20 times each arm.*

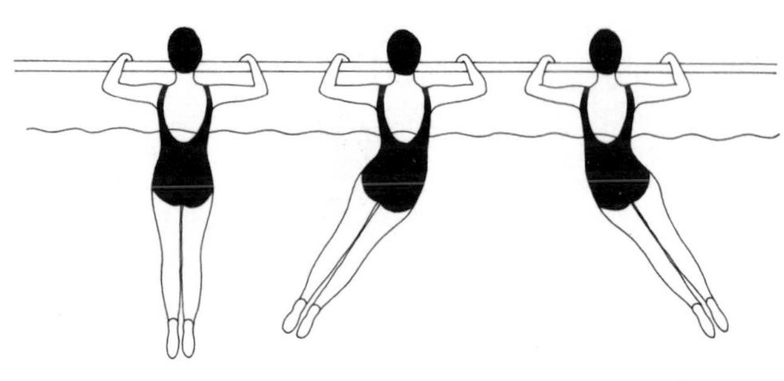

Waist Swing – Hold rail, keeping legs straight and toes pointed, swing each side from the waist, torso firm, for 2 minutes.

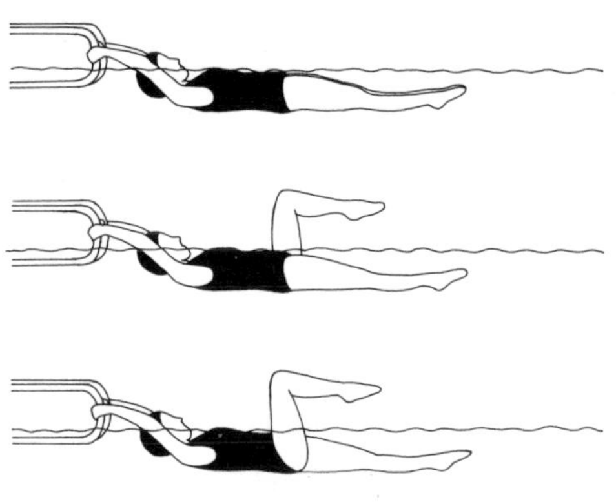

Bicycle Kick – Lie on back, hold ladder or edge. Bicycle kick lifting feet out of water, knees high and push hard on downward kick. *30 kicks or more.*

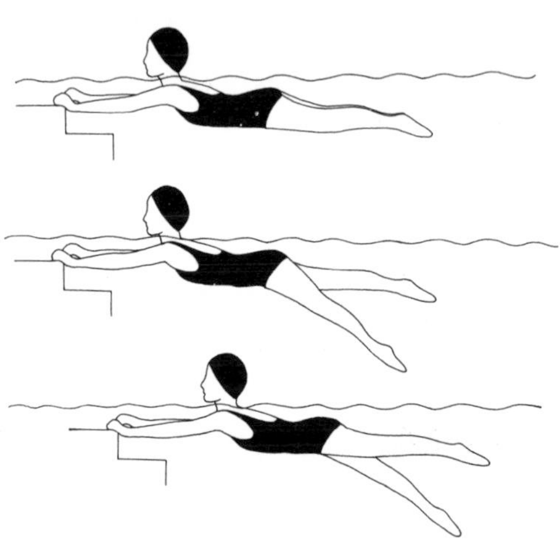

Leg Kicks – Hands on ladder or edge. Float in a horizontal position. Holding knees straight, kick legs fast and hard for 2 minutes. Rest. *4 times.*

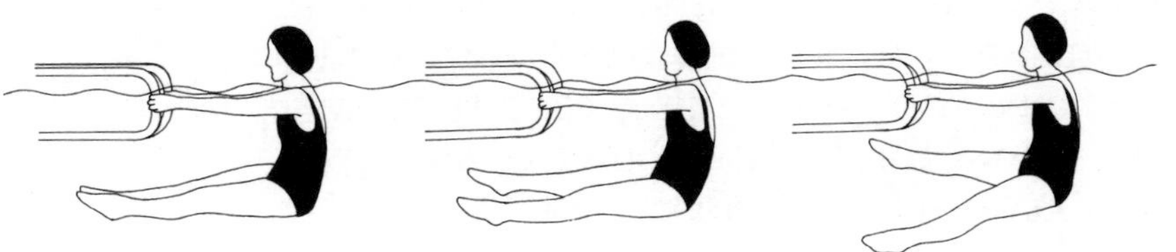

Water Scissors – Grasp ladder, sit in water, arms straight, legs together. With a jump of the body, open legs wide to a scissor, hold, draw together. *Quickly 30 times.*

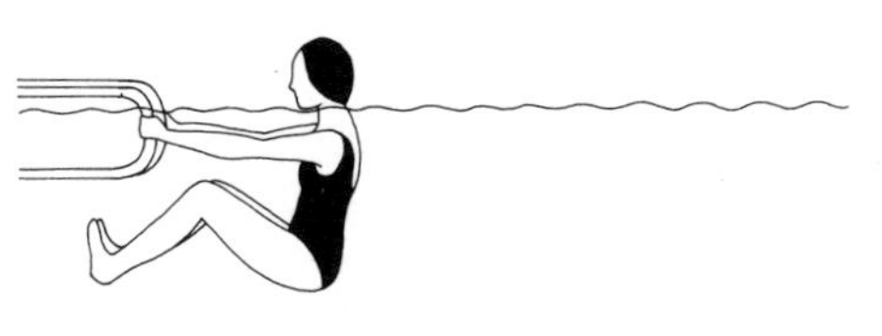

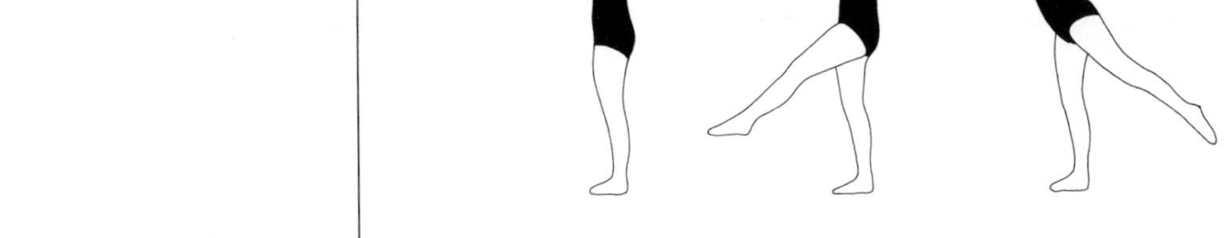

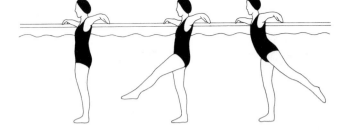

Leg Swing – Stand with one hand holding rail, other arm straight. Swing one leg up high in front, then back really stretching. *20 swings*. Reverse sides.

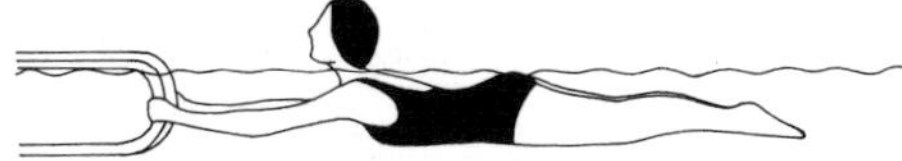

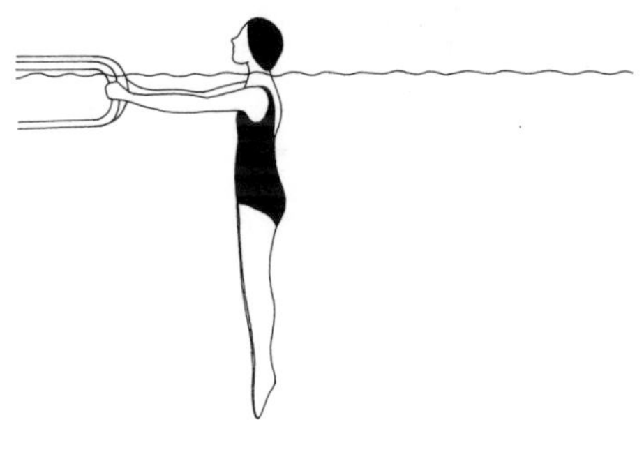

Leg Thrust – Face ladder or edge, hold. Sit in water, bend knees, feet slightly apart. Thrust legs back to prone position. Balance a few seconds; slowly return. *25 times.*

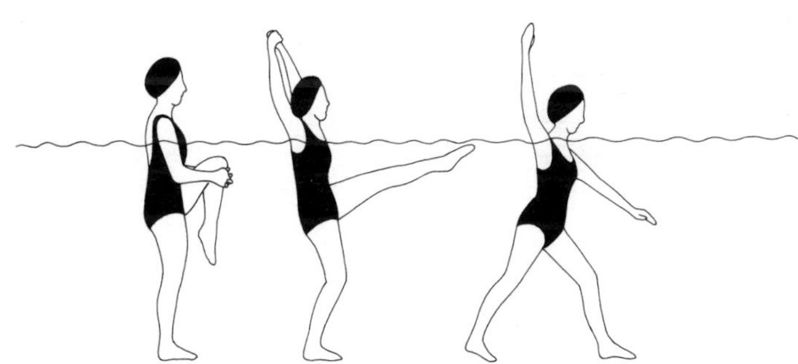

Giant Walk – Bring a knee to chest, clasp with arms. Stretch leg high in front, arms clasped overhead. Take a giant step forward swinging one arm down over front leg, other arm back to balance. Repeat with other leg. Walk for 3 minutes.

BED

If you have trouble getting up in the morning, these exercises are for you. Prime requisite is a firm mattress. Although most exercises are performed lying down, they require more muscle effort than you would think. They build up energy for the day but are also good relaxers after work.

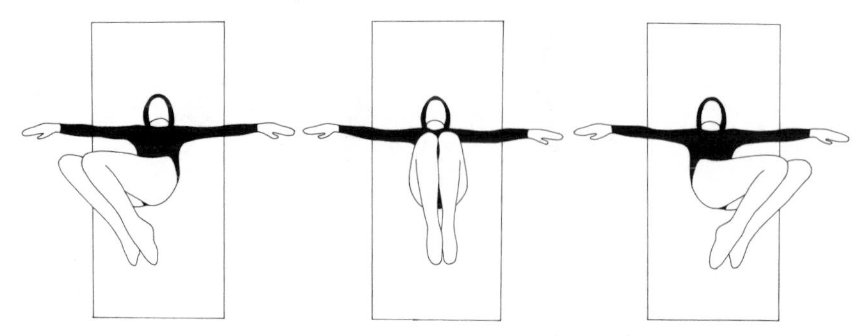

Waist Turn – On back, arms stretched out. Bend knees, lift feet. Keeping knees firmly together, swing legs from left to right aiming to touch bed. *20 times.*

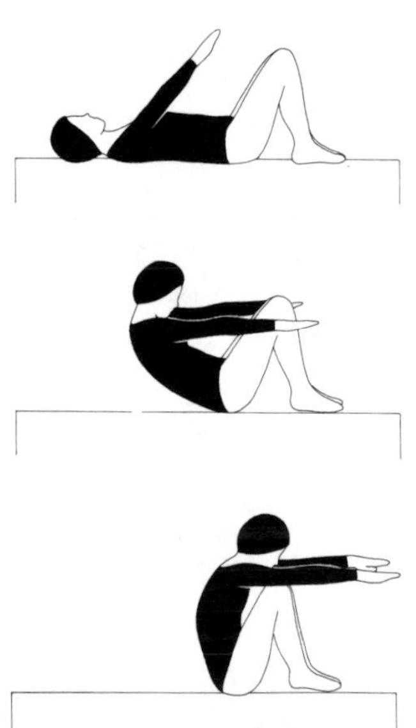

Stomach Tug – Lie on back, knees bent, feet flat, arms out in front, a little apart. Pull up body so chest touches thighs. Lower slowly. *10 times.*

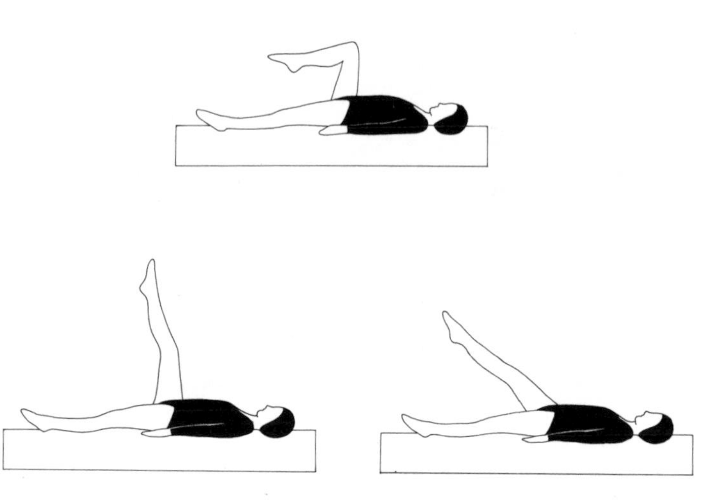

Leg Control – Lie on back, arms at sides, palms down. Bend one knee at right angles, count 3. Stretch to ceiling, count 3. Lower to bed, keeping straight. *6 times each leg.*

Bed Scissors – Lie on side, head supported by elbow. Raise upper leg as high as possible, hold, lower slowly. *10 times*. Reverse sides.

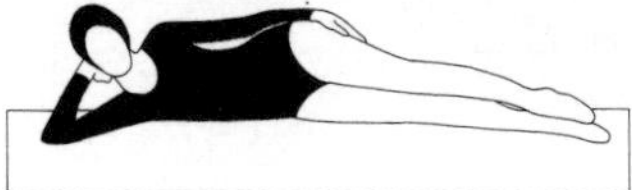

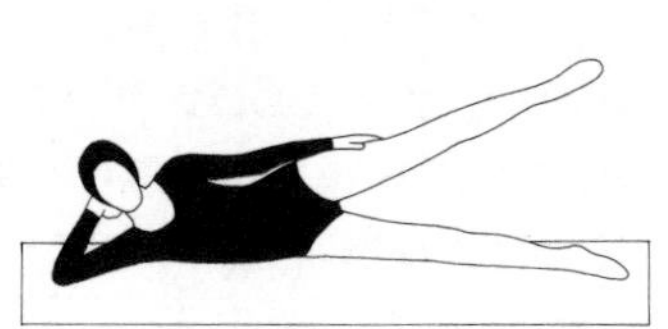

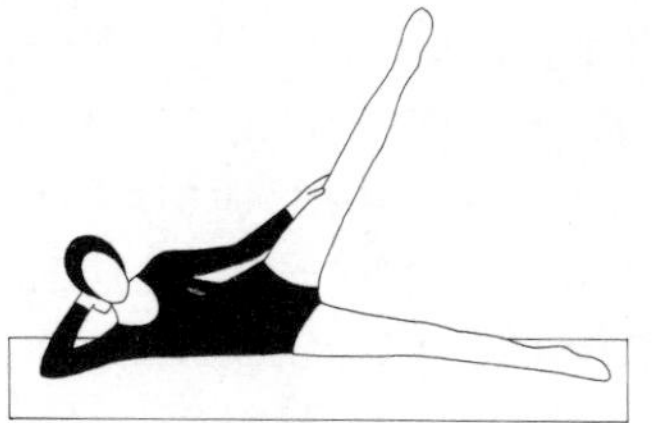

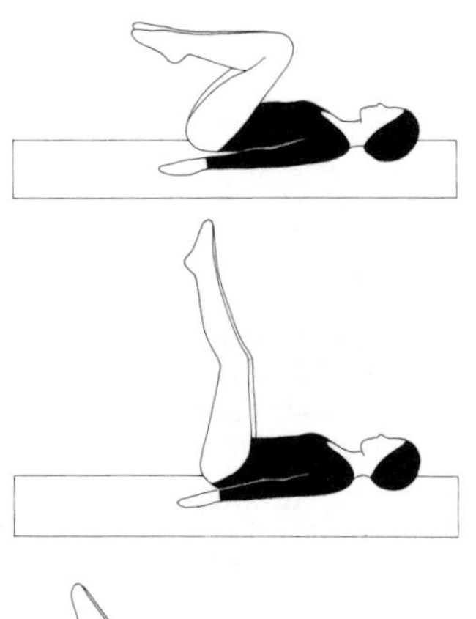

Leg Stretch – Lie flat, arms by sides, palms down. Bend knees against chest. Stretch legs high and straight, lower slowly without bending knees. *10 times*.

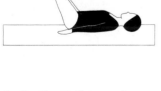

Arm Crossover – Lie on back, arms at sides. Lift arms and cross over face, swing back to stretch out flat. *20 times, alternating arms*.

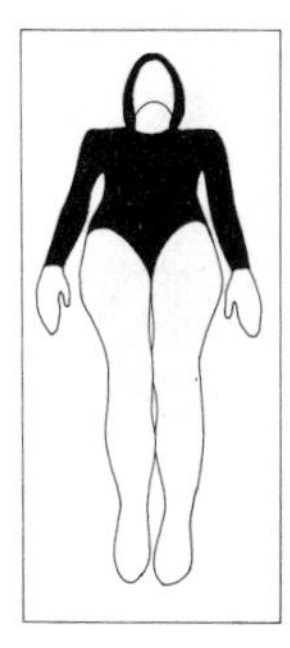

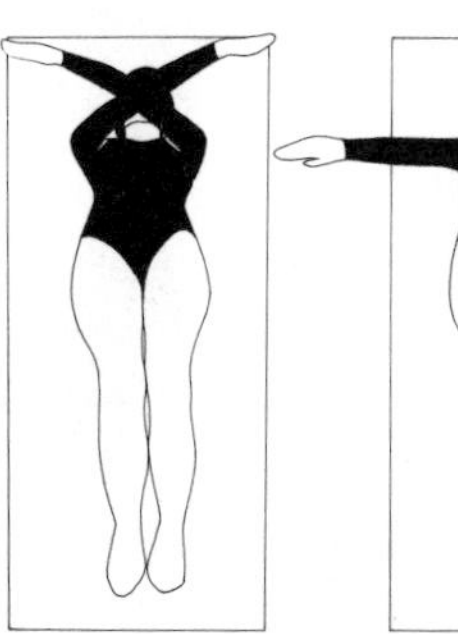

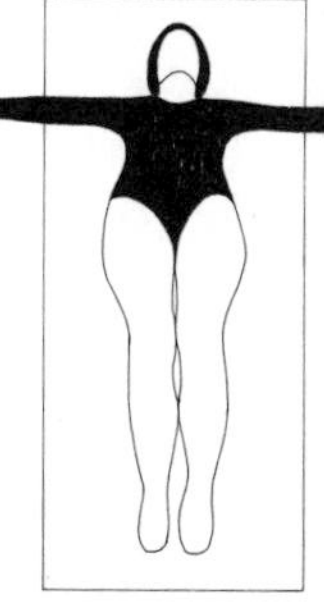

Air Walking – Lie face down at end of bed, feet on floor. Grasp mattress. Raise one leg slowly to horizontal position, hold. Lower gradually. *10 times each leg*.

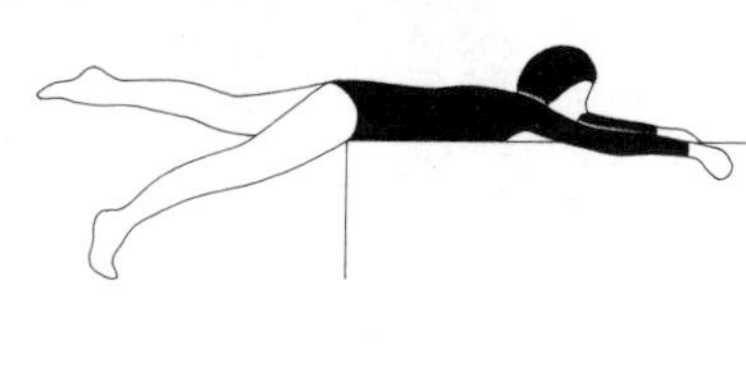

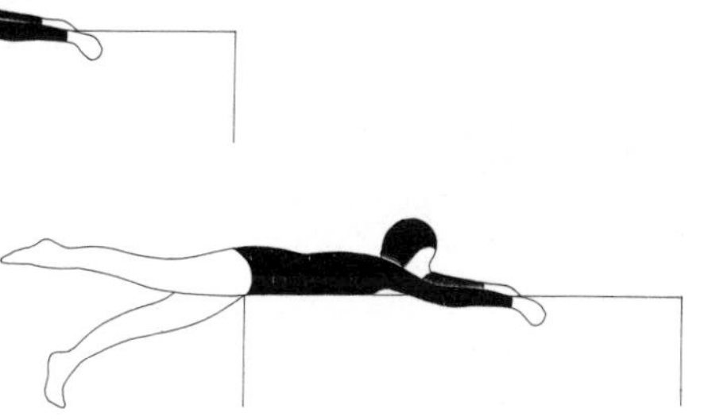

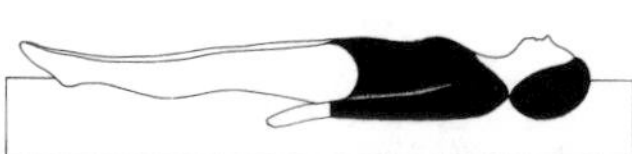

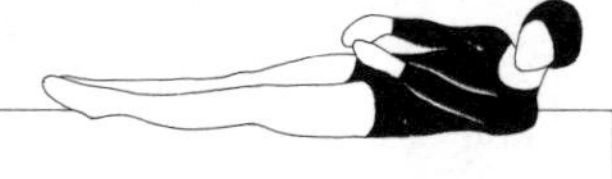

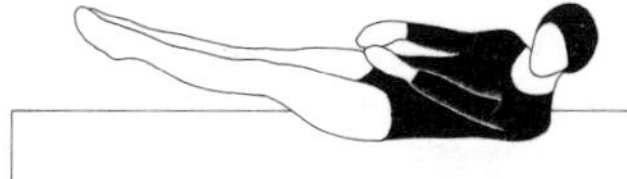

Almost Up – Lie on back, arms at sides. Raise head, then shoulders, also raising arms to clasp over abdomen. Slowly lift legs together. Balance, count 5. Relax. *10 times*.

SCULPTURE

Pioneered by Dr Bess Mensendieck, this is based on the simple premise that by learning to do everyday movements in the proper way one can reshape the body within limits of frame. Movements do not require outward exertion but are muscle controlling schemes motivated by mental concentration. At times limbs are used, but slowly. All ages and figures can benefit from this type of reshaping programme.

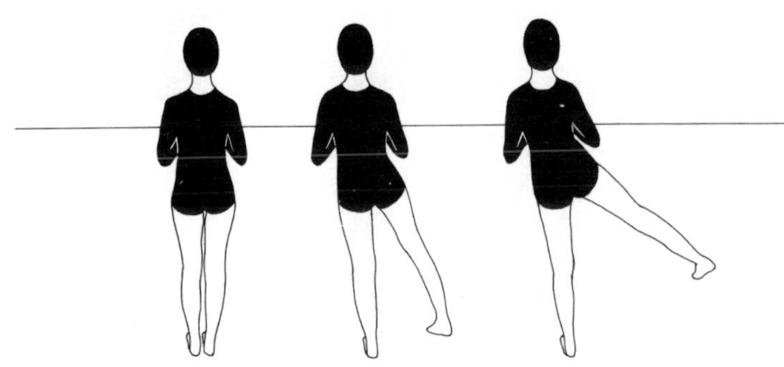

Leg Pendulum – Stand balanced, hold support if necessary. Slowly draw up right leg from hip, draw in stomach. Using right buttock muscle, move right leg backward then up, keeping leg straight. Release buttock muscle slowly lowering leg; then release muscle of right lumbar region, lowering foot. Relax. *3 times each leg.*

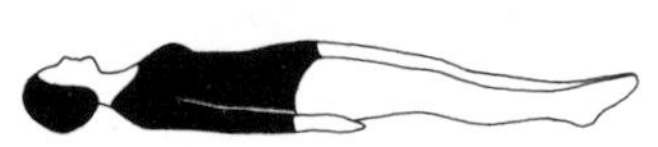

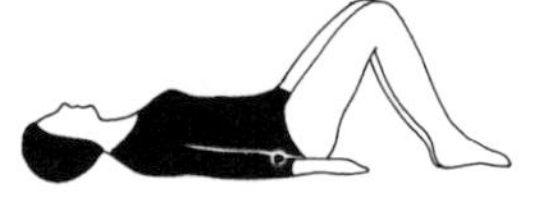

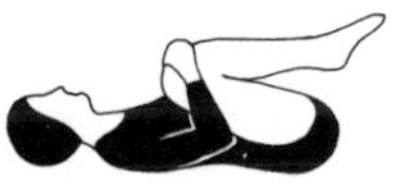

Body Fold – Lie at rest, body supported at all parts on floor. Bend knees so feet are close to buttocks. Bring knees up to the chest, folding body through muscle contraction in back and stomach. Clasp hands around knees if necessary, count 6. Relax. *5 times.*

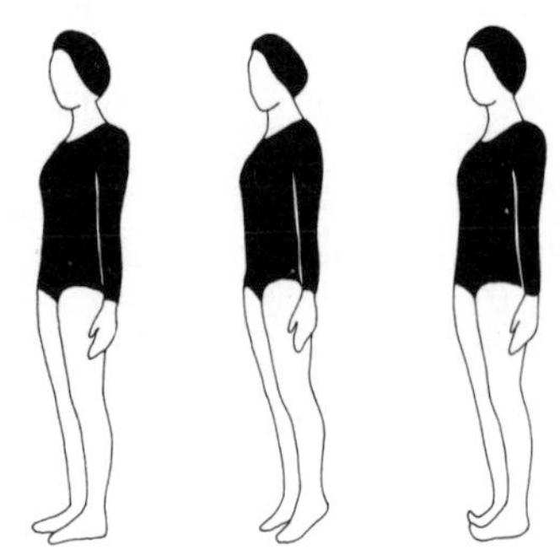

Heel and Toe Raising – Stand balanced. Using calf muscles, slowly raise heels, transferring weight to balls of feet along inner margin. Hold buttock muscles and those of inner thighs. Count 6. Release. *3 times.* Rest. *3 more times.* Rest. Now using stretcher muscles of the toes, try to raise all toes straight upward. Sometimes only big toe will respond at first. Make the others do so through will power. Count 6. Relax. *3 times.* Rest. *3 more times.*

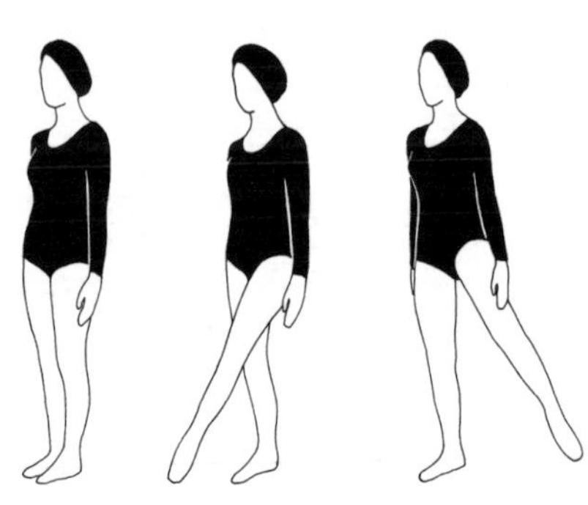

Leg Arcs – Stand balanced. Using muscle in lumbar region, draw left leg up so heel is off floor. Use left buttock muscle to slowly move leg backwards, at same time drawing in the abdomen. Make an arc to the side. With thigh muscle bring leg back to original position. *3 times each leg.*

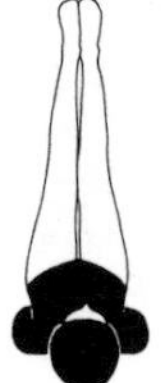
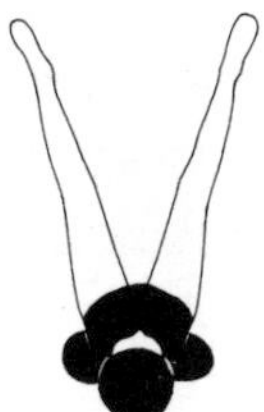
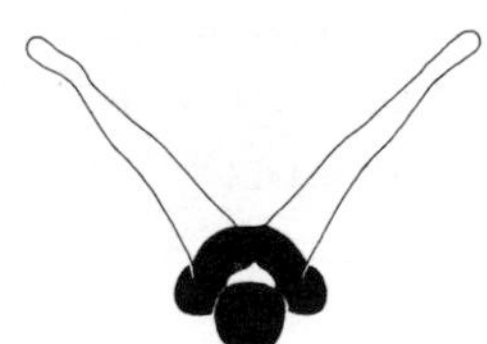

Leg Spread – Lie at rest, arms by sides. With knees straight, lift legs holding close together until at right angles to torso. Slowly open legs wide as possible. Count 6. Return together, relax. *5 times*.

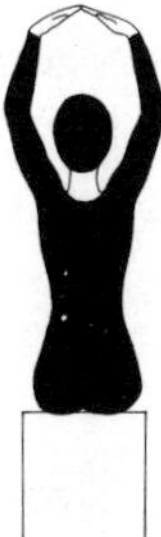
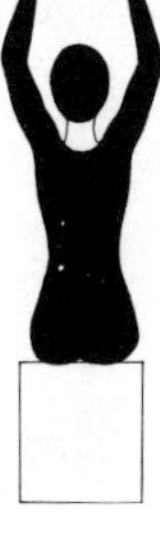
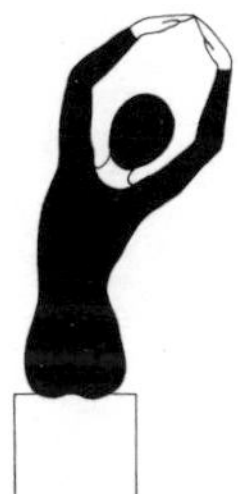

Trunk Bend – Sit balanced, make this posture a habit: sit near front edge of chair on sitting bone, feet flat, parallel and slightly apart. Arms loosely by side. Draw abdomen in and up, beginning near groin and continuing up to chest; use ball of each foot and sitting bone for support.
Now raise both arms overhead, palms facing; stretch elbows as much as possible. Slowly bend over by stretching opposite side of trunk; consciously stretch up before bending. Count to 6 at limit. Return to upright position. *3 times*. Relax. Reverse sides.

Buttock Control – Assume correct balance, which you must consciously adjust to whenever standing: feet parallel, a tiny bit apart, pressing forwards on ball of each foot, weight evenly distributed. Using muscles in front of thighs, pull up knee caps. From small of back, slowly stretch spine upwards, lifting head straight as though a thread were pulling from the top. Shoulder blades back and down. Arms loose at sides – with inside of elbows and palms facing body.
Place palms over buttocks. Slowly draw buttocks towards each other, when as tight as possible count 6. Release. *3 times*. Rest. *3 more times*. Sometimes one muscle pulls faster and better. Consciously make both sides work evenly. Check in rear mirror in the nude.

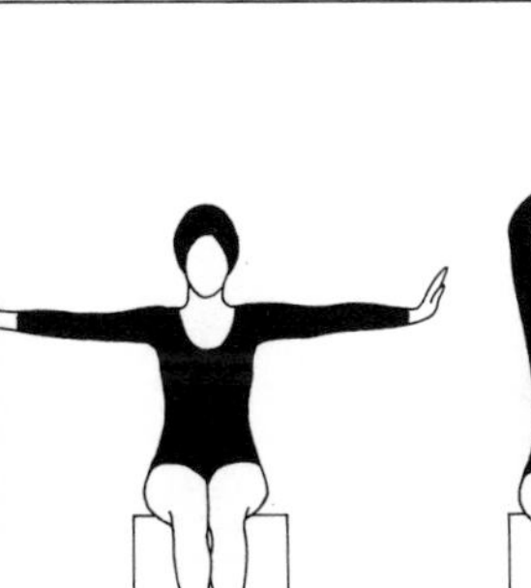
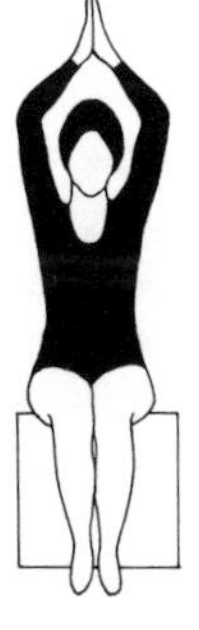
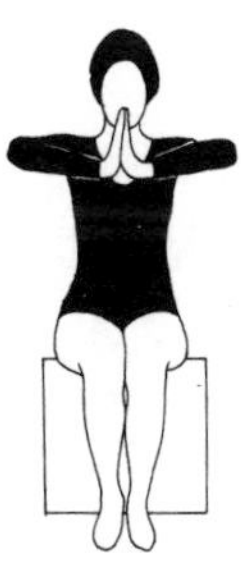

Bosom Lift – Sit balanced. Lift arms slowly to side, then up and over head, elbows as straight as possible, palms together. Using muscles to lower shoulders and arms, push elbows out until shoulder level. Count 6. Relax. *3 times*. Rest. *3 more times*.

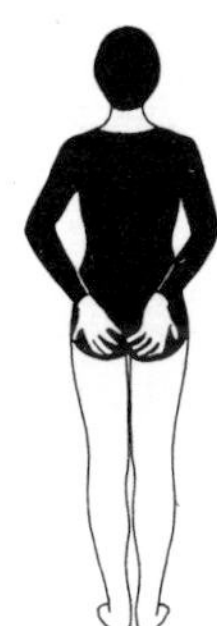
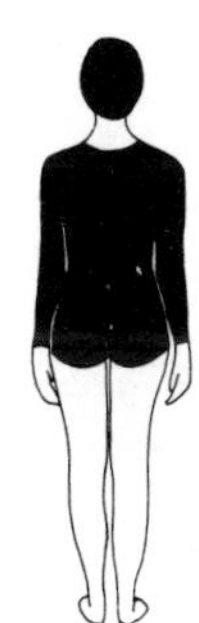

ISOMETRIC

There is very little movement to these exercises and anyone can do them anywhere. The principle is that muscle can be toned by setting one strength against another. Consider these as bonus exercises, to be done at odd moments during the day; at work, on the bus, in bed, and after the bath.

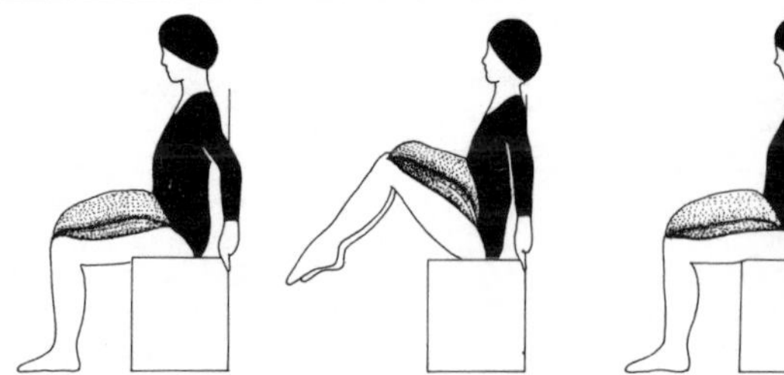

Cushion Squeeze – Sit with cushion on lap. Grip sides of chair. Bend knees, raise thighs trying to squeeze cushion against stomach. Count 10. Relax to count of 3. *3 times.*

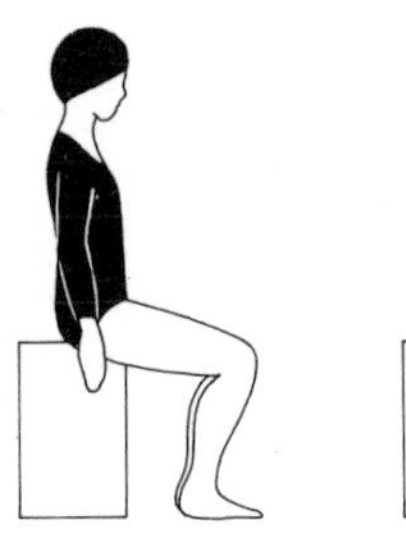

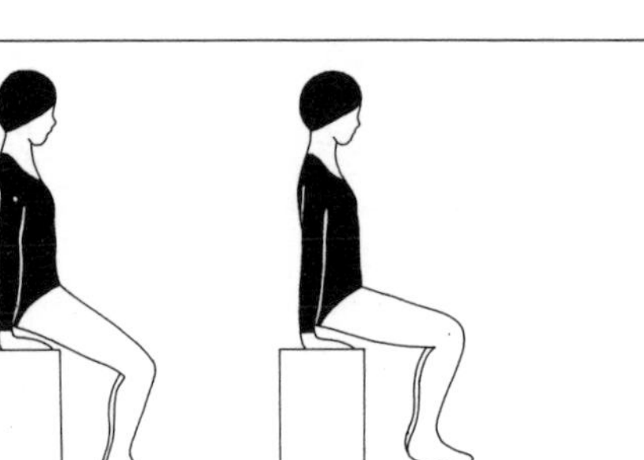

Chair Lift – Sit on armless chair, palms flat on seat, arms straight. Lift buttocks and thighs off chair, feet off floor. Count 6. Relax to count of 3. *10 times.*

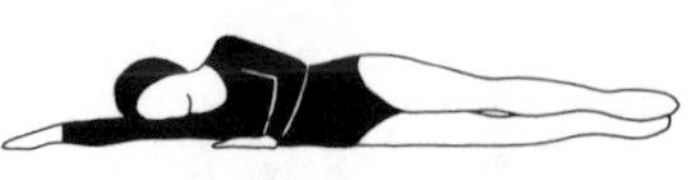

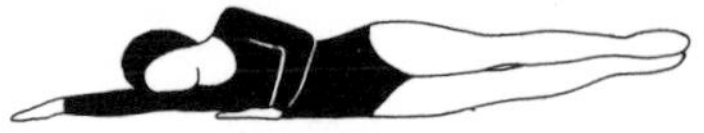

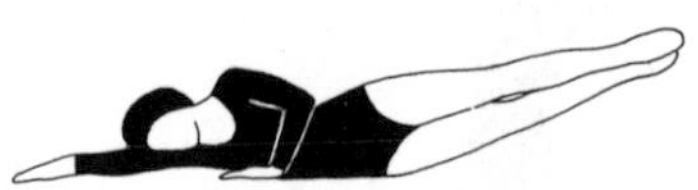

Bed Support – Lie on one side with feet tucked under bed edge. Stretch one arm under head, lift legs to touch underside of bed, keeping them rigid. Count 6. Relax to count of 3. *5 times each side.*

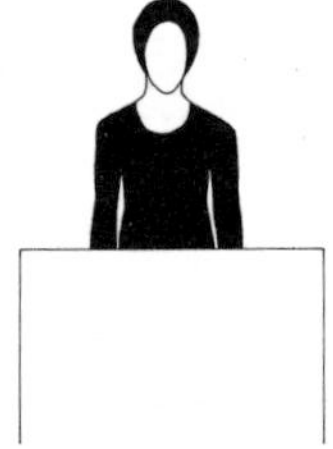

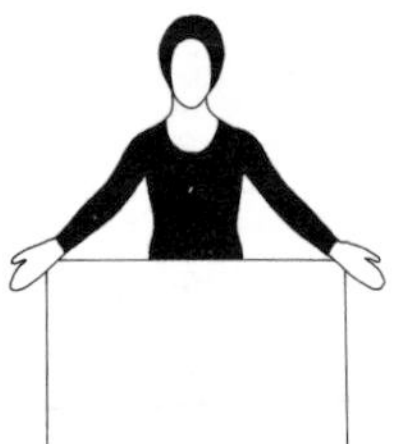

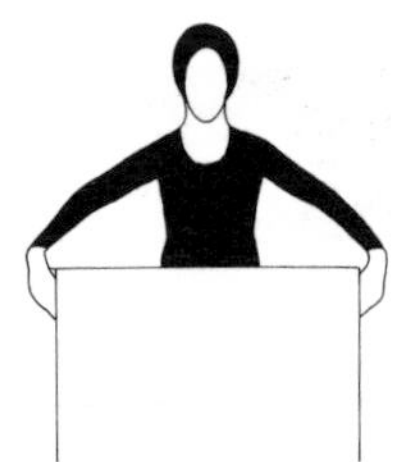

Desk Work – Sit, arms at sides. Lift arms to clutch edges of table and squash together. Count 6. Relax to count of 3. *10 times.*

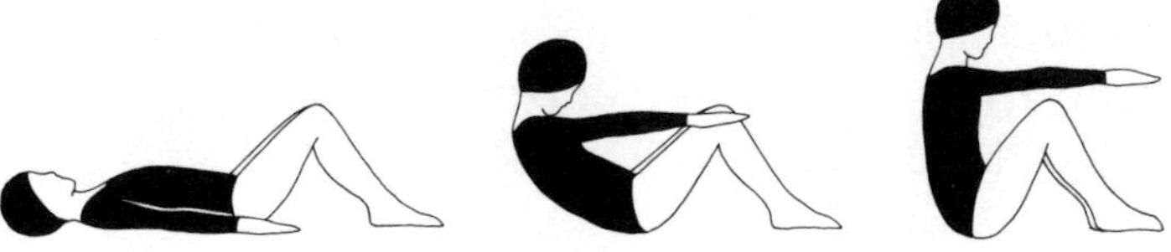

Floor Contact – Lie, knees bent, feet firm. Pushing floor away with feet, raise body bringing arms to knees then beyond. Count 6. Relax to count of 3. *10 times.*

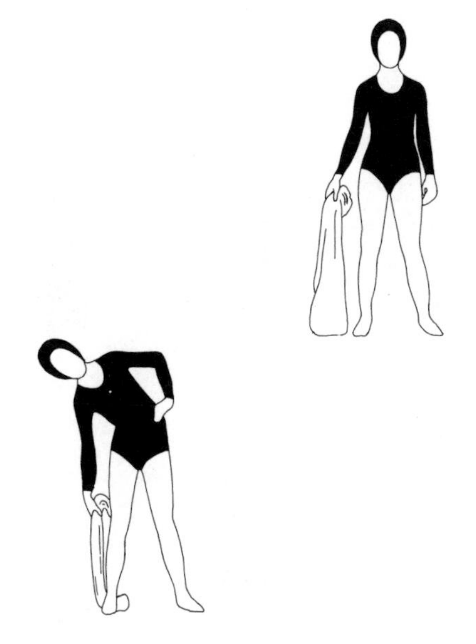

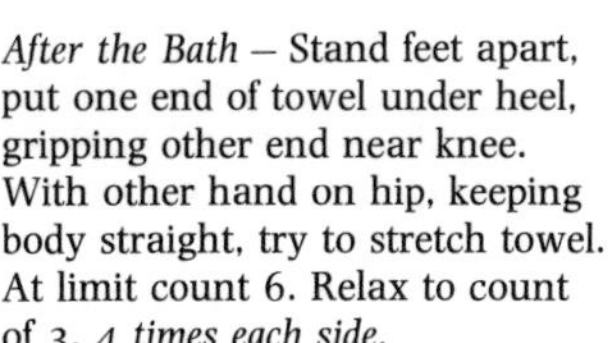

After the Bath – Stand feet apart, put one end of towel under heel, gripping other end near knee. With other hand on hip, keeping body straight, try to stretch towel. At limit count 6. Relax to count of 3. *4 times each side.*

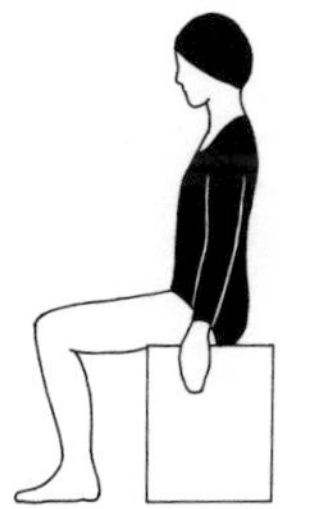

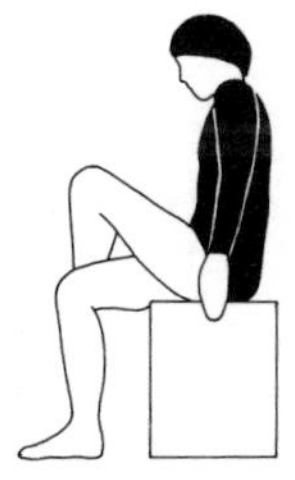

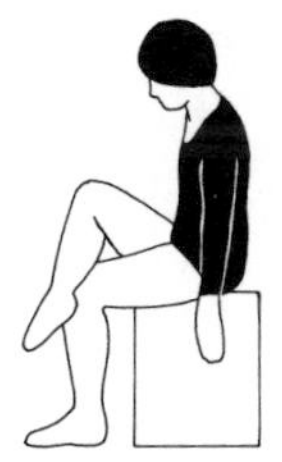

The Cross-over – Sit, hands gripping chair. Cross one leg high over thigh and lean in that direction as though pushing chair away. Count 6. Relax to count of 3. *6 times each leg.*

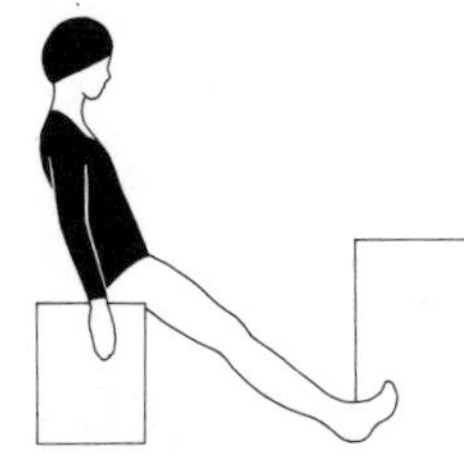

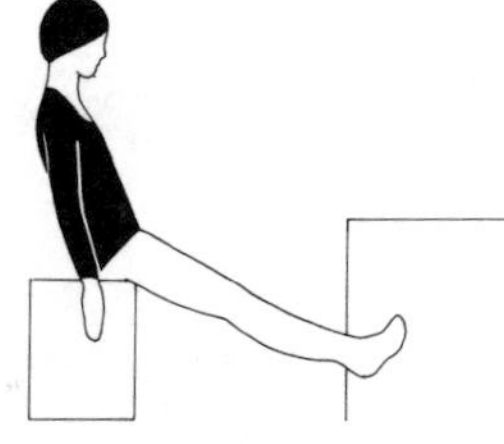

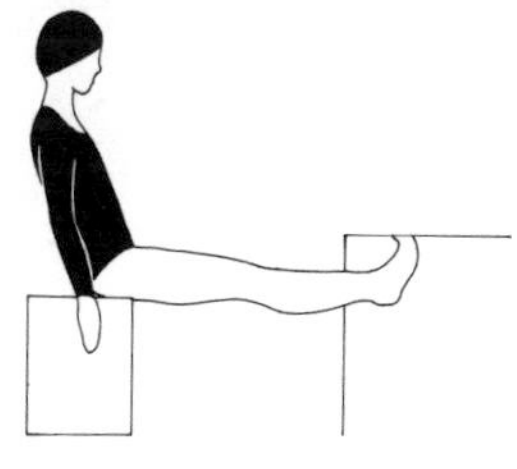

Table Push – Sit a little away from table. Stretch legs under it, toes touching. Press feet upward as if to lift table. Count 6. Relax to count of 3. *6 times.*

YOGA

Yoga benefits both mind and body. Technique depends on breathing, posture, relaxation. Never strain to accomplish an exercise; with each repetition you'll get better. And as you get better try to hold positions longer. This is modified yoga, adapted as daily exercises for figure streamlining.

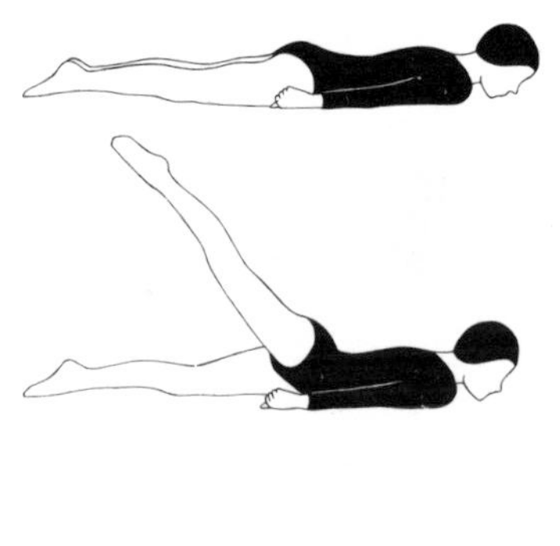

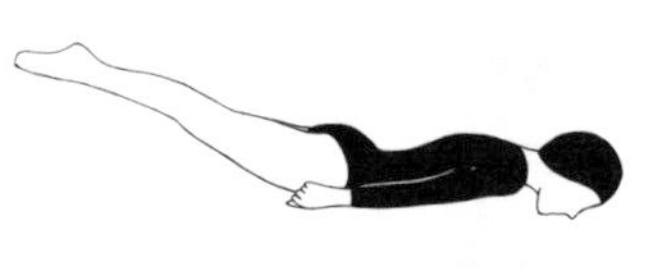

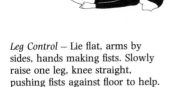

Leg Control – Lie flat, arms by sides, hands making fists. Slowly raise one leg, knee straight, pushing fists against floor to help. Hold 10 seconds. Relax. Starting from same position, legs together, knees straight, raise both legs. This is the locust position. Hold 10 seconds. Relax. *Each movement 3 times, alternating legs.*

Shoulder Stand – Lie flat, slowly raise legs over torso. Tighten stomach muscles, raise legs high, supporting body on hands. Push up; slowly lower knees to forehead. Return torso, legs to floor. Hold 1 minute, work up to 3.

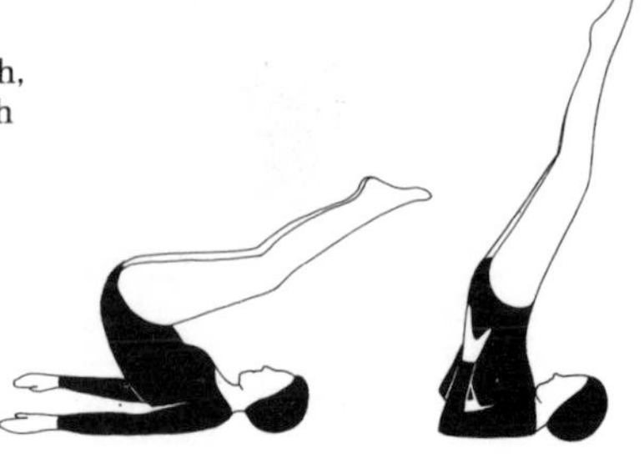

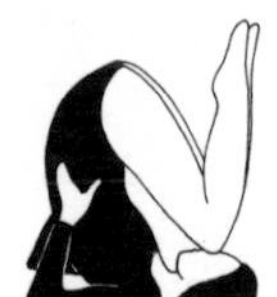

Chest Expansion – Stand straight, arms in front, keeping elbows straight move arms behind back, clasping hands, lean back. Let neck go limp, drop head forward, hold arms high. Hold 5 seconds. Bend forward, hands still clasped. Relax. *3 times.*

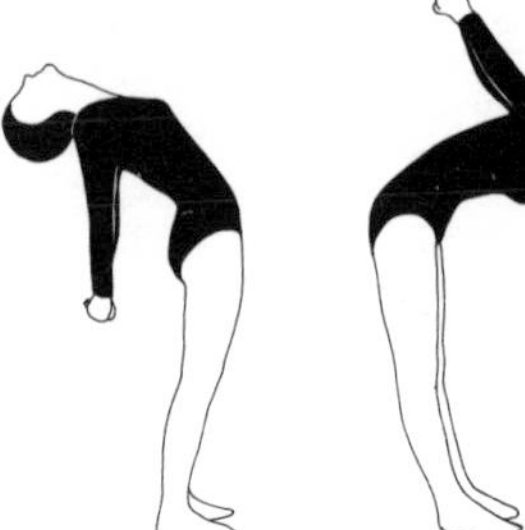

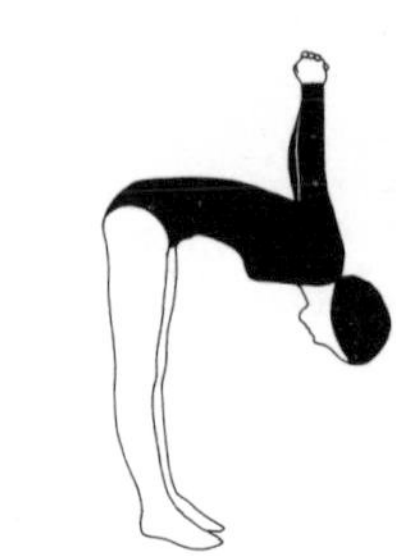

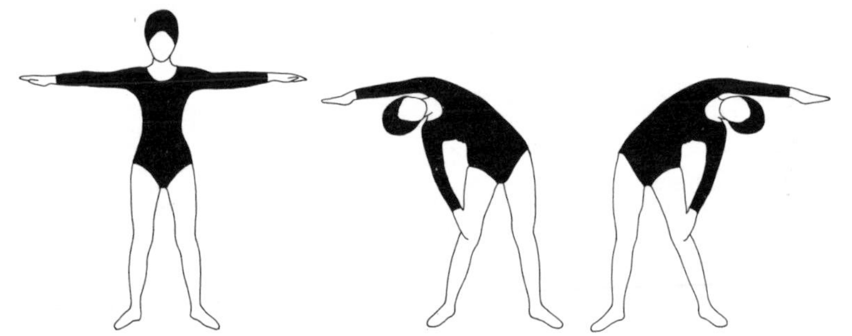

Triangle Bend – Stand erect, feet apart, arms extended. Bend slowly to one side, bringing one arm high over head; slide other arm down corresponding leg. Hold 10 seconds. Relax. *3 times on each side.*

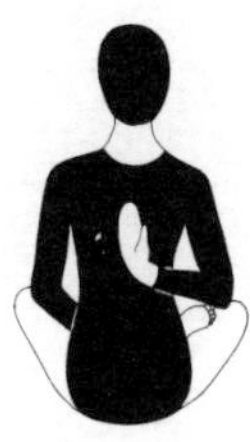

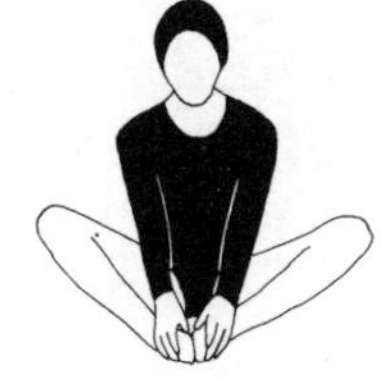

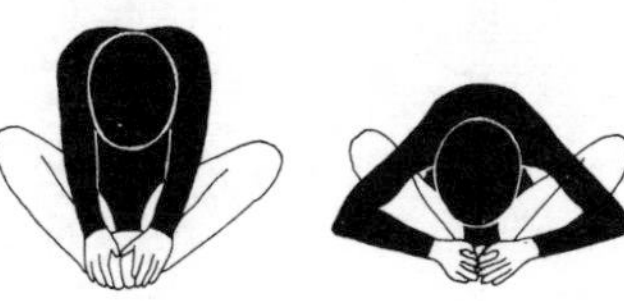

Forehead-Heel Stretch – Sit, legs widely bent, soles together. Clasp hands over feet (not toes), bend forward slowly aiming forehead towards heels. Hold 10 seconds. Relax. *3 times.*

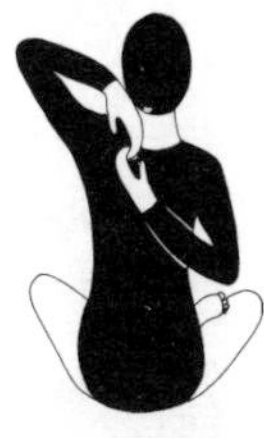

Stretching Spread – Sit, legs spread wide, knees outward, palms on inside of knees. Raise arms, bend forward, sliding hands down outerside of legs, try to clasp ankles. Hold 10 seconds. Relax. *3 times.*

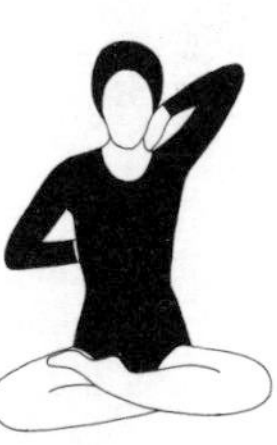

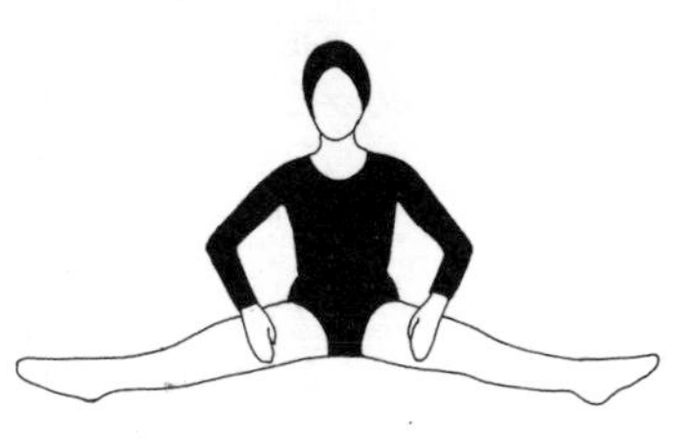

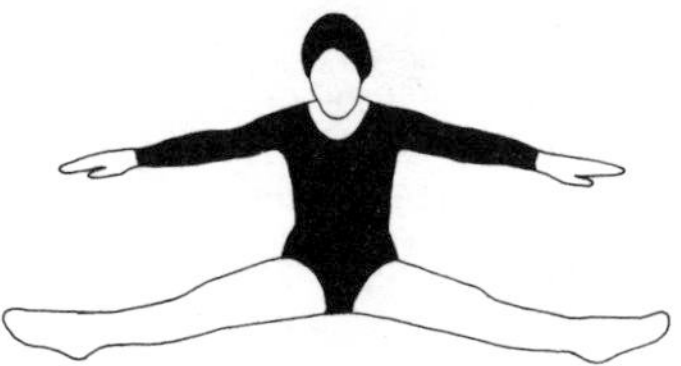

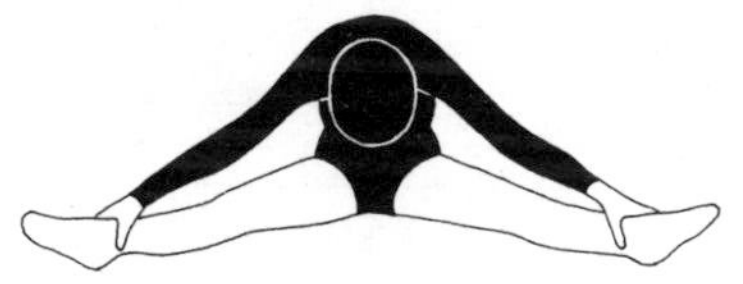

Backward Handclasp – Sit cross-legged, one foot on opposite thigh. Bend right elbow so hand touches spine. Raise left arm, bend back. Inch hands towards each other, clasp fingers. Hold 10 seconds. Relax, reverse hands. *3 times.*

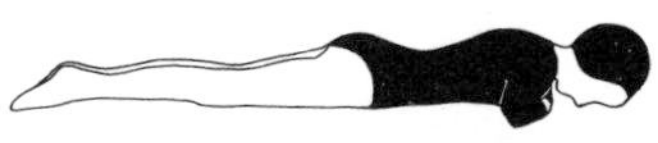

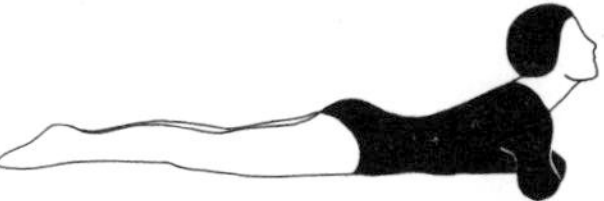

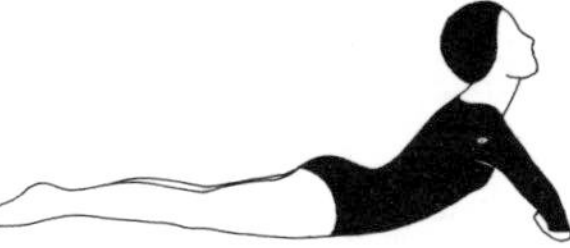

Cobra Arch – Lie face downwards with chin on floor, elbows bent but raised a little, palms flat. Slowly raise head then shoulders, pushing on palms, raise chest and upper abdomen. Head far back. Hold 10 seconds. Relax. *3 times.*

MODERN

At first an endurance test, as controls and concentration are equal for these exacting movements. Developed by Lotte Berk, this system emerges as the most contemporary, well geared to modern thinking and agile bodies. Based on Hatha yoga, ballet and orthopaedics, most routines are done with the pelvis rolled in, accent on lower torso and thighs.

Warming Up – Stand legs apart, hands above head, bend over and down pushing bottom out. Return, down again, curling further, pushing arms through legs. *10 times, work up to more.*

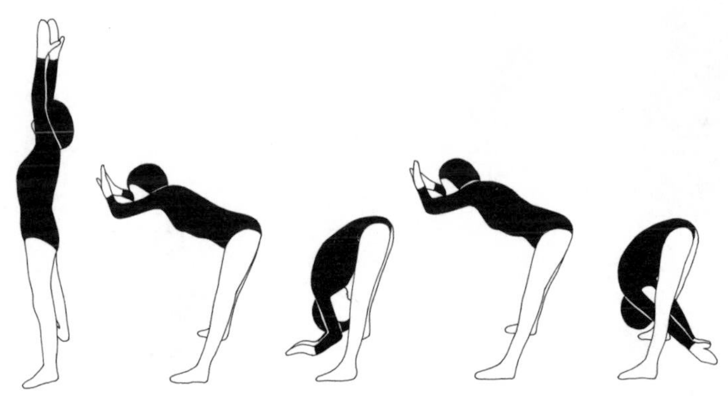

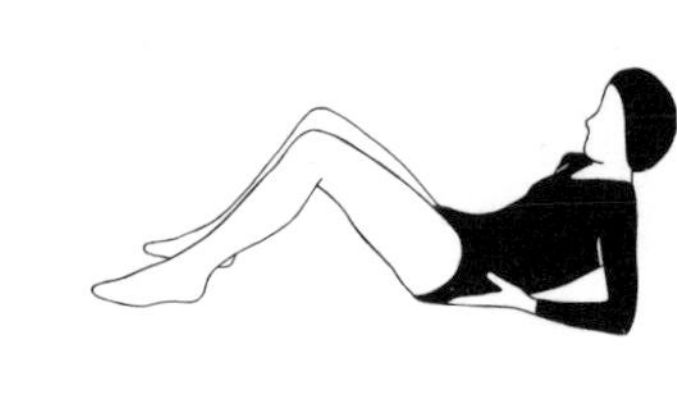

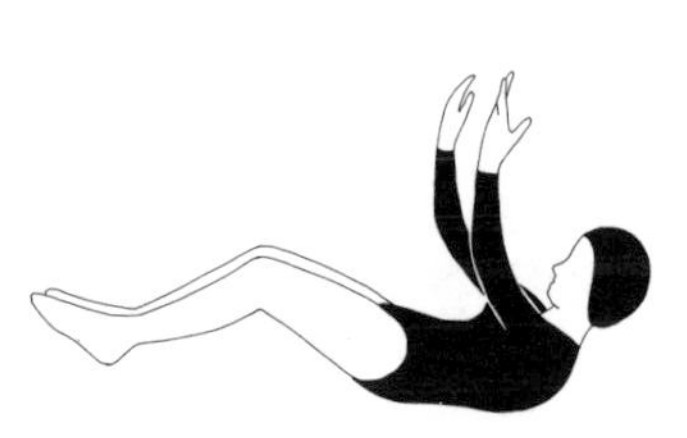

Central Control – Half lie knees bent, elbows supporting. Roll pelvis in, bring arms in front clicking fingers, one, two, three, at the same time raising feet a little off floor. Return. *6 times, work up to more.*

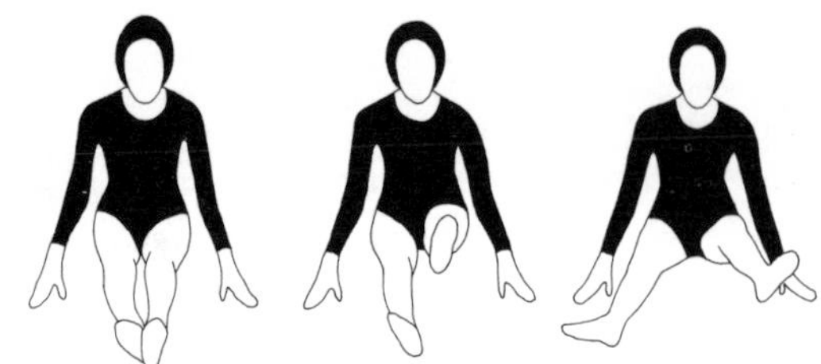

Foot Circles – Sit, legs stretched out, pelvis rolled in, rest on hands. Lift leg, twist foot in wide circle around ankle. Make 20 circles. Reverse feet.

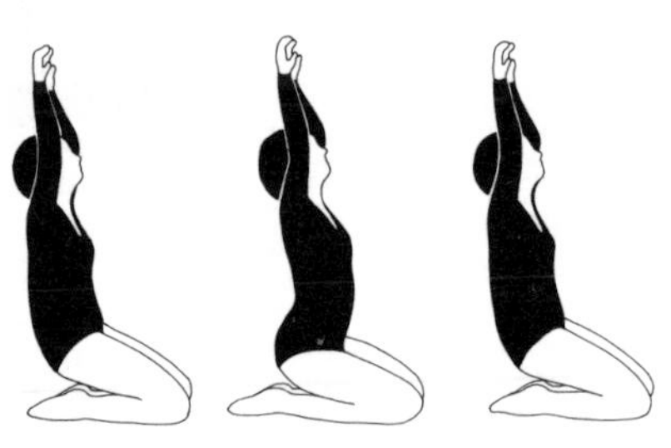

Pelvis Roll – Kneel, knees a little apart, hands linked over head. Roll pelvis in, then with hips and shoulders in a straight line, lean slowly backwards, lifting a little off heels. Roll the pelvis forward, once, twice, hold. Relax. *5 times, work up to more.*

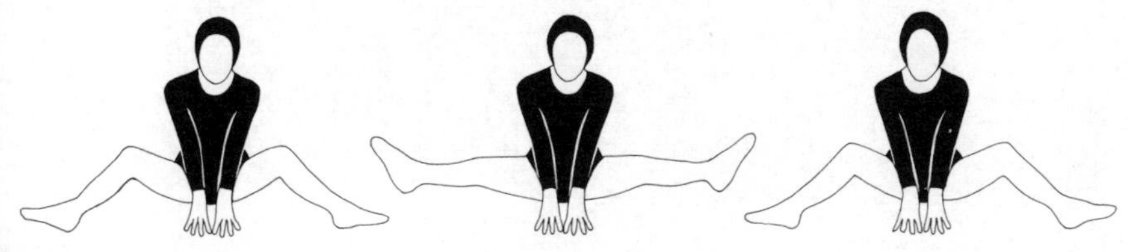

In the Air Stretch – Sit, legs wide apart, arms between legs, palms flat. With weight on hands, lift legs a fraction off floor. Bend legs, stretch, bend, stretch. *10 times rhythmically*. Relax. Repeat.

Crouch Bounce – Stand sideways by a support, crouch low, heels together, pelvis rolled in, back straight. Hold, bounce up and down lifting buttocks from heels. *10 times, work up to more.*

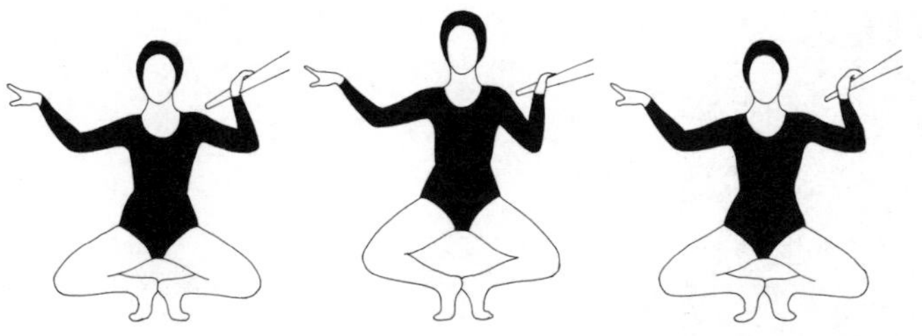

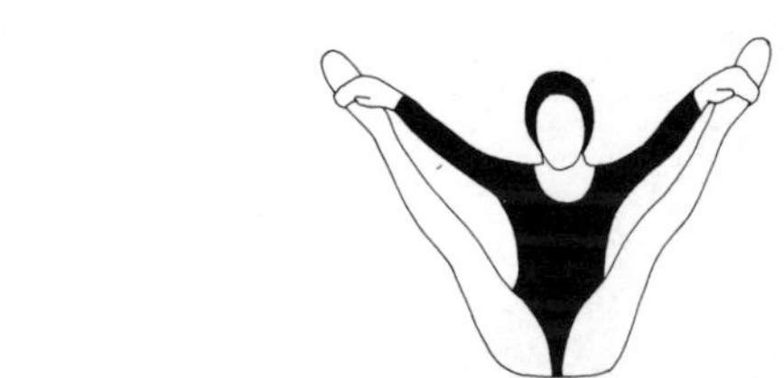

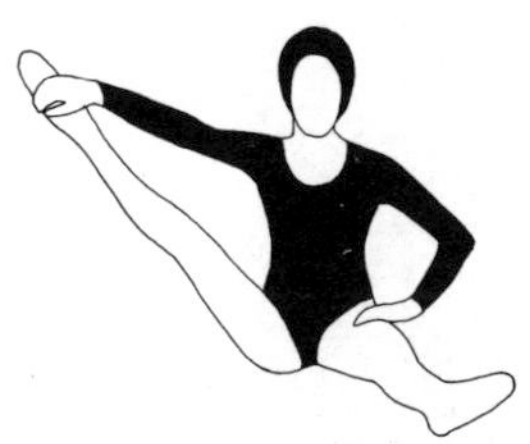

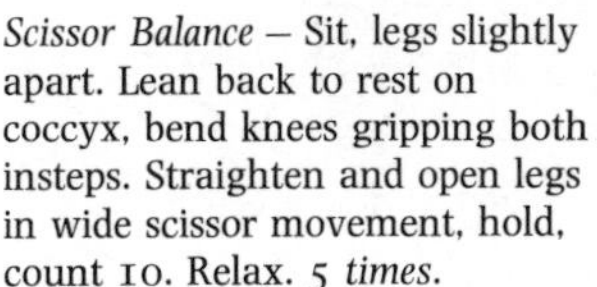

Scissor Balance – Sit, legs slightly apart. Lean back to rest on coccyx, bend knees gripping both insteps. Straighten and open legs in wide scissor movement, hold, count 10. Relax. *5 times.*

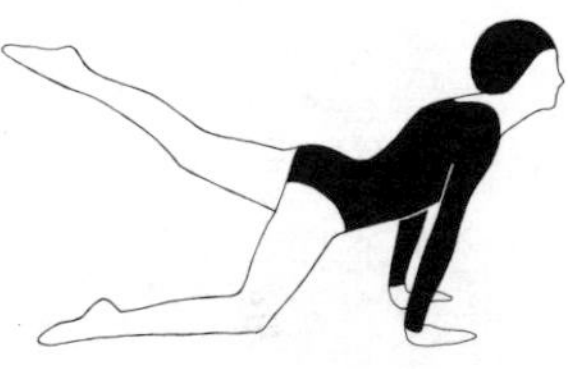

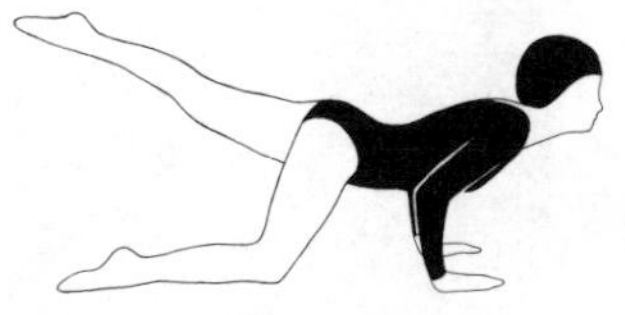

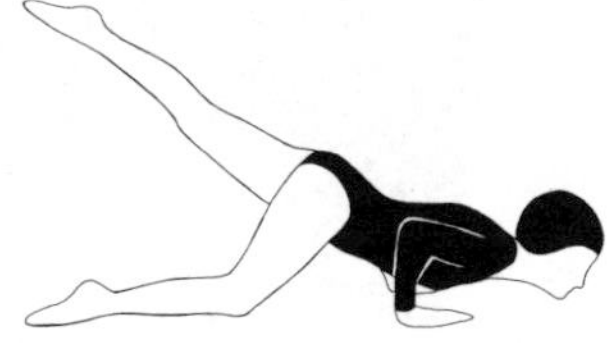

Kneeling Seesaw – Kneel on all fours, arms apart, palms flat. Control pelvis, arch back, lift a leg. Seesaw body by bending and straightening elbows. *10 times, work up to more.* Reverse legs.

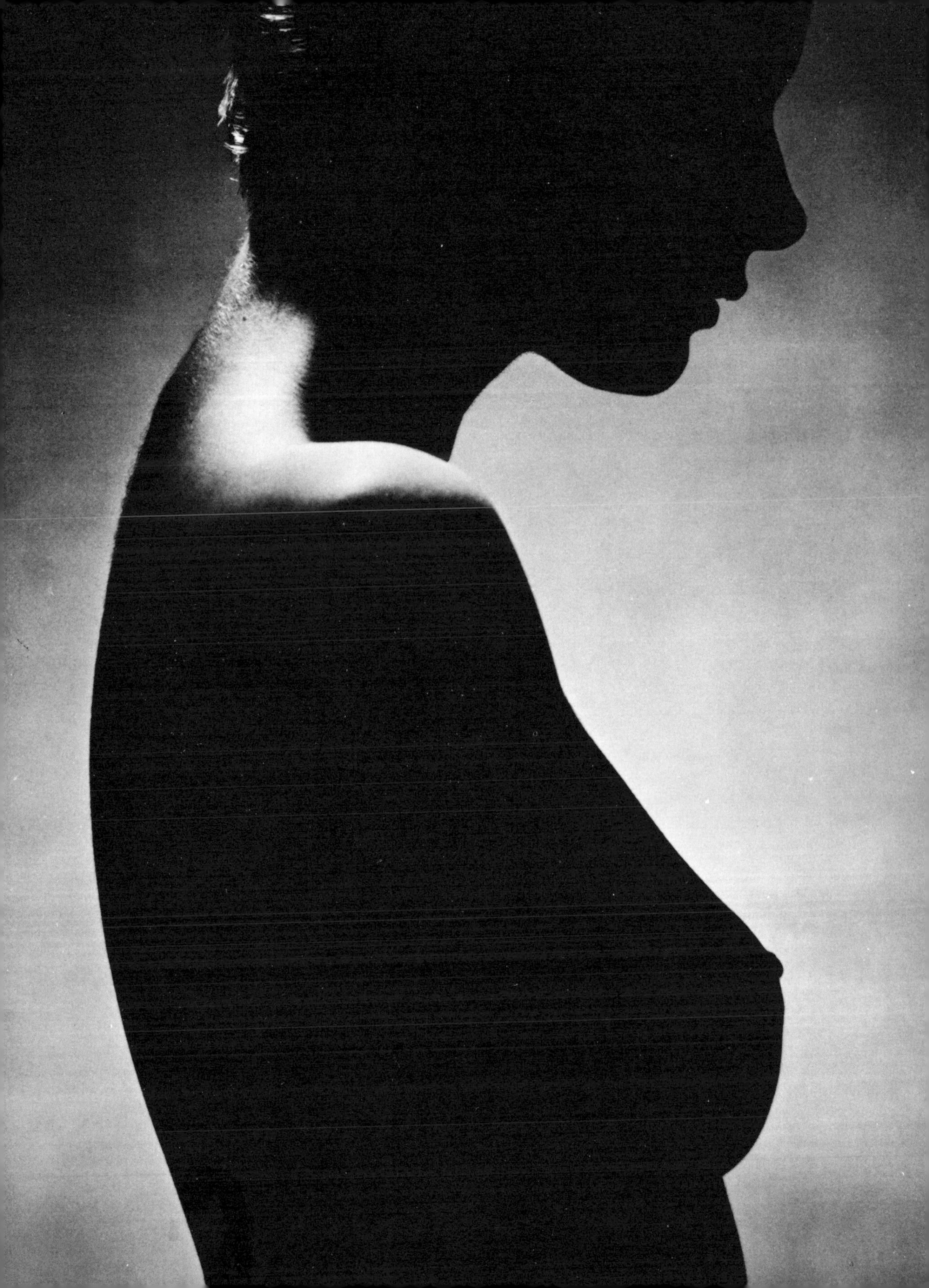

5

SEXUALITY

Sexuality is intrinsically linked with health and beauty. It should describe one's whole being as a woman, but it has come to be thought of as the degree of ability in direct sex functions. Orgasm is still to many women an achievement but it is part of the all-encompassing sex cycle that is a powerful tonic to looks and health. If you make love you will glow and look more beautiful. If you make love you are more aware of your body. Sexuality is knowing your body, liking it, taking care of it. Most women know every pore on their face and what to do about it, but have no idea of the shape of their bosom nor how to take care of it.

We are no longer governed by our reproductive system: the physical and emotional implications of periods, cramps, unwanted pregnancy, premenstrual moods and the menopause can all be handled with confidence and knowledge. The stress effects produced by ovulation are real and biochemical in origin. Knowledge of hormones has changed life for all of us and in this connection the life and beauty of a woman can be divided into three eras. As a girl approaches eleven or twelve, oestrogen and progesterone surge from the ovaries; during the mature years production is steady; as she nears fifty and the menopause production gradually slows down. These hormones are responsible for sexual characteristics: development of the breasts, shaping of the hips, the appearance of pubic hair and the onset of menstruation. For the whole of a woman's reproductive life hormones are produced in a cyclical pattern, usually within a four-week period. They affect looks, skin, hair, vitality, the health of the ovaries and uterus, the menstrual cycle, the state of the vaginal tissue and the structure of the breasts. They have a stabilizing influence on the emotions. Hormones control what is visible and invisible, adding up to the sum total of individual sexuality.

THE BOSOM

More women are concerned about the health, shape and size of their breasts than any other part of their anatomy. If a woman feels they are larger or smaller or rounder or more pear-shaped than others, she can become concerned and the self-consciousness may remain throughout life. Some women feel so strongly that their whole life is affected and under these circumstances, plastic surgery should be considered. Many doctors are sympathetic to the idea, particularly in the case of the flat-chested woman who thinks this is the cause of much of her emotional unhappiness.

The breasts are fundamentally two mammary glands meant for suckling the young. They usually extend from the second to the sixth rib on either side of the breast bone and over the chest muscles. They are contained in fatty tissue, which determines the shape and size. The fine covering of skin is connected by fibrous tissue which decides your bosom type as bouncy or firm. Internally the bosom can be affected by several factors. As it is controlled by hormones, breasts change during the menstrual cycle; they may appear larger or fuller just before menstruation, they may also be a little sore. Crash diets and overeating can also alter their shape; and so can gravity if the pull of the breasts is allowed to go unchecked. Going bra-less is not a health hazard unless your breasts are very heavy, in which case a posture problem may develop. Some women claim their muscles are forced to work harder and so breasts actually take on a better, firmer shape. However unless you are watchful about exercise or conscious about muscle control during the day you can preserve the shape of your breasts better if you use some support.

Apart from plastic surgery, there is little one can do to noticeably change size and shape but it is possible to improve the way breasts hang, their texture and resiliency, with improved posture, exercise, water therapy and oil massage.

Posture – slouched shoulders and hunched backs produce sagging breasts. Improved posture can make the biggest improvement; this does not mean shoulders back and bosom obviously thrust forward. It involves lifting the bosom up from the diaphragm, stretching the vertebrae from the pelvic muscles, and lifting the head as though it were being tugged skywards with a string.

Exercise – the pectoral muscles at the sides and curving underneath the breasts cradle, control and uphold a good bosom but only as long as they are firm and well-toned. Do a couple of exercises a day; these are simple and effective and although the bosom will not show immediate improvement, muscles will slowly strengthen to give the breasts a better placement on the chest cage.

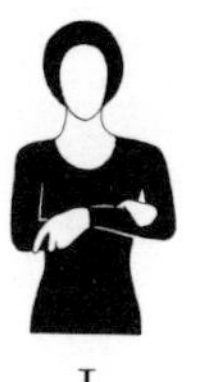

1

1. Forearm Push: fold arms, grasping each forearm below the elbow with the opposite hand. Push hard towards the elbows without moving the hand up the arm. Feel a pull in the pectoral muscles. Do 20 times.

2. Arm Stretch: stand with elbows bent at shoulder level, the backs of the hands facing the body. Push arms back unbending to slowly stretch straight, keeping arms at shoulder level. Back and forth 10 times.

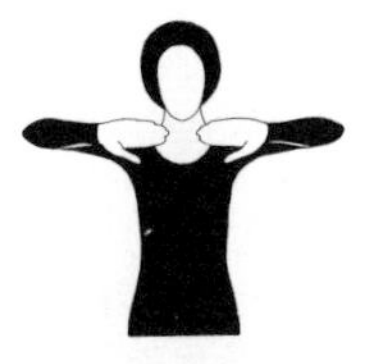

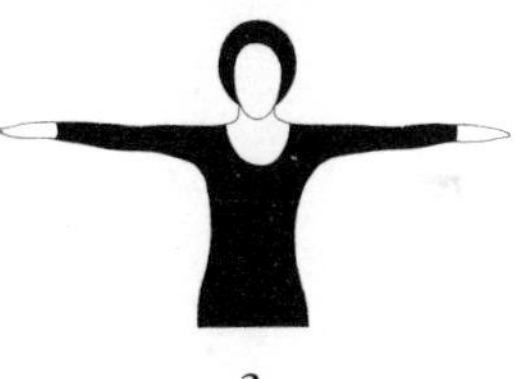

2

3. Swimming Stroke: stand legs apart, don't bend knees, lean forward as far as possible with one arm stretched out. Now bring the other arm up in the crawl swimming stroke movement. Continue, building up to 10 strokes per arm.

Water therapy – cold water stimulation can tone the breasts. After bathing, turn the shower on cold, full force, and spray directly on each breast, two minutes each side. If you don't have a shower, splash with cold water. When bathing, keep the warm water below breast level.

Massage – for improved texture, massage body moisturizer, lotion or oil into the breasts; always apply a liberal coat of sunscreen lotion before tanning.

Make-up – to create the illusion of depth and curves, brush blusher down your cleavage; a frosted blush for evenings.

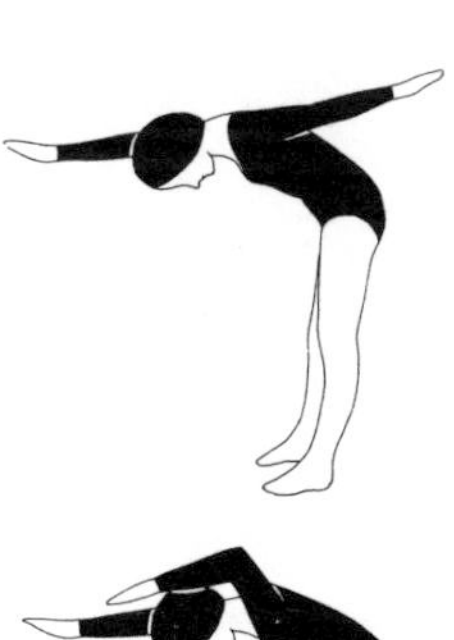

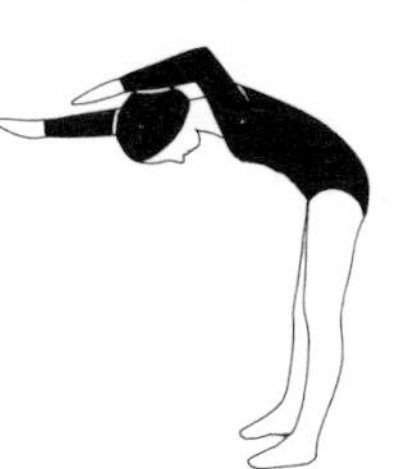

3

Irregularities in the breasts are a cause for concern. Breasts are often sore and painful, particularly prior to menstruation, and to touch appear to be full of undulations. Doctors emphasize that if a lump is painful it is rarely malignant and is probably due to one of the following conditions:

CYSTS AND FIBROADENOMAS: These are definitely non-cancerous, but cause obvious breast lumps and swellings. Cysts occur because the liquid that is secreted by glands in the breasts has not properly drained through the breast ducts. They are usually regular in shape, mobile when handled – move under the skin. They frequently crop up just before menstruation and disappear by themselves after bleeding has started. They can be removed by draining them under local anaesthetic, which is considered less of a physical or psychological trauma than surgery – which is also sometimes used.

Fibroadenomas are growths of the fibrous tissue that holds the breast together. They may occur in just one part of the breast or in several spots on both breasts. They should be reported to a doctor who will remove them if they are uncomfortable. Some women suffer from chronic cysts or fibrous growths. These should be constantly checked even though neither condition becomes cancerous.

CANCER: This is the big fear – cancer is now the leading cause of female deaths in the 40 to 44 age groups and the primary cause of cancer deaths among women of all ages. All women can develop breast cancer but some seem more susceptible: those in the mid to late forties who never had children or did not begin having them until after 30, whose mother or sister has had the disease, who are overweight. There are indications that women who are married have a slightly lower breast cancer rate than those who are single, also those who have breast-fed several children have fewer breast malignancies than those who have not. The evidence is statistical only and there is no certainty of developing cancer even if you fit into all the risk categories. One thing is certain: if left untreated, breast tumours can spread rapidly invading lungs, skeleton, liver or brain.

Despite years of research, the cause of breast cancer remains unknown. Reports indicate that there is no correlation between cancer and the Pill. Diet has been cited as a factor, based on statistical evidence showing breast cancer's greater prevalence in countries where people eat large quantities of animal fat. Injuries – bumps and bangs on the bosom – do not initiate the disease.

Early detection is vital; when malignancies are small they are completely curable. It is a woman's responsibility to keep watch over herself. Breast lumps are sometimes found by doctors during routine examinations but most changes of tissue are spotted by accident or during self-examination. Finding them in the early stage can be a problem because cancerous growths rarely cause pain or feel sensitive to the touch.

Three techniques are used, often in combination to ensure detection: physical examination, thermography, which is a method of measuring heat given off by a tumour, and mammography, an X-ray technique which can spot very small tumours before they can be felt even by an experienced examiner. One of the best methods is a type of mammography known as xeroradiography, which reveals tiny dots of calcium that are commonly present in breast cancer.

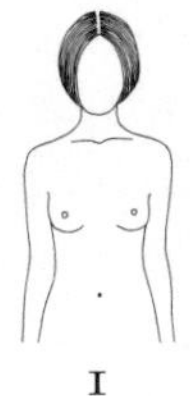
1

SELF-EXAMINATION OF THE BREASTS: The importance of monthly self-examination of the breasts cannot be over-emphasized. Many women know they should examine themselves but do not because they are scared of what they might find. Don't worry if, on first examination when you are not familiar with the feel of your breasts, they appear to be full of irregularities, bumps and nodes.

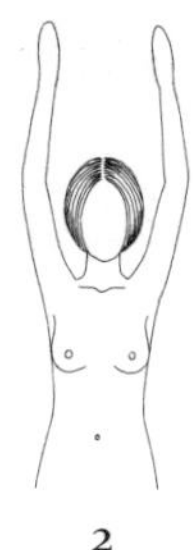
2

The earlier you start examining your breasts the better. Sixteen is not too young; this does not mean that a young woman should start worrying about cancer; it simply helps her become familiar with the feel of her breasts and establishes a habit of self-examination.

Examination should be done in the week following menstruation and continued for six days. It is a ten-minute procedure. A woman who is familiar with the feel of her breasts in their normal state should be able to detect any thickening. Do it after a bath, as this is relaxing and allows the superficial blood vessels of the breasts to dilate and thus become easier to observe. If you do find anything, see a doctor without delay.

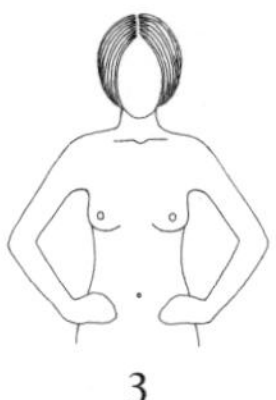
3

1. Sitting or standing in front of a mirror, take a good look at your breasts, get to know their shape, the tracery of the blood vessels. Be alert to any unusual puckering or dimpling, any change in the look of the nipple, or the appearance of bigger or more vessels.
2. Stretch arms above the head, observe any changes.
3. Place hands on hips, check the shape and fall of the breasts.
4. Fold arms, push hands against the area between wrist and elbow so that the pectoral muscles flex under the breasts; observe.

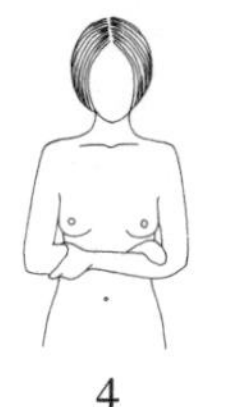
4

5. Lie down, place one hand behind the head, then with the fingers of the other hand, flattened, gently feel the breast, starting at the nipple and working outwards in concentric circles; be careful not to miss any spots; be very aware of any swellings. Repeat with other breast.
6. Check the armpits by raising one arm over your head. Insert the fingers of your other hand well into the armpit and with flattened fingers press it against the chest wall, checking for irregularities. Do the same on both sides. Armpits are as important as the breast area because they contain both the lymph glands and the tail of the breast.

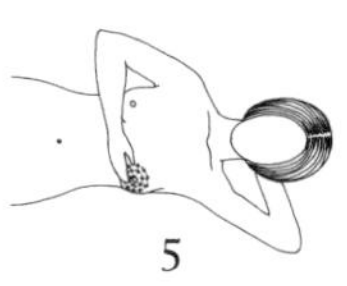
5

When a lump is found some women try to ignore it in the hope it will miraculously disappear. Frightened women often wait as long as a year: don't, it could be fatal. And remember that statistics indicate that 65% to 80% of all breast lumps are not cancerous.

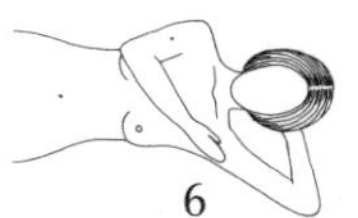
6

On examination doctors can often determine the type of growth. If it hurts it is unlikely to be malignant, also if it appears to be unanchored it is usually all right. A needle biopsy can be used – a needle is inserted and fluid or cells withdrawn for examination. However some growths are too small or too hidden to be checked by these methods and so a surgical procedure is necessary. The lump is cut out and immediately checked; within minutes the surgeon can tell if cells are cancerous.

If the result is positive, something has to be done as soon as possible. Many surgeons feel that the only prudent method is immediate surgery and frequently take the precaution of asking permission from the patient to perform a mastectomy (removal of the breast) if cancer is present. This, they say, reduces both the risk and the expense of two operations. Even so, most women would rather know beforehand; a few days doesn't make any appreciable difference in growth, though a few weeks can.

A woman with breast cancer should know what options she has. The size of the lump is the determining factor. The choices are: radiation only, lumpectomy (the cutting away of only the lump), simple mastectomy (the removal of only the breast), radical mastectomy (the removal of one breast and the nearby regions) or double radical mastectomy (the removal of both breasts and their regions). It is usual for mastectomies to be followed by radiation treatment, which can be painful and irritating.

Efforts are being made to improve the ways in which radiation alone can be used on a cancerous spot to avoid mutilation, but this therapy is still debatable. Ultra-sonic treatments are being investigated, but are still in the exploratory stage. The current choice is a decision about the extent of surgery. Many doctors feel that complete amputation is not always necessary. Research has shown that where lumpectomy (removal of the lump only) was performed, cancers have not spread to the lymph nodes. In this respect it is considered as effective as more radical operations and less damaging psychologically. Other doctors point out that these were lucky cases. Partial mastectomy is also possible which, while more extensive than lumpectomy, still spares most of the breast. The arguments against these procedures is that most cancers have been growing from six to eight years before they are discovered. By that time invariably they may have spread in microscopic clusters elsewhere in the breast.

THE SEX ORGANS

The two ovaries are the source of female germ cells (ova) and the female hormones oestrogen and progesterone. They are each the size of a bean, supported by ligaments and touched by the fallopian tubes, the ducts for the passage of ova to the uterus (or womb). The uterus has a narrow neck, the cervix, dipping down into the top end of the vagina, which is about three to four inches long, opening at the vulva, the surface sex organs where the clitoris is the most sexually receptive area. The whole system is T-shaped, the bar of the T being the fallopian tubes, the stroke being the uterus and vagina.

This area controls general health patterns and emotions. We are very dependent on the hormone production and any lack or excess can have far reaching effects. Our reproductive capacity depends on the menstrual cycle; our sexual responses on its stimuli. Regular gynaecological check-ups are important and should not be reserved only for when obvious symptoms appear. Most women are bothered by varying degrees of vaginal discharge or vulva irritation, some are harmless secretions, common and normal, others need attention.

VAGINAL INFECTIONS: A group of low-grade infections are prevalent but neither dangerous nor likely to spread; they should be controlled and cleared up by medication if they persist. They are not necessarily contacted through sexual activity but produced by the body's own flora. Many women have one or more of them on different occasions and they may occur simultaneously in what is called a mixed infection. Self-help involves avoiding hot baths as the fungus thrives on warmth; keeping the body as cool and dry as possible. Cotton underwear or no underwear helps prevent infections by allowing air to circulate more freely to the outer vaginal area. Constant douching can also destroy the beneficial flora and upset natural balance. The occasional use of mild douche powders, or a little salt in warm water, is acceptable.

Moniliasis – also known as leucorrhoea, vaginal fungus, yeast infection or 'whites'. Discharge is white and thick; can provoke vaginal and vulva itching, areas may become reddened, the vagina sometimes has white patches. Local vaginal creams or suppositories are effective.

Trichomoniasis – produces an abundant malodorous, yellow or greenish-white discharge. Can cause inflammation, itching, soreness and bleeding of the vagina. It is passed back and forth between sexual partners although the male usually does not have symptoms. Treatment involves oral medication to be taken by both partners.

Bacterial infection – discharge is white or yellow, heavy and viscous. It covers the vaginal walls and may cause burning or frequent urination. Can be cleared easily with medication.

Cervicitis – inflammation of the cervix, often associated with a vaginal infection. Symptom is painful and frequent urination. It can be treated with oral antibiotics. Drink lots of water, especially after intercourse.

GONORRHOEA AND SYPHILIS: Both are sexually transmitted and can be extremely harmful if not treated in the early stages. The incidence of gonorrhoea has trebled in the last ten years, and the problem for women is that they have no obvious symptoms until the disease is quite far advanced. If there is any possibility you may have been exposed to it have a test every six months. A sample of discharge from around the cervix is taken to the laboratory for culture.

The early symptoms of gonorrhoea usually include an inflammation of the urethral lining, causing a discharge and frequent burning urination. These are usually mild, and invariably passed as a transient bladder irritation. Later on, infection induces an abundant yellow discharge. The real trouble begins when the virus invades the fallopian tubes causing inflammation and the development of pus within the ducts. At this stage there is often copious discharge, fever, lower abdominal tenderness following the menstrual period and pelvic pain during intercourse. This invasion of the fallopian tubes must be treated within 36 hours after the onset of pain, otherwise the result might be scarring and blocking of tubes finally to cause permanent sterility. Penicillin remains the most effective drug for treatment, and is also used for checking the progress of syphilis.

Syphilis is considered a three-stage disease that spreads over many years. It starts with the intrusion of an infectious organism into the skin or mocosal tissue. The area becomes red and swollen, then ulcerates turning into a painless sore; the adjacent lymphatic glands usually become swollen and hard. This is the primary stage of the disease and at this point it is highly contagious. The sore heals within six to ten weeks and although a skin rash erupts, it often goes by unnoticed.

Syphilis can be detected early, within weeks of contact by a blood serology test. If not treated during the first phase of development, the infection makes its way into the bloodstream. This stage can last from ten to fifteen years but is no longer contagious and presents few overt symptoms. In the third and final stage, the virus attacks vital organs.

VAGINAL WARTS AND HERPES: Warts often occur between the vagina and rectum, beginning as little grains of tissue. They can be treated in a doctor's surgery by the application of a solution that causes them to fall off within two or three days. If they are allowed to develop surgical procedures may be necessary. The herpes group of viruses is responsible for cold sores and fever blisters, but when they appear in the vaginal area they are of a different genre and are linked with the possibility of cancer of the cervix, so should be thoroughly checked.

OVARIAN CYSTS: These are growths on the ovaries which occur frequently. The most common type is soft and 3 to 4 centimetres large, and will often regress within two or three menstrual cycles. Ovarian cysts that are larger and persistent require surgical intervention. In rare cases, cysts will rupture, bleed or cause problems. Surgery gives immediate relief. Young women are frequently afflicted. While they usually cause no problems, they may lead to emergency situations if left undetected. Fertility is not affected.

CANCER: Cervical cancer is 100% curable if found early. It is practical to have a smear every six months. For this, cells are gently scraped from the cervix with a wooden spatula and are sent to a laboratory for examination. Results are available in about a week. If positive, it is usually considered necessary to have a hysterectomy, which is the removal of the uterus and fallopian tubes together with the ovaries. Because the cancer is usually localized within this area, there is rarely a chance of it having spread. A hysterectomy is also performed for some infections that cannot be helped in ways other than surgery. Hormonal substitutes are given to compensate for loss of natural production.

D AND C (DILATION AND CURETTAGE) OPERATION: This is one of the most common operations performed on the female sex organs and can be used in the diagnosis of many different conditions as well as part of treatment. It is sometimes known as scraping.

In a D and C, a fine metal rod is first inserted into the opening of the cervix, to measure how far in it is possible to put the dilators – a series of curved metal rods of progressive thickness which the surgeon uses one after the other until the cervix is open enough to provide a passageway into the uterus. This part of the operation is called dilation.

The curettage involves the introduction of an instrument called the curette, which is passed across the lining of the uterus to scrape away sections of it. This does no harm because it does not remove any tissue that is not normally shed automatically. The lining of the uterus is naturally lost every month in a period. There is no incision, no stitches.

The operation is done to check on the health of the uterus should any infection or fibroid build-up be suspected. It is often used as a treatment after a miscarriage, to ensure that all the debris is cleared away. In the same way it is used to terminate pregnancy. Often the first period after a D and C is a specially heavy one.

MENSTRUATION

A 28-day cycle is average; longer and shorter cycles within a year are perfectly normal, while many women never have a cycle longer than three weeks or shorter than 30 days. Duration and quantity of blood loss also varies, but it should be more or less the same each month. The cycle is controlled from the hypothalamus which responds to nervous stimuli and nudges the pituitary gland into the action of sending out appropriate hormones at the appropriate time of the month. The first one is released into the bloodstream at the beginning of menstruation, going straight to one of the ovaries to ripen an egg. Simultaneously the ovary produces oestrogen which goes to the uterus to prepare the endometrium (the inner lining) for the arrival of the mature egg.

About 14 days after the start of menstruation, the mature egg moves from the ovary through the fallopian tube to the uterus. This is known as ovulation and is the time of possible conception. Meanwhile in the follicle that held the egg in the ovary, another hormone is being produced, progesterone, which also goes to the uterus to assist in making it the perfect environment for a fertilized egg. If the egg is fertilized new hormones are summoned by the pituitary to aid in pregnancy. If it is not the unwanted lining disintegrates and is shed together with the unfertilized egg as the menstrual flow. Then the whole process starts again.

It is a highly complicated, sensitive and responsive activity, based on interrelated endocrinal activity. Because it is controlled by the hypothalamus where emotional stress is also registered, any upset readily disturbs the cycle – enough either to bring on or delay menstruation. Persistent excess bleeding or pain should be medically checked.

DYSMENORRHOEA (PAINFUL PERIODS): The most common cause of menstrual distress is hormonal imbalance. There are two types of period pains: spasmodic and congestive dysmenorrhoea. Spasmodic sufferers get sharp uterine cramps as the periods start. This often afflicts young women and may be eliminated after having a baby, as one cause is believed to stem from pain when the egg and menstrual blood pass through a tight cervix. If it continues, it can be helped by introducing oestrogen, at times in the form of the Pill.

Congestive dysmenorrhoea often intensifies with age and successive pregnancies. Symptoms heralding menstruation include depression, lethargy, water retention, head or backache, tender breasts and constipation. Hormone therapy is indicated, probably progesterone which can be given in pessaries or suppositories. Treating with the Pill does not always work out in this case, as the Pill contains progestogen, which is a synthetic substance and does not necessarily act like progesterone.

AMENORRHOEA: This is the absence of periods and thought to depend on psychological elements due to some kind of response to stress in the hypothalamus. A drastic change in life patterns can cause it, some medications such as tranquillizers, while a few women have it after stopping the Pill. Sudden weight gain or loss are other causes, particularly anorexia. It always requires medical attention; currently hormone therapy is considered the best treatment.

MOOD CHANGES: Researchers report that from 25% to 95% of all women suffer mood changes prior to having a period, mostly depression, irritability, anxiety and low self-esteem. Usually this occurs 4 days before and during the first 4 days of menstruation. Moods are predictable through the whole cycle and are due to hormone levels. During the first half of the menstrual cycle, most women feel alert, happy, out-going and competent. These feelings reach their peak at the time of ovulation, which is also when libido is at its height. During the second half women feel more passive and self-centred, while just before the period begins they become tense, anxious and sometimes aggressively bad tempered. The emotional changes parallel hormone changes; oestrogen production increases up to ovulation, afterwards progesterone levels begin to rise and both hormones circulate; then a few days before menstruation, both levels drop.

CONTRACEPTION

Today women have reliable and hygienic control over the number of children they have. There is a choice of contraceptive alternatives:

THE PILL: The most reliable form of reversible contraception. Used correctly it gives 100% protection against pregnancy; it does not interfere in any way with the sexual act. It alters the body's hormonal mechanism by combining progestogen with relatively small doses of oestrogen and inhibiting ovulation. The early pills had a high oestrogen content but this has been greatly reduced because it was considered responsible for some side-effects. Progestogen pills are often misleadingly referred to as mini-pills. These work by bringing changes in cervical mucus making it hostile to sperm penetration.

The Pill has had a bad reputation for causing weight increase, but the low-level oestrogen varieties limit this. Should weight go up by over seven pounds, check with a doctor. The most troublesome occurrence when the Pill is first taken may be break-through bleeding. It should cease, but if it continues after two months, a change of preparation is advisable. The Pill should not be self-prescribed; a clinic or a doctor can decide which type of pill is best for your particular metabolism.

All the pills are taken in the same way: one each day for 21 days then dropped for 7. Some packs contain dummy pills so that one is taken every day. It is important to take the pills in correct sequence. During the fourth week, light menstrual-type bleeding occurs, but this is not a true period. The progestogen pills have to be taken throughout the cycle and timing needs to be precise because coverage is of limited duration.

The biggest fear is side effects. A few hypersensitive women may experience a rise in blood pressure but the incidence of thrombo-embolic trouble has decreased since the withdrawal of high-oestrogen pills. However, there is a definite risk and the Pill should not be taken by any woman with a known predisposition to thrombosis. Pill taking should also stop for six weeks before surgery. It is also advisable to terminate three months prior to an anticipated pregnancy.

IUD (INTRA-UTERINE DEVICE): This is a small device in the shape of a loop or coil, usually plastic or plastic and copper, inserted into the uterus. How it prevents conception is not fully understood but it permits intercourse at any time. It is specially fitted and can be left in place for several years with regular medical check ups. Many women expel them and some suffer heavy periods. Coils can come out unnoticed during the first few months especially during a period. Conception can take place with the IUD still in position in which case it must be removed immediately otherwise it may harm the foetus. Most coils are not given to childless women because they can be painful to insert and more likely to be ejected, but the copper IUD usually known as the Copper-7 is an exception as it is smaller, easier to insert, and less likely to be expelled.

DIAPHRAGMS AND CAPS: Mechanical devices, effective if used properly. They should be left in for at least six hours after intercourse. They are dome-shaped rubber preventives, fitted after examination at a clinic or by a doctor. Instruction is given on how to insert and remove, which can be messy. Diaphragms should be checked once a year for fit and impermeability. They should preferably be used with a spermicide.

CONDOMS: An ancient method and effective if condoms are properly manufactured. They are made of rubber and simply collect the semen. Apart from possible rubber allergies, they have the drawback that the rhythm of love-making has to be interrupted to put them on, and there is the possibility of leakage, particularly if the penis is not withdrawn immediately after climax. For maximum reliability use with a spermicide.

RHYTHM METHOD: This relies on restraint in not having intercourse during ovulation which lasts about a week in between the cessation of the last cycle and the beginning of the next. It is difficult to estimate, as it varies so much. Timing by temperature is not always reliable.

COITUS INTERRUPTUS: This means withdrawal of the penis just before ejaculation and is not for the sensitive. It is also messy and can be a strain on sex and relationships.

SPERMICIDE CHEMICALS: These include creams, pastes, jellies, foaming tablets and pessaries, which have to be put into the vagina just before intercourse. They are not very satisfactory if used on their own.

STERILIZATION: An operation on fallopian tubes which stops eggs passing from ovaries to the womb. The normal menstrual cycle continues, but the operation is hardly ever reversible. It is a more serious operation than that for men (vasectomy) which involves a minor procedure on ducts leading from the testicles which prevent ejaculation of sperm with seminal fluid.

PREGNANCY

The best age for a woman to have a child is between 20 and 35. In younger mothers there is a much bigger chance of premature birth, while older mothers risk chromosomal errors including Down's Syndrome and mongolism. In this respect, the breakthrough is a process called amniocentesis – a technique of examining the chromosomes of the unborn foetus. A needle is inserted through the abdominal wall of the mother to draw off a sample of the amniotic fluid surrounding the baby. This enables such abnormalities as mongolism to be diagnosed. The sex of the unborn child can also be determined, which is important for families with sex-linked disorders.

Preferably a man should beget children before he is 45.

Ideally there should be an interval of at least two years between children, otherwise the younger one may be of lower intelligence.

Don't take drugs during pregnancy. That includes aspirin, nose drops, even supplementary vitamins, unless medically prescribed.

Don't smoke; studies indicate that smokers tend to have smaller babies, which means they are more susceptible to disease.

Avoid X-rays during pregnancy, including dental ones; make sure teeth are attended to early in pregnancy.

Every woman should see a doctor as soon as she feels reasonably sure she is pregnant. Regular check-ups will be arranged, the date of confinement estimated, and then it is up to you to take good care of your body.

Diet – a diet rich in protein, vitamins and minerals is important to the infant's health as well as your own. Pregnancy is never the time to lose weight though sometimes the more solid areas will slim down due to the fact that deposited fat is mobilized during pregnancy and put at the disposal of the growing foetus. Try to stay within a 2,000 Calorie a day regime, concentrating on meat, fish, poultry, fruit, fresh vegetables, cheese and wholegrain breads and cereals. No fried food, few fats. There is no need to drink extra milk, sufficient calcium is found in the other foods. Avoid sugar, white grains and breads; no alcohol. One of the early symptoms of pregnancy is an aversion or craving for certain foods. Control any desire for sweets, ice-cream or sugary confections. Don't eat raw, rare or undercooked red meat; it can adversely affect the foetus.

Exercise – swimming and walking are the best forms; add to that, housework, if necessary. Wear low or medium heeled shoes, and put your feet up should they be inclined to swell. If there is a tendency to varicose veins, wear a supporting stocking. Do one or two foot exercises a day. Keep breast muscles strong by wearing a fully supporting brassiere and during the last few months at night as well as during the day. Bathe the bosom with cold water night and morning. Do a simple exercise to strengthen pectoral muscles.

Rest – plan two rest periods a day, one before the midday meal and a longer one before dinner. Put your feet up, completely relax if you can.

Skin – this is twice as active which means it can improve more quickly and often does. It usually needs more cleansing, more frequently. Pigmentation marks sometimes appear but vanish when the baby is born. Some doctors advise patients to take vitamin D.

Stretch marks – they are less likely to occur if you don't get overweight and keep active. Rub in olive oil or lanolin cream. Weight should not increase more than ½ pound (240 g.) a week.

Nails – can prove difficult, need regular hot soakings in oil and nightly massage with a rich cream.

Hair – it will probably look marvellous during pregnancy but may fall out after the birth. This is usual beginning around the third month and not later than the seventh after confinement. If it is an excess amount or appears to be getting progressively worse, consult a trichologist.

Fifty per cent of conceptions are achieved within six months of trying and 80% within a year. If you have trouble conceiving, don't wait too long before seeking medical advice. Factors preventing pregnancy can be complex but many are straightforward and can be put right easily. Subfertility requires checking of both partners for mechanical or physical blockage of either sperm or ovum availability or effectiveness.

Spontaneous abortion occurs in 10–20% of all pregnancies. The majority should not be averted, particularly if they occur once or even twice during the first three months. The reason may be that the foetus is not perfectly normal. If miscarriage is repeated, especially after the initial three month period, the reasons should be medically ascertained.

ABORTION

Clinical abortion is available in almost all the major nations of the world. It is a relatively riskless procedure if done under the proper conditions; termination is technically simple and unlikely to lead to damage of the uterus which might affect later pregnancies. Up to three months and sometimes a little beyond an abortion is performed by doing a D and C operation and scraping the womb of the early foetal growth; it involves overnight hospitalization. More advanced pregnancies can be aborted by inducement and generally a salt solution is injected into the uterus bringing on contractions and abortion; several days are required. The decision to have an abortion is not a matter of medical uncertainty but one of morality. However, emotional upset is proving not to be nearly as high as was either expected or women were led to believe; it is more likely to bring relief.

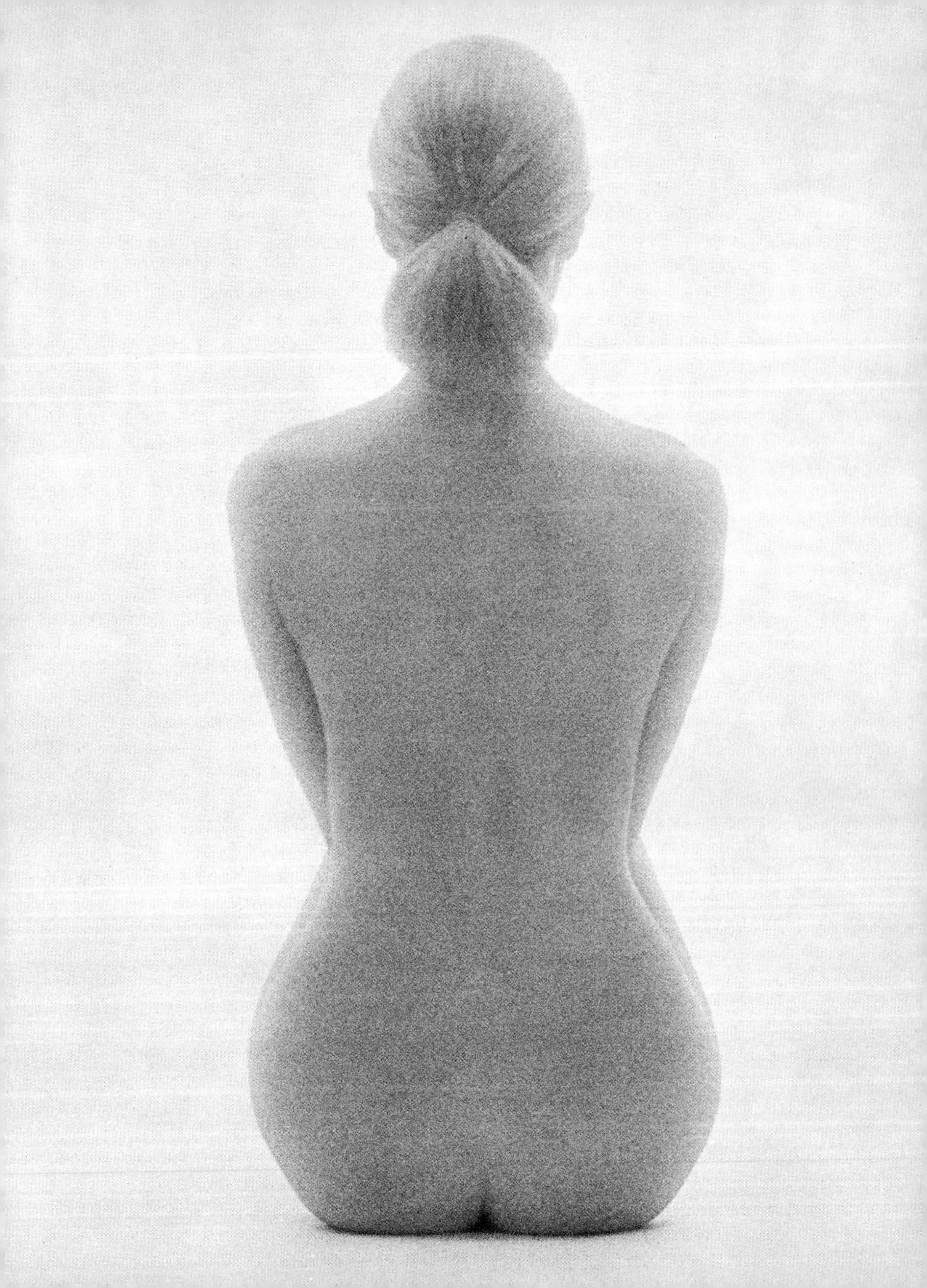

6

SKIN

The skin is a very complex structure. Four things affect it: genetics, environment, age and attention. Skin renews itself with biochemical efficiency and invariably responds well to treatment. A good skin is unblemished and uniform in colour, whether dark or light. It is firm, smooth and resilient. We are apt to think of skin in terms of the face only, but all body skin (except that of palms and soles which is hairless, thicker and tougher) is the same and will react in the same way. Every woman can have a great skin at any age, it's just knowing how to care for it.

Skin is the body's largest organ, 2 millimetres thick, weighing approximately 6 lbs (3 k.) with a hardworking life of its own. It is a protective covering, guarding the body against bacteria, chemicals and foreign objects. It breathes, contains blood vessels, sebaceous gland ducts, nerves and hair follicles. It acts as a thermostat, retaining heat or cooling the body with its sweat glands. It absorbs the shock of blows to the body and through its receptive sensory organs, keeps you in touch with the world.

It is made up of two main layers: the epidermis which you see, and the dermis. The outer layer protects by sealing in all the body's fluids and keeping out potentially harmful things. The inner layer supports, nourishes and supplies it with that most essential commodity – moisture. In structure the two layers are dissimilar. The epidermis consists of several rows of living cells covered by compact sheets of dead cells (sometimes referred to as the keratin layer). It is constantly growing and about every twenty days new cells are born at its base. They quickly die and the dead cells are then pushed to the surface by the arrival of the new ones underneath and are continuously shed. Every new top layer is another chance to have a beautiful skin. Even if you remove a portion of the outer layer it will grow back as good as new. The living reproductive cells are nourished through the blood vessels, but the dead cells have only one requirement: water. It will plump, soften or smooth. The amount of water the outer layer holds determines the skin's texture and to some extent its contour. It receives a steady supply of water from the dermis, but this is limited and frequently not enough.

The epidermis also holds the skin's pigment; the darker the skin, the greater the pigmentation. Oil and sweat glands belong to this layer, though they are actually situated below, communicating through ducts that end on the surface. Oil glands greatly influence the skin's condition.

The inner layer helps determine contour and is responsible for tone and resiliency. It is all living, though it cannot replace itself and only grows until maturity. Damage to this layer results in permanent degeneration or scarring. It consists of bundles of tough supporting tissue (collagen) interlaced with elastic fibres and blood vessels that transport water and nutrients, and set complexion tone. The emotions often affect these vessels. Embarrassment can cause them to flood resulting in a blush; panic can cause them to empty, leaving the skin dead white. If you feel bilious, you can turn green as the yellowish bile from the liver is transported to the surface.

Care of the skin requires a nutritious diet, plenty of water, fresh air, exercise, sleep and minimum stress. The skin needs to be protected against the environment – sun, wind, cold – by using barrier creams. Poor health habits, too many fats and sugars, too many stimulants like coffee, are bad for the skin; so is excess smoking, excess alcohol. Weight fluctuations should be avoided as, after sun, they are the prime cause of wrinkled skin. When you gain weight the skin has to stretch and this puts strain on the elastic fibres of the inner layer. When you lose weight the skin does not always spring back to its original shape, particularly if the loss has been quick and drastic. Apart from wrinkles, visible scars remain – stretch marks – and they are seen mostly on upper thighs and stomach. (They can sometimes be alleviated by rubbing in pure coconut oil or cocoa butter, particularly as a preventive measure during pregnancy.) Fat pads are extremely important to the skin's appearance; they lie directly beneath the skin and separate it from the deeper muscle and bone. Their function is to cushion and support the skin, to supply the sebaceous glands and to act as a vehicle for the oil-soluble skin vitamins A, D and E. Loss of almost all fatty tissue through extreme dieting or disease can alter the appearance and quality of skin very quickly.

A wholesome diet is essential. It is important to get enough proteins, vitamins and minerals; lean meat, fish, poultry, eggs, fresh vegetables and fruits; avocado, cucumber and cabbage are particularly recommended. Vitamin A is the skin's most needed vitamin, but it is widely available in everyday foods and excess can be detrimental. A supplement of C and E can do no harm. It is generally accepted that vitamins A, D, E and K can be absorbed through the skin, though how much, under what circumstances and to what value, varies with the source. The case for vitamin E is debatable. Dermatologists are dubious about its supposed skin-regenerating claims, but some people burst a 200 mg. vitamin E tablet and squeeze oil directly on the skin, saying it thickens it, dries up whiteheads and helps erase wrinkles.

Hormones play a tremendous part in the condition of the skin. The hormonal balance is responsible for the coarsening of pores at puberty: the sex hormones stimulate the sebaceous glands; these enlarge and so do the ducts and the pores. Over-stimulation can lead to acne. The hormones involved are oestrogen and progesterone, the female ones that make the skin finer, less oily, less porous, and androgen the male hormone that makes the skin coarse, oily and porous. We have a mixture of all but in varying proportions. Large doses of oestrogen can provide a smoother, better skin, but are not advisable in adolescence or during child-bearing years. The Pill has a high oestrogen content, but its effect on the skin is individual; most women report there is no noted change, some say skins improve, others that it worsens. There is no evidence to support the idea that sexual activity affects the skin for the better. Skin changes are often apparent during or after pregnancy, but that's the change within you and nothing to do with your sex life.

The ageing of skin is a gradual process, but it can be slowed down and reversed within limits. Regardless of how much care is given, minor structural changes will eventually occur, but the more serious skin problems are caused by neglect and abuse. The most important structural changes are cellular build-up, dryness and pigment increase; they cause problems in texture, contour and colour. Older skin produces a different type of epidermis cell that tends not to shed so easily when dead. Because of this, the sheets of dead cells mount up, giving the skin a coarse, leathery look. These older cells do not hold water so well and unless moisture supply is constant and increased they can become dry and shrivelled. In addition there is a decrease in oil gland function which further aggravates the moisture problem. Pigmentation increases with age. This is not noticeable in black, brown or even dark olive skins, but fair skins darken a shade or two and not always evenly. Discoloration may appear as blotches or as freckle-like areas on hands and face commonly called liver-spots, although nothing to do with the liver – the sun is the culprit, for it dries and discolours.

Ageing changes the inner layer. As the supporting tissue degenerates, the elastic fibres lose their effectiveness and the skin is unable to maintain its normal resiliency. Wrinkles, lines and creases appear; the skin of the eyes and neck is the most vulnerable. Finally the blood vessels respond to age by expanding, sometimes causing the complexion to take on a ruddy look, sometimes breaking to form red spider lines and spots.

SKIN TYPES

What your skin needs in the way of treatment and preparations depends upon its type – and that depends upon texture, colour and condition. There are three textures – oily, dry and balanced (often known as normal); many skins are a combination of oily and dry. Colour influences texture while any skin can have a sensitive or blemished condition. To determine skin type, cleanse skin thoroughly and using a magnifying glass in strong light, examine it closely.

TEXTURE:

Oily – Caused by overproduction of sebum by the oil glands. Affects darker skins mostly; but even a light skin is inclined to go sallow. Skin shines constantly, is coarse and has enlarged pores. It is often plagued with blackheads, occasional break-outs and is the skin most prone to acne. It stays younger-looking longer, has few wrinkles and usually improves with age. Trying to remove all oils from the skin only encourages greater gland activity. It is important to remove only excess oil from the surface, leaving a sufficient amount to ward off any over-activity. Too enthusiastic a treatment with harsh soap or cleansing lotion will often dehydrate the epidermis, leaving skin in a flaky condition.

Dry – Three different things cause dry skin: dehydration, insufficient amount of oil secretion and ageing. It affects 85% of all light-skinned women. Skin is generally of a fine texture, but looks and feels tight and drawn. It chaps, flakes and peels easily, and even at an early age may show wrinkles and lines, particularly around the eyes and mouth. Contributory factors to this condition are: use of wrong cosmetics, strong soaps, exposure to sun and wind, indoor heating and air-conditioning. One of the most important steps in dealing with a dry skin is to try and avoid further dehydration by sealing in moisture. The lack of natural oils must be compensated by rich external lubrication.

Balanced – Exists when oil, moisture and acidity are harmonious. It is ideal but rare. Skin is fine textured with no visible pores, smooth to touch, neither wet nor greasy. It has a tendency to become more dry with time, so it needs assistance to retain the status quo.

Combination – This is really skin in transition between dry and oily state. It gives off too much oil in the T-area of forehead, nose and chin; the rest is dry particularly around eyes and on cheeks. The dry and oily areas have to be treated separately.

COLOUR: The colour of the skin depends on the degree of pigmentation. Light skin tones are graded from pale to pink, beige to rosy; dark skin tones go from olive to caramel, brown to black. The general term 'black' covers a much wider range than does 'white'. One dermatologist differentiates 35 variations of basic shading for black skins, 10 for white. There is no basic difference in structure and quality – therefore no difference in skin-care regimes. Black skin is usually more oily and has more sweat glands. However it still suffers the effects of dryness, which shows in its ashen cast in cold weather. In general the darker the skin, the slower the ageing process. The reason is a combination of heredity and habitat. The sun is the great enemy of light skins which usually have dry tendencies so lines are created faster. The evenly distributed pigment in dark skins acts like a sun filter and its more oily surface acts as a shield keeping moisture in. Dark skins, even black skins, can tan and burn, but they do so less drastically and more evenly than light ones. Dermatologists say that black skins are less likely to develop acne or skin cancer.

CONDITION: *Sensitive* – Usually dry skin plus. Fine textured often with a transparent look, the upper layer being particularly thin and sensitive and likely to develop broken capillaries. Reacts quickly to both external and internal influences – sun, wind, emotions, food, drink. Needs usual dry-skin care plus extra protective lubrication. Watch for any allergies.

Blemished – Usually oily skin plus. Troubled with pimples, sometimes to the intensity of acne. Needs usual oily skin care plus attention from medicated preparations that dry and heal – and professional advice.

BASIC CARE

Body skin usually can be taken care of by retaining moisture through a body lotion, using oil in the bath if skin is dry and by rubbing away the flaking skin. Facial skin is more vulnerable but consistent care can give lasting results. It need not take more than three minutes morning and evening but is vital. The key to good skin is activity; you must keep the renewal rate of skin cells as high as possible. The only way to do this is by regularly keeping the skin clean, moist and thinned of its dead-cell build-up. It's easy to get into the habit, and once attained it is hard to break. The preparations only influence the epidermis, but that's enough. The steps to good skin are: cleansing, freshening, moisturizing, conditioning, exfoliating (thinning) and stimulating. The first four are daily procedures, the other two are weekly unless you have a special problem – then more often. Check this chart for treatment necessary for each skin texture; check below for complete details. Warning: corrective skin care is minimal. If you try to do more you can possibly harm the skin.

SKIN TREATMENT SCHEDULE

	OILY SKIN	DRY SKIN	BALANCED SKIN
Twice daily (morning and evening)	cleanse with soap or rinsable cleanser – and water astringent light moisturizer	cleanse with mild soap, rinsable cleanser, cream or lotion – and water diluted toner rich moisturizer	cleanse with soap or rinsable cleanser – and water toner light moisturizer
Daily	eye cream emollient for throat area	eye cream rich emollient conditioner	eye cream light emollient conditioner
Weekly	exfoliation treatment (twice a week is better)	exfoliation treatment (more if dry skin builds-up)	exfoliation treatment
Weekly	stimulation and clearing masque (twice a week is better)	stimulation and clearing masque	stimulation and clearing masque

CLEANSING

It is necessary to remove stale make-up, pore-deep grime as well as some natural secretions which can cause skin problems. How you do it is important: cleansing incorrectly is worse than not cleansing at all, as the skin's natural moisturizers and oil protectors can be removed in the process. Cleanse twice a day, always in the morning and at some time in the evening, not necessarily just before going to bed.

There are four types of cleansers: oils and greases, creams, soaps and rinsable cleansers (creams and lotions). The greases and creams dissolve make-up but are not so adept at removing dirt or themselves. Tissuing off is not enough, a freshener is always needed. There is no substitute for soap and water. Even if you're fair skinned and fragile, cleansing creams and oils do not provide the kind of cleansing soap can and there are many mild soaps suitable for the face. Rinsable cleansers are the next best solution for older and particularly dry skins, and although these may be creams and lotions, they should be rinsed, not wiped, off.

Many women never use water in the belief that it is bad for the skin. It is not true. Frequent and excessive contact with water can cause dry and chapped skin, because in time it will remove most of the skin's moisturizers, but you are hardly likely to soak your face that long. The entire cleansing routine should not take more than two minutes and should be done no more than twice a day.

Procedure:

Use cream or oil for make-up removal, particularly for eyes; tissue off.
Wet skin with lukewarm water.
Using soap or rinsable cleanser, work up a quick lather for 30 seconds.
Rinse with warm water till soapy traces have gone; three times is usual.
Pat with towel to absorb residue water, don't rub.

FRESHENING

Fresheners do the important job of rinsing off all traces of cleanser and pore dirt and restoring the skin's acid mantle. They also help stimulate local circulation and refine skin texture. Freshener, toner and astringent are the three names for the preparations used and are basically the same product in graded strengths depending on the alcoholic content. Astringents are the strongest and are recommended for oily skins; fresheners and toners for dry and balanced skins. Medicated lotions are astringents with more alcohol and the addition of anti-bacterial agents.

Procedure:

Apply straight after cleansing; saturate cotton pad with freshener, wipe over skin thoroughly.

A between-cleansing clean-up can be done by wiping face with a freshener; recommended for very oily skins.

Natural Aids:

A teaspoon of cider vinegar added to $1\frac{1}{2}$ cups of water. Use as liquid toner.

Rub skin with a slice of raw potato.

Rub with a slice of lemon, or splash with lemon juice and water.

Cucumber freshener: squeeze juice of 2 cucumbers, heat to boiling point, skim away froth, bottle and refrigerate.

Sprinkle a few drops of camphor in the last cleansing rinsing water.

MOISTURIZING

Helps to offset the evaporating effects of the environment. Moisture is not actually fed to the skin, but preparations form a protective film holding in the skin's moisture. Moisture is the single most important ingredient in skin chemistry. Dry and older skins which don't have as much moisture as they need, are additionally helped by an emollient that attracts moisture from the atmosphere, holds and feeds water to the skin. A moisturizer smoothes and plumps skin surface, improves the feel and fills in the gaps giving a good base for make-up. If used without make-up a heavier type is best. Most creams and lotions moisturize, as they trap water.

Procedure:

Best time to apply is directly after a bath or face-washing; even after drying with a towel, skin is damp and retains some moisture – that is the time to seal it in.

Dot on forehead, nose, cheeks and chin; smooth emulsion all over face and throat, using upward strokes and finger-patting around the eyes.

Wait for moisturizer to be absorbed before applying make-up.

If weather is harsh, reapply to driest and most vulnerable areas.

Natural Aid:

Milk of almonds: skin 1 oz. (30 g.) almonds by dipping alternately in boiling and cold water. Grind until a powder, add drop by drop $\frac{1}{2}$ pint (3 dl.) of distilled water, continuing to blend until liquid is milky; strain.

CONDITIONING

Its purpose is to keep skin soft and supple as well as smooth; most effectively done when you are sleeping or resting and the skin is relaxed. Dry skins need a deep lubricating cream that stays on overnight or for several hours during the day. Balanced to dry skins require a lighter emollient; oily skins are better with just a moisturizer. Combination skins should have each area treated separately. Ideally conditioning should include the use of an eye cream since the area around the eyes lacks natural oil and is very prone to dryness and wrinkling. A light-weight emollient is as effective as a special cream.

Skin needs to be conditioned every day. It is impossible to correct a neglected or damaged skin overnight by applying a thick layer of emollient. A thin film adheres and is adequate; the rest is waste. All preparations of similar consistency give much the same results; the important difference is the concentration, which determines whether a product is light or heavy. An emollient can be used as a daytime barrier cream against inclement weather.

Procedure:

Apply after cleansing and freshening.

Pre-wet skin by covering with a wet facecloth; this increases effectiveness of conditioner.

Finger-pat eye cream around eye area.

Gently massage conditioner into skin. This is an opportunity to firm and contour the face and throat. Too much manipulating of facial skin is not good so do it quickly. Use both hands, fingertips only, many strokes.

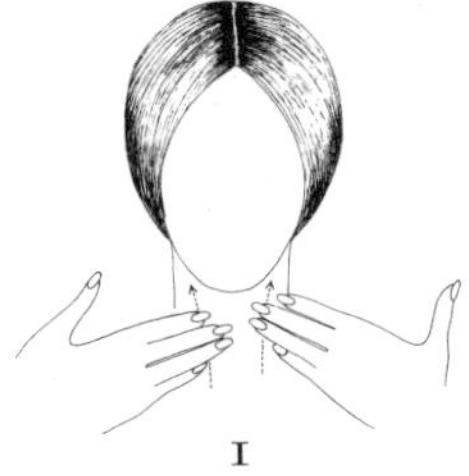

1

Skin Contouring – the same movements should be used for all skin care.

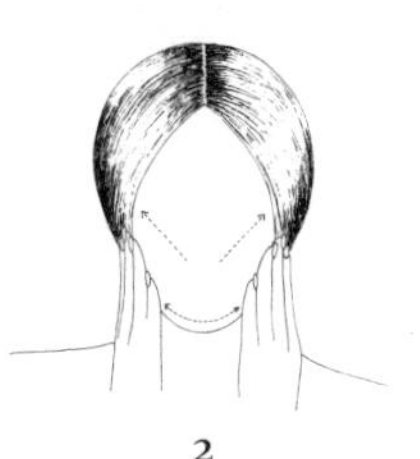

2

1. Neck: use long alternating strokes from collar bone to jawline.
2. Cheeks: from centre line, smooth upward and outward from chin to ears, nose to temples; stroke the nose bridge downwards, sides outwards.
3. Forehead: stroke upward, in high arcs to the hairline.
4. Eyes: using one tip, finger pat, starting in the centre between eyes, making a semi-circle going outward both above and below eye.

Leave conditioner on a few hours or overnight.

Before applying make-up, cleanse, freshen and moisturize.

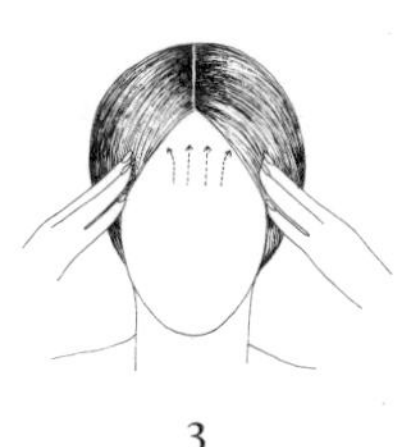

3

Natural Aids:

For extremely dry skin, melt a teaspoon of butter and beat in 2 tablespoons of milk; apply liberally and leave a few hours.

Apply a thin film of petroleum jelly for dry and balanced skins.

Any vegetable shortening makes an effective weather barrier.

20-minute honey conditioner: moisten face, massage in raw honey; rinse away with warm water.

Honey-and-cream: mix 1 teaspoon honey with 2 tablespoons light cream; beat together, apply, leave for 20 minutes, rinse away.

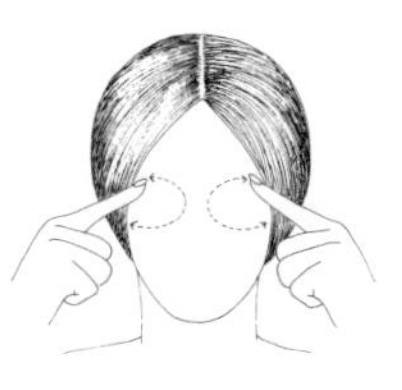

4

For dry skin – oil of avocado, almond, wheatgerm or olives.

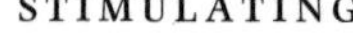

STIMULATING

This is the way to give the skin a quick pick-up, to exercise it by activating circulation and bringing nutrients and oxygen to the surface. It is usually done through masques, sometimes through steam facials. Nearly all masques contain a high percentage of water; the rapid evaporation that follows application causes them to be cooling, soothing and contracting. This is often reinforced by the addition of sharp aromatics and alcohol. When the masque is taken off, the blood vessels expand and the skin looks rosier; fluid from the enlarged vessels plumps up the inner layer, smoothing the skin and compressing the pores. There is a definite improvement in the appearance of the skin, and although this 'masque effect' is transitory, the skin is exercised and stimulated.

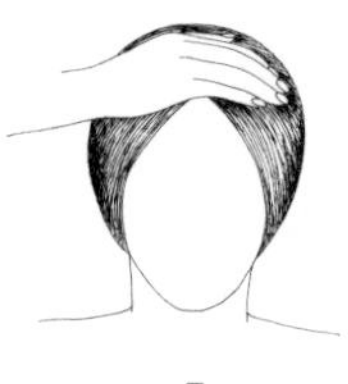

1

In addition, masques may have one or more corrective effects on the skin. They usually contain materials that act as cleansers and purifiers, drawing out dirt, toxins and grease. All masques rely on a drying process; they are divided into rinse-off and peel-off types. The rinse-off ones are the better cleansers; many contain clay or silicas (forms of sand) with the ability to suck out oil and dirt. Some masques contain gums and proteins. Peel-off preparations usually contain rubber, wax or some type of plastic. They work like a sticky piece of Scotch tape removing surface dirt and a few dead cells; they are not such good cleaners as the rinse-off ones, but equally good stimulators. Oily skins need a masque twice a week, dry and balanced skins, once.

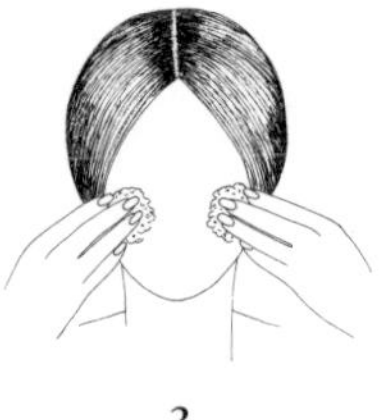

2

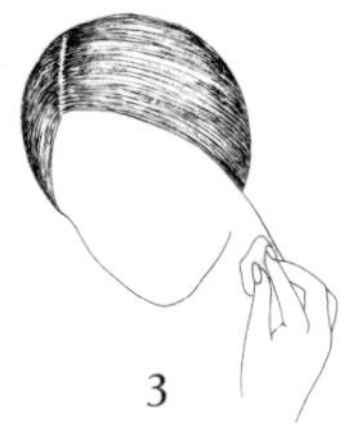

3

Procedure:

This is a facial: here are the professional steps. It takes about half an hour.

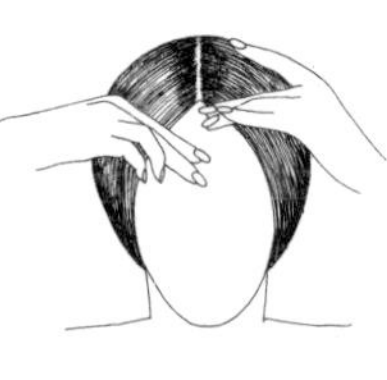

4

1. Smooth hair away from face and tie back.
2. Apply a cleanser using motions illustrated for skin contouring (page 119). Tissue or rinse off depending on cleanser.
3. With cottonwool pad, apply freshener to remove last traces of cleanser.
4. Dot light moisturizer on forehead, cheeks and chin; blend in.
5. Rinse with clear lukewarm water.
6. Apply masque all over face and throat; leave a free circle around the tender eye area.
7. Cover eyes with cottonwool pads soaked in milk or a non-alcoholic freshener. Leave masque on and relax lying down for 20 minutes.

8. Remove all traces of masque, blot face and throat with towel; finish with a thin film of moisturizer.

Natural Aids:

The following facial applications should be left on for a minimum of 20 minutes, then thoroughly rinsed off with water.

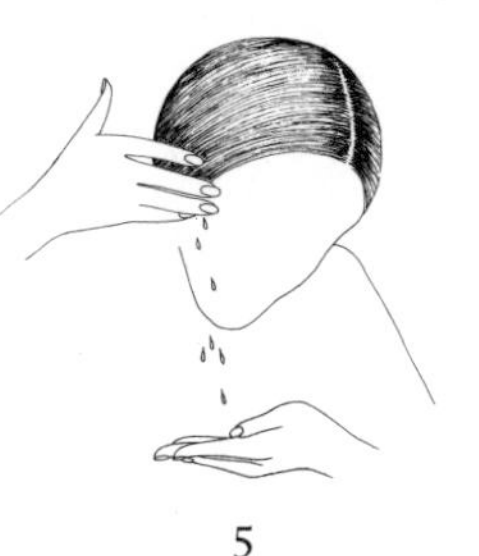

5

Crushed strawberries used alone or mixed with oatmeal.

Ripened pears give an astringent action to oily skin.

Apply juice from a few green cabbage leaves.

Cucumber masque: grind or mash enough to cover face; refreshing.

Brewers' yeast facial: 1 teaspoon of powdered yeast and 2 teaspoons warm water; adjust consistency so it spreads like a paste.

The beaten white of an egg – with the optional addition of $\frac{1}{4}$ teaspoon lemon juice or cider vinegar; good for oily or balanced skin.

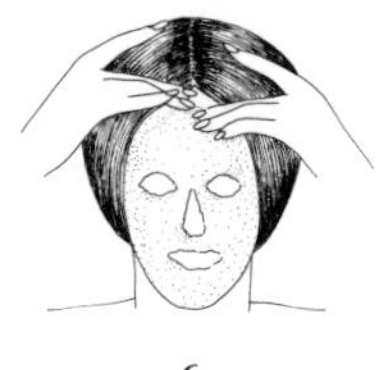

6

Another version of an egg-white facial is to beat it with a tablespoon of skimmed milk.

An egg yolk, a few drops of cider vinegar and a little vegetable oil; good for dry skin.

Honey masque: 2 tablespoons honey and $\frac{1}{2}$ teaspoon of lemon juice or cider vinegar.

Steam Facial

This is a method of stimulation; steam encourages the pores to push out dirt and impurities, it promotes perspiration and stimulates circulation. Sensitive skins or those with broken veins must not be treated.

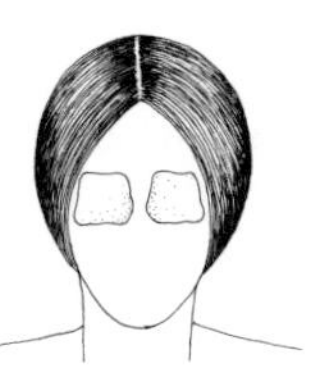

7

Steaming with a herb infusion is most beneficial. Pour boiling water over herbs in a bowl; make a towel into a head tent and steam face over bowl for 10 minutes. Blot dry, freshen, then moisturize. The following can be used individually or combined.

For cleansing, soothing: camomile, lady's mantle, nettle, rosemary, thyme.
For tightening: peppermint, elderflower, tincture of benzoin, gum arabic.
For drying: yarrow.
For healing: leek, comfrey, fennel.

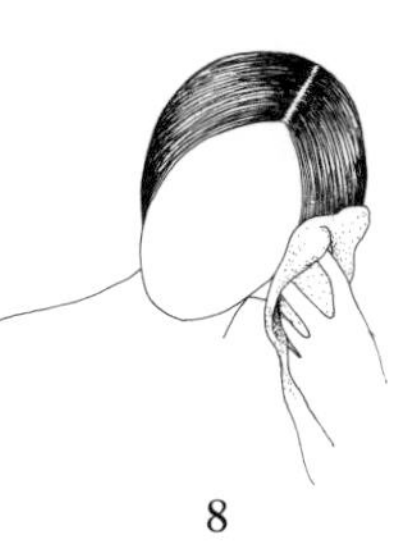

8

EXFOLIATING

This takes cleansing a step further and is the removal of dead surface cells (flakes) from the skin. It is one of the most important skin-care procedures and one of the least known. The skin's texture and contour are both improved; the thinned skin feels smoother, appears more translucent and has a lighter and more uniform colour tone. Pores look smaller and an additional benefit is that the outer layer is more easily moisturized after the dry hard surface cells are removed. Slough-off products can be lotions, gels or creams, sometimes with visible abrasive ingredients like grains. Some astringents act as very mild exfoliators. Young skin may be thinned simply by rubbing with a rough facecloth wrung out in lukewarm water. Older skin requires heavier thinning, using a preparation and a complexion brush, sponge or textured cloth. It is really a mild peel and should be done once a week, sometimes twice if skin looks scaly. Deep peels are drastic remedies to get rid of lines and blemishes; they are done by physicians or specialized cosmetologists.

Procedure:

Thinning is done immediately after cleansing.

Apply preparation according to instructions.

Remove by wiping or brushing off, using circular movements for forehead, chin and cheeks, vertical movements for nose, facial borders and neck; use water if necessary to clear skin.

Moisturize immediately.

Guard against early sun exposure.

Natural Aids:

Sprinkle ordinary salt on a wet facecloth; rub face lightly, rinse away; not for delicate skin.

Papaya mint tea removes skin debris; pour 2 cups boiling water on 2 tea bags, steep for a few minutes; soak a facecloth in the tea, wring out, apply to the face holding cloth against skin. The tea must be hot to be effective; keep heating, and renewing cloth. Continue for 15 minutes.

SUNTANNING

The right amount of sun can help you to look wonderful – tawny, glowing, healthy. Too much sun and you will be doing your skin irreparable damage and depleting your body of vitamin B. Prolonged exposure, year after year, is responsible for both premature ageing of the skin and many skin cancers. The damage is cumulative. It is only about one per cent of the sun's radiation that affects the skin and all the burning and tanning is caused by the invisible short-wave ultra-violet rays.

Activity takes place on two different levels in the epidermis. First, the pigment-bearing cells, tucked away on the underside of the epidermis, are activated by the ultra-violet rays – only the shortest of these rays are strong enough to penetrate the cells making them produce melanin (the brownish pigment). The effect cannot be seen for about two days, but it is this action that produces a long-lasting tan. Meanwhile the longer-wave rays work on the melanin granules that already exist in the upper layers of the epidermis, turning them a dark brown. The reason why the long-lasting tan is slow in coming is that the lower melanin granules gradually work their way to the surface. Tan disappears not because it 'fades' but because the pigmented cells flake off. To preserve a tan, involves controlling the natural shedding of cells. This can be done by using oil in your bath and a body lotion afterwards.

A suntan is a defence mechanism. The granules of melanin act as a screen on the surface, filtering out harmful rays and protecting the delicate underlayers. If this were the only effect of the ultra-violet waves, there would be few problems, but they also release a chemical that penetrates the skin's inner layer. It is this that causes the blood vessels to dilate, accounting for a lobster red colour. Some hours later the dilated vessels allow serum to enter the tissues. This leads to swelling, pressure and irritation on nerve endings; peeling follows and in severe cases, blisters. Damaged cells work their way to the surface, become harder and thicker, forming a tough layer. This is the second line of defence for the skin, as it reflects and scatters light, but also makes the skin look leathery and dry.

Whether you live under the sun all the time, or whether it is a transient exposure, protection is essential. If you want to acquire a tan, you also need patience. Sunburn protectors come in varying strengths, the most effective being the opaque sunblocks. These reduce the likelihood of damage, but also reduce the likelihood of tanning. Some sun lotions are only moisturizers or greases which attract the rays and prevent drying. Be cautious, read labels. Quick natural protectors are cocoa butter, or a mixture of salad oil and cider vinegar.

A protective screen should be used all over exposed areas. The most vulnerable parts are the face, nose, shoulders, upper chest, midriff, backs of knees and backs of hands. If you are in the sun for the first time for several months, take it slowly. The first day sunbathe for only half an hour in the morning, keep in the shade until the late afternoon, then take a little more sun. Increase your time in the sun each day; avoid midday rays, strong reflection from the water and the combination of sun and wind.

Some skins burn and dry, others tan. Generally the colour of skin and eyes determines the effect of the sun on the skin. The lighter, the more cautious you need to be. The very fair skinned with little melanin can't expect a deep tan ever; redheads who sit in the sun often go freckled. Both types should use a strong sunblock. It has been reported that some people susceptible to sunburn have been able to take more exposure by supplementing the B vitamin of PABA (see Vitamin Chart, page 32) to the degree of 1,000 milligrams a day; also by applying it as an ointment, delicate skins can tan.

Olive to caramel skins need a sunscreen only, a stronger one if you don't want to deepen the tone. Brown to black skins require a mild sunscreening lotion, one that simply moisturizes and lubricates with emollients. It is true that dark skin does not burn as easily as fair skin, and can take more exposure, but this does not mean that it should not be helped. Any skin dries out in the sun without lubrication.

Artificial tanning by means of a sun-lamp is a practical way to build up a tan slowly, or to keep a healthy colour. It is preferable to go to a clinic where lamps are used under supervision. The temptation at home is to take an extra minute, which can be very harmful indeed. Half a minute is ample for fair skins with a gradual increase in time according to skin colour. Goggles are essential as concentrated ultra-violet rays can harm the eyes. There is no need to use any protective cream, but apply an emollient or oil afterwards to alleviate drying.

If you get a sunburn and it is red and painful, try these remedies: equal parts of baking soda and water, patted onto sunburn and left on for half an hour, rinsed off with tepid water. Beat the white of an egg with 1 teaspoon of castor oil, smooth over skin as a lotion. Cover with a mashed pulp of cucumber. Soothe with a strong solution of ordinary tea or sage tea. A diluted solution of vinegar and water brings relief. Mix ¼ cup buttermilk with 2 tablespoons rose water, splash over skin and wait until it dries, rinse off.

SKIN BLEMISHES

Skin is subjected to various growths and infections which look ugly and can develop into serious disorders. Here are the most common problems:

ACNE: One of the most distressing skin disorders, and primarily affects young skin. If neglected it can cause extensive inner-layer scarring. Acne is caused by sex hormones. Diet, once thought to be so important, is only a minor consideration – though too fat a diet can aggravate the condition. The male hormone, testosterone, is mainly responsible, because its production is apt to be inconsistent at puberty. The sex hormones stimulate the skin's sebaceous glands and regulate oil output. Overactivity results in excess oil secretion and thickening of the pore openings. The pore becomes blocked and in addition fatty acids are produced by enzyme action. The result is a pimple, a whitehead (a waxy point with no surface outlet) or a blackhead. At this point infection often sets in and pus ruptures the wall of the oil gland, the infection spreading to the inner layer. This inevitably results in a permanent scar.

Since one cannot eliminate the cause of acne, treatment is limited to measures that suppress infection and keep it from breaking out in the oil gland. Although a healthy diet, good skin hygiene and medical preparations are of some help, antibiotics are now considered the basis of therapy. These remove the bacteria that cause infection; cortisone is used but sometimes this has undesirable side effects. Oestrogen, the female hormone, can be given to balance the excessive output of testosterone, but caution is necessary particularly in young women. Natural sunlight and ultra-violet treatments often help, so does superficial X-ray therapy.

BLACKHEADS: These are oil plugs in the pores that blacken on exposure to air – the colour has nothing to do with dirt, it reflects oxidization. They are the most common form of skin blemish, sometimes become infected and turn to acne. Regular, proper cleansing helps prevent them and alleviate mild ones. Removing the firmly entrenched plugs is often better done by a professional. The procedure is to open the pores first through steaming or hot compresses. Pressure around the opening is applied either with a special instrument or clean fingertips (never nails). This forces out the blackhead. Some cosmetologists use a suction technique. Afterwards skin must be dabbed with alcohol, then wiped with an astringent to close the pores. At home use hot compresses soaked in a mixture of 1 teaspoon of sodium bicarbonate in 1 cup hot water.

BROKEN VEINS: The legs and face are usually affected. The faintest tracery is the most difficult to get rid of. There are technical ways of draining veins with a special needle and a chemical fluid. It often requires a series of treatment sessions over a period of time.

DERMATITIS: This is a general term that covers inflammation of the skin caused by physical or emotional means. Eczema and psoriasis come into this category and are said to have emotional or nervous origins.

Medical treatment can control them during flare-ups, but cannot control the source. The conditions often come and go, but do not leave scars.

MOLES: These patches of dark pigment can look unattractive particularly when raised or sprouting isolated hairs. They can be removed quickly and painlessly. Don't pluck or pull at hairs, if necessary cut them close to the skin. The slightly raised mole, particularly if it has been there from childhood, is usually harmless. But if a flat mole suddenly becomes darker or larger or more raised, or if it bleeds, go to your doctor at once.

PIGMENT BLOTCHES: If you have been careless about the sun, you have probably acquired a few brown spots varying in size. Removing them is not easy, and many bleach creams are too harsh for safety. They can be removed by planing or deep peeling. Should any pigmentation appear in the form of rough red spots, professional advice is absolutely necessary, as they can become malignant. Skin cancer is every bit as serious as any other kind; certain types stay localized but others spread rapidly to the lymph nodes and on throughout the body. Red patches can be treated in the early stages by cutting, burning, scraping, freezing, acids or X-ray.

WARTS: When they are small, warty growths can be removed easily by scraping them off the surface; this usually leaves no scar. The larger ones must be cut or burned off and sometimes a scar results.

WHITEHEADS: These appear as tiny white beads of waxy matter just under the skin and have no way out to the surface unless helped. A tiny opening has to be made and the application of oil helps to force them out.

SKIN PEELING

There comes a point where certain old skins or blemished skins cannot be helped except by literally getting rid of the old skin and growing a new one. This is a drastic measure, but it can be done. It is entirely different to plastic surgery which corrects contour problems. Peeling is aimed at improving the skin's texture. There are two methods: chemopeel, which involves the use of chemicals to burn off the outer layer, and dermabrasion which planes it down. Both are medical procedures.

CHEMOPEEL: Sometimes called chemical surgery. It is used to treat skin scarred by acne and other blemishes, but the results with ageing skin can be dramatic. A caustic is used to destroy all the epidermis and part of the inner layer. This not only gets rid of the old surface skin which is thickened, large-pored and wrinkled, but also all the things attached to it such as warts, rough spots, pigment blotches. The removal of a portion of the inner layer stimulates growth of new tissue and helps to rebuild the skin effectively. It is a very delicate operation with success depending on precision control and timing. The whole face, usually together with neck area, is treated at the same time to avoid tide marks. Localized touch-ups can be done later if necessary. The degree of penetration of the chemical determines the depth of peeling.

It is not as painful nor as uncomfortable as you might expect, but the caustic does cause intense inflammation. This looks horrific and is often combined with swelling. Understandable when you consider that at the end of the peel there is no outer layer of skin and only two-thirds of the inner one. A new epidermis grows gradually and completely; initial protection from all outside elements is essential. The final covering is smooth, unblemished and fine-textured. The inner layer is a little thicker than before, firmer and more resilient; it has the effect of plumping up the skin.

It takes about three to six months to see the complete visual improvement. There is one drawback: the new skin often has an artificial look about it. This is primarily because the inner layer consists entirely of scar tissue, lacking the tone and depth of the original skin. It is also less durable and can relapse within one to ten years depending on how well you treat it. The operation can be repeated to maintain the effect.

Some complications can occur; the most common is the formation of more pigment than before. This may be due to a strong reaction to the caustic or to early exposure to the sun. The reverse can happen – no pigment and the skin is left ruddy.

DERMABRASION: This is often the preferred method to reduce scars, or acne, remove surface blemishes and reduce fine wrinkles. The upper layer of skin tissue is removed by an electrically operated rotating wire brush or steel burr. The depth of planing depends on the severity of the case; it can also be done in isolated areas. A scab forms very quickly, which is first softened by a prescribed ointment, then with lukewarm water. It usually comes off within a month and at first the face looks badly burned, but in time the redness diminishes. Protection from sunlight is essential for six months. Fine dermabrasion is often used in conjunction with a face lift.

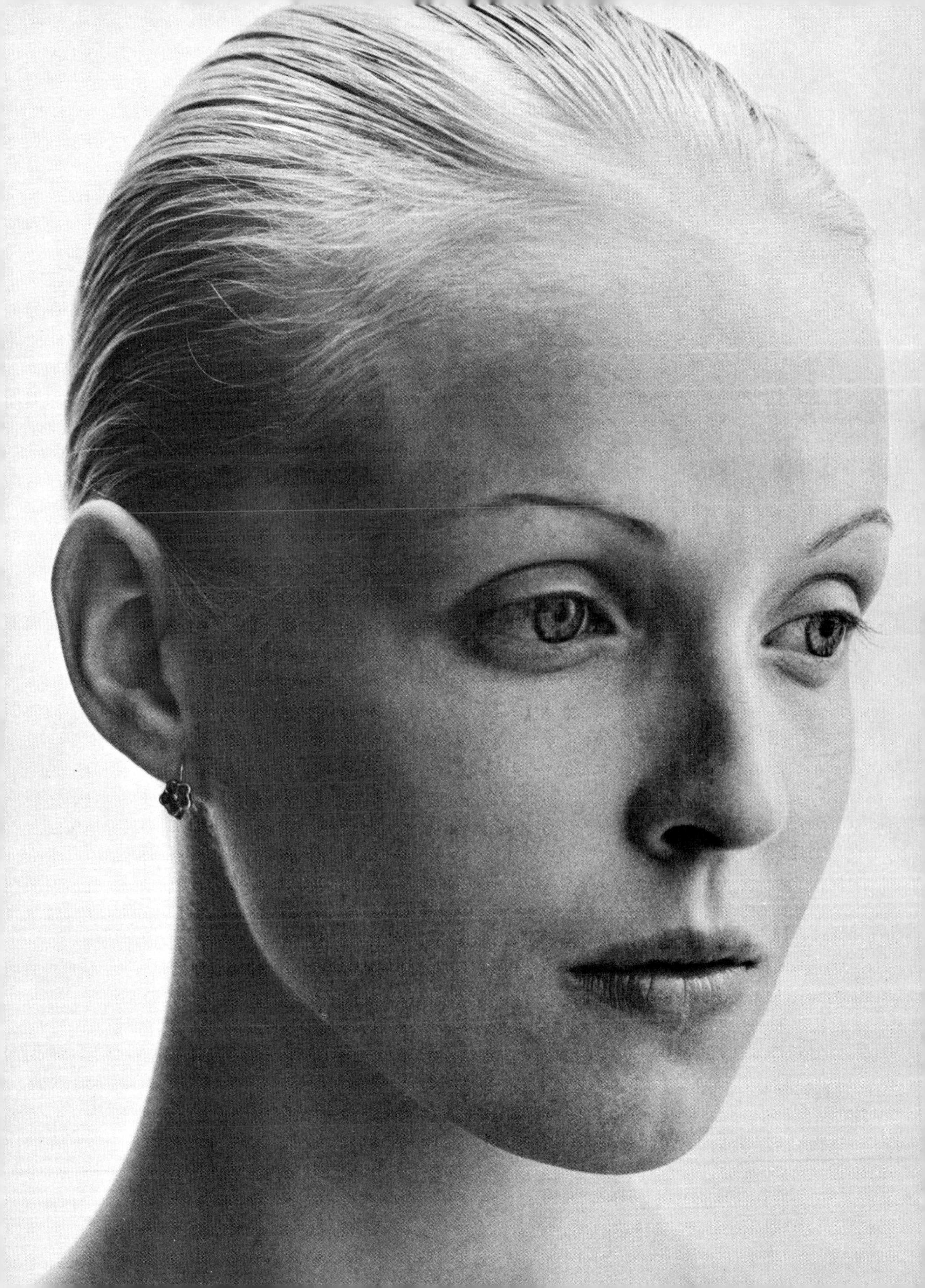

7

THE FACE

The most important bone of the face is the frontal bone. It forms the forehead, eye sockets and bridge of the nose. The size and angle vary tremendously and primarily contribute to the individuality of each face. The cheek bones form a flat area below the eye sockets and determine the moulding and planes of the face. The other bones are the nose bones – two small ones which link with the frontal bone – and the upper and lower jaw bones which hinge together close to the ears and hold the teeth. The ear has no bone structure and is made up of cartilage and muscle.

The eyes are delicate and intricate, depending for effectiveness not only on the condition of the eyeball but on muscles and nerves.

The muscles of the face are very intricate, giving mobility to every single inch of it. The most important, from the beauty point of view, are the zygomaticus muscles which extend across the cheeks from the temples to the corners of the mouth, keeping the contours of the face firm. All these muscles determine the expression of the features. Chewing exercises the face. Smiling and laughing, although they may add a few lines around nose, eyes and mouth, also exercise cheek muscles and pull the corners of the mouth in an upward direction, preventing the face from sagging.

The face will age long before the body. Its muscles react negatively to stress, emotion and tension. It is easy to get into the habit of grimacing, frowning and raising eyebrows and this leads to lines and wrinkles that become more definite each year.

LATEGAN

EXERCISE AND CONTROL

Like any other part of the body, the face and interrelated neck structure needs exercise and muscle control to keep it in good shape and condition. Control is primarily awareness. It does not mean immobility but being more conscious of the changing movements of your face when you are talking and listening; try not to exaggerate expressions.

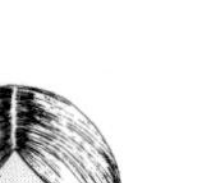

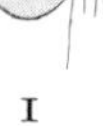

1

FACIAL EXERCISES: To improve and maintain the characteristics of a youthful contour and covering. They may look weird, for they are face-pulling gymnastics that manoeuvre the face to correct it, but you will quickly see that when you do them, certain lines and wrinkles are momentarily ironed out. Done with regularity, they are very effective. Do them in the bath or in front of the mirror before making up.

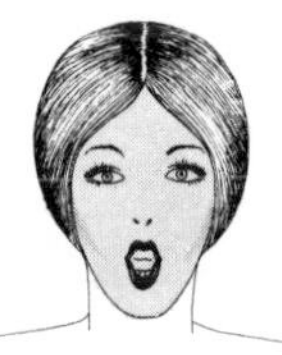

2

1. *Mouth and Cheeks* – Purse lips and at the same time fill cheeks with air. Place the 3 middle fingers of each hand on each cheek, either side of the mouth. Press fingers in against the blown-out surface, but don't let the air out. Count 10. Relax. Repeat 10 times. Work up to holding to the count of 30.

2. *Mouth, Cheeks and Eye Area* – Open mouth wide as if screaming, open eyes wide and staring at the same time. Count 3. Repeat 10 times. Then repeat, turning face first to the left, then to the right – 5 times each side.

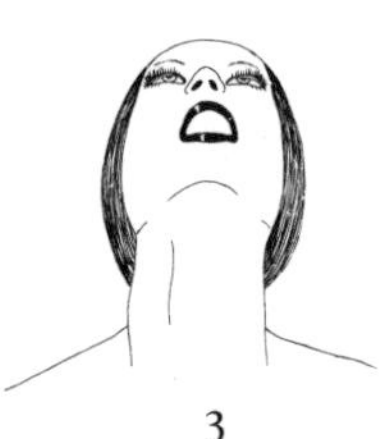

3

3. *Mouth and Jaws* – Open mouth wide, fling head back. Open and close mouth moving the back teeth. Open and close 10 times.

4. *Forehead* – Using palm of hand, push scalp back from the hairline smoothing out any furrows. Count 3. Repeat 10 times.

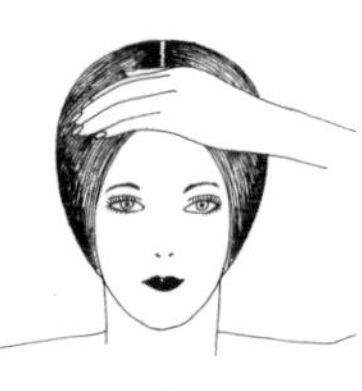

4

NECK EXERCISES: Bad muscle habits in the neck cause crêpiness and lines. When neck muscles are properly toned, the skin is held smooth and taut. When they are not, the horizontal lines crease and the contours sag. The neck is not an isolated area, but part of good posture, vital in keeping the throat area smooth and agile. Most women do not realize how little control they have over the set of their heads, or in moving from side to side. These exercises help to give you control by freeing the neck from tension, loosening and lowering the shoulders, elongating the neck muscles. It is important to be aware of what the neck is doing, how it is being held. Feel it; feel the distance between neck and ears; feel the shoulders hanging freely without knotted-up tension.

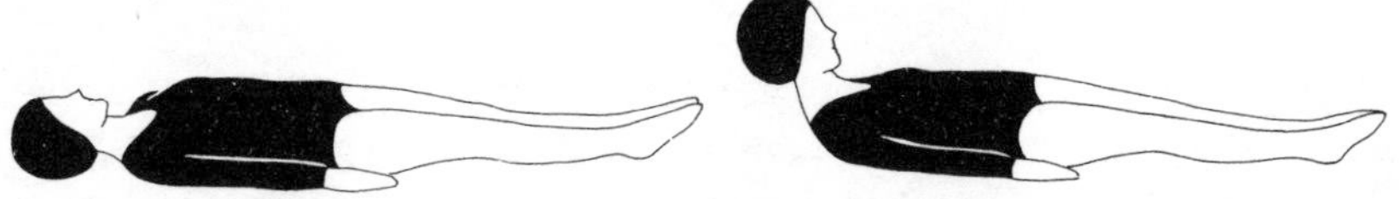

1. *Neck Stretch* – Lie down (on the bed), arms by sides, legs straight and together; slowly raise head and neck, stretching the neck as you raise it. Lower slowly. Do 5 times, work up to 20.

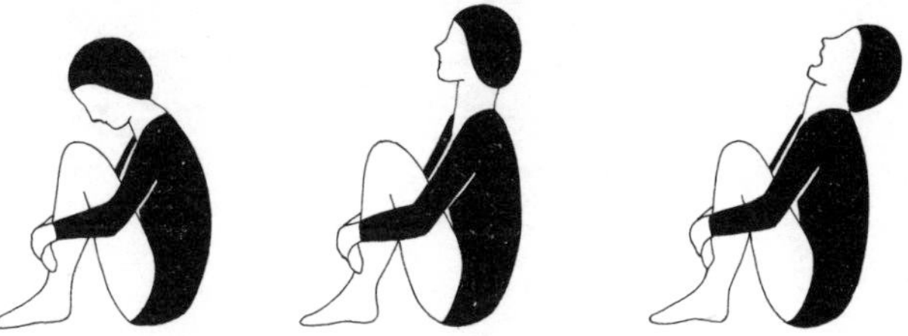

2. *Muscle Toner* – Sit (can be done on the bed also) with knees up to chest. Stretch neck up, shoulders down. Now tilt head forward; slowly pull head back as far as possible, open and close mouth slowly, 3 times. With mouth closed, bring head forward. Repeat 5 times.

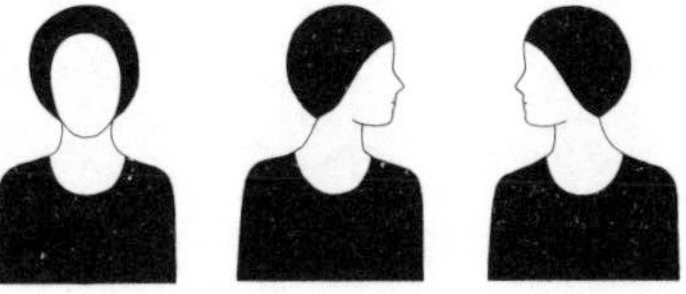

3. *Neck Control* – Sit (on the bed) cross-legged, palms flat just behind buttocks; shoulders down, back straight. Without moving the torso at all, turn chin slowly over each shoulder, keeping neck stretched high. Repeat 5 times each side.

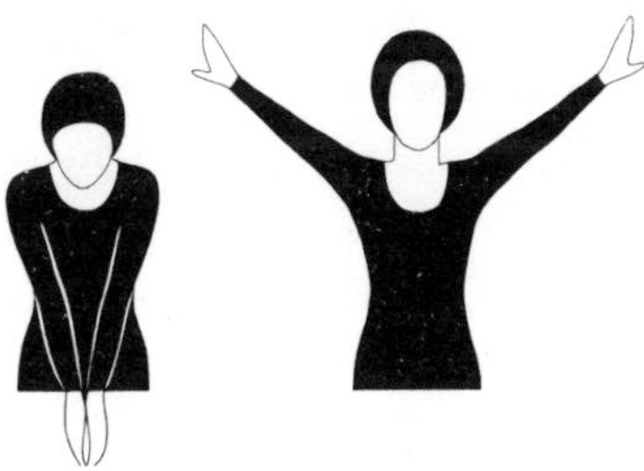

4. *Shoulders Free* – Stand with feet a little apart, arms in front with backs of hands touching, head lowered. Slowly lift head, stretch arms up and back, fingers apart, palms facing back, neck stretched. Repeat 10 times.

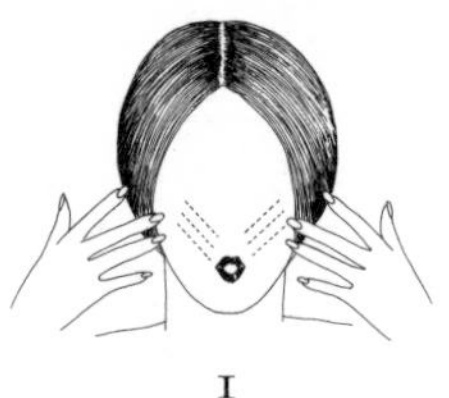
1

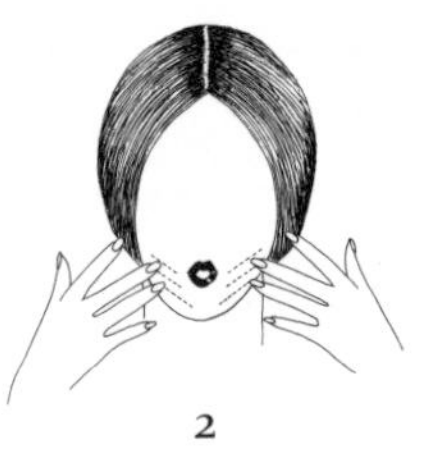
2

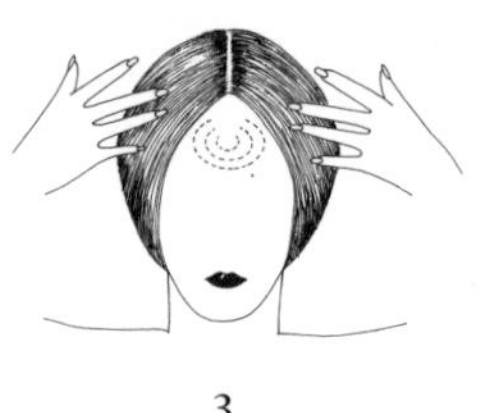
3

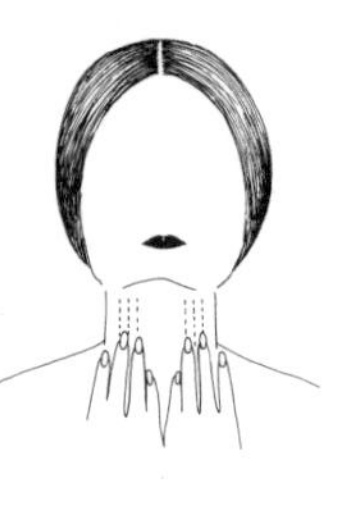
4

FACIAL AND NECK STROKING: This is much lighter than massage and is done with the tips of the third, fourth and fifth fingers; glide them across the skin with the lightest touch. This gentle stroking directs the skin into smoothness, no pulling or pushing. Heavy massage can be destructive, and these almost undetectable movements get better results if done consistently. Aim for 8 to 20 minutes a day. Best place: in the bath, in bed, watching television.

1. *Cheeks and Mouth* – Purse lips in an O-shape, breathe normally. With three fingers (first, second and third) stroke upwards from the outer corners of the mouth, making a V-shape up across the cheeks. Stroke slowly, 6 times.

2. *Chin and Mouth* – Purse lips; with the tips of the three end fingers stroke upward from the centre of the chin out to the hollow cheeks. Do 6 times.

3. *Forehead* – Mouth normal, lips together. Starting at the centre, stroke outwards in a circular movement, back in at the top. Repeat 6 times.

4. *Throat and Underchin* – Mouth together, trace fingers up from collar bone brushing off the edge of the chin; movement should be slightly outwards, fingers starting at the bottom, palms down. Repeat 6 times.

EYES

The eyeball is circular, roughly one inch in diameter, but only about one-twelfth of it shows. The part you see through is the black pupil, where light passes through to the back of the eye. Pupils appear small in daylight and wider at night because the surrounding coloured iris contracts and expands; it shrinks when it is dark allowing the pupils to expand and let in more light. The cornea is the eye's transparent surface and is a kind of lens that enables it to focus. Further back is a lens that refines what the cornea absorbs. This is slim and relaxed when eyes look into the distance, and thicker when viewing something close up. Eventually an image reaches the retina at the back of the eye which in turn passes it to the brain. All of this happens in a split second.

An eye is functionally mature at ten years of age and usually no serious changes occur in it until after forty. A healthy eye can focus easily at its nearest point as well as adjusting to distance. The focusing power depends on the anatomical arrangement of the cornea and lens, and refractive errors are usually genetically determined. Dysfunctions such as short and long sightedness and astigmatism usually occur because the lens is the wrong proportion for the eyeball. No permanent damage

Opposite: Guy Bourdin, 1973
Overleaf: Norman Parkinson, 1972

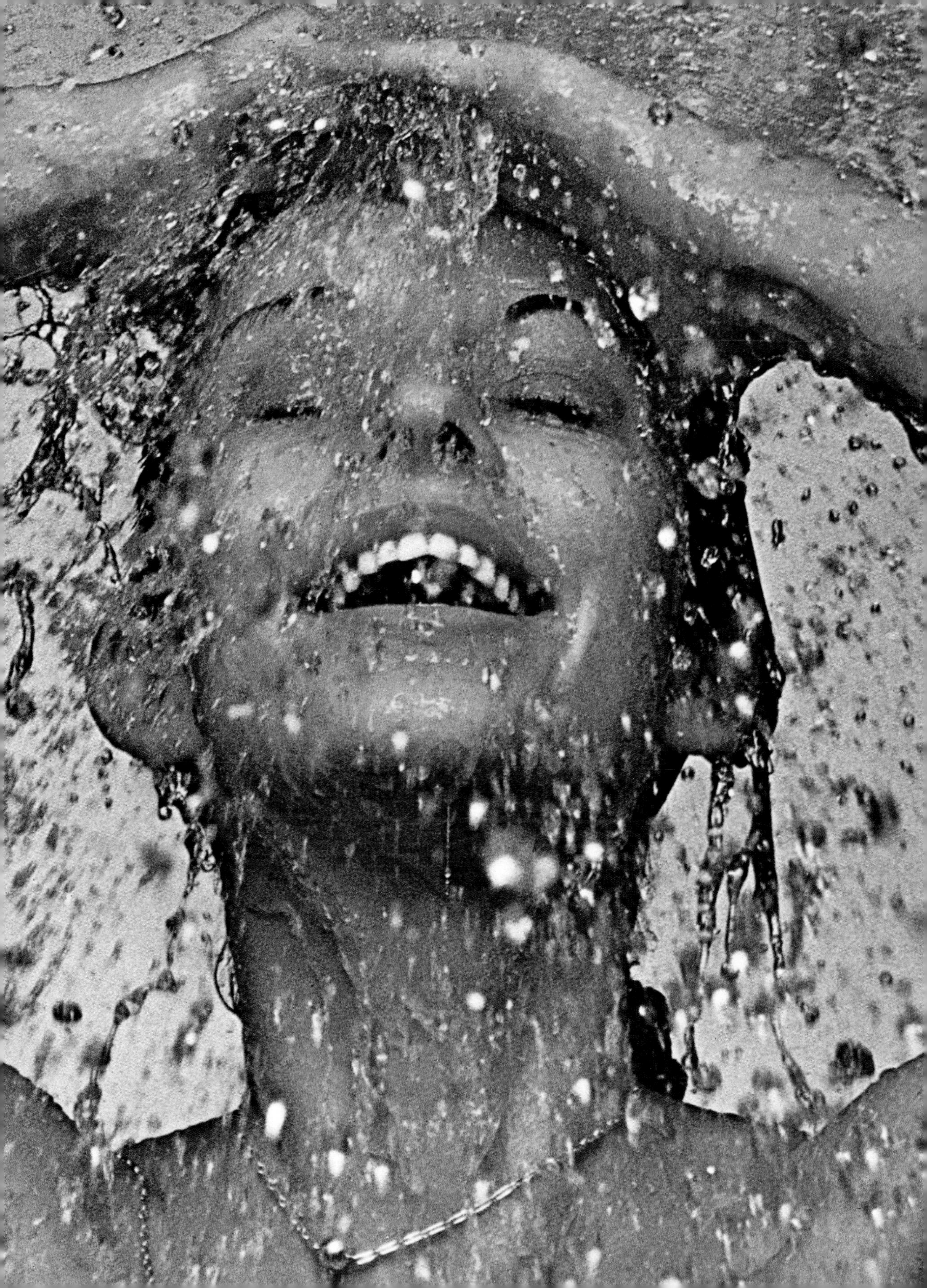

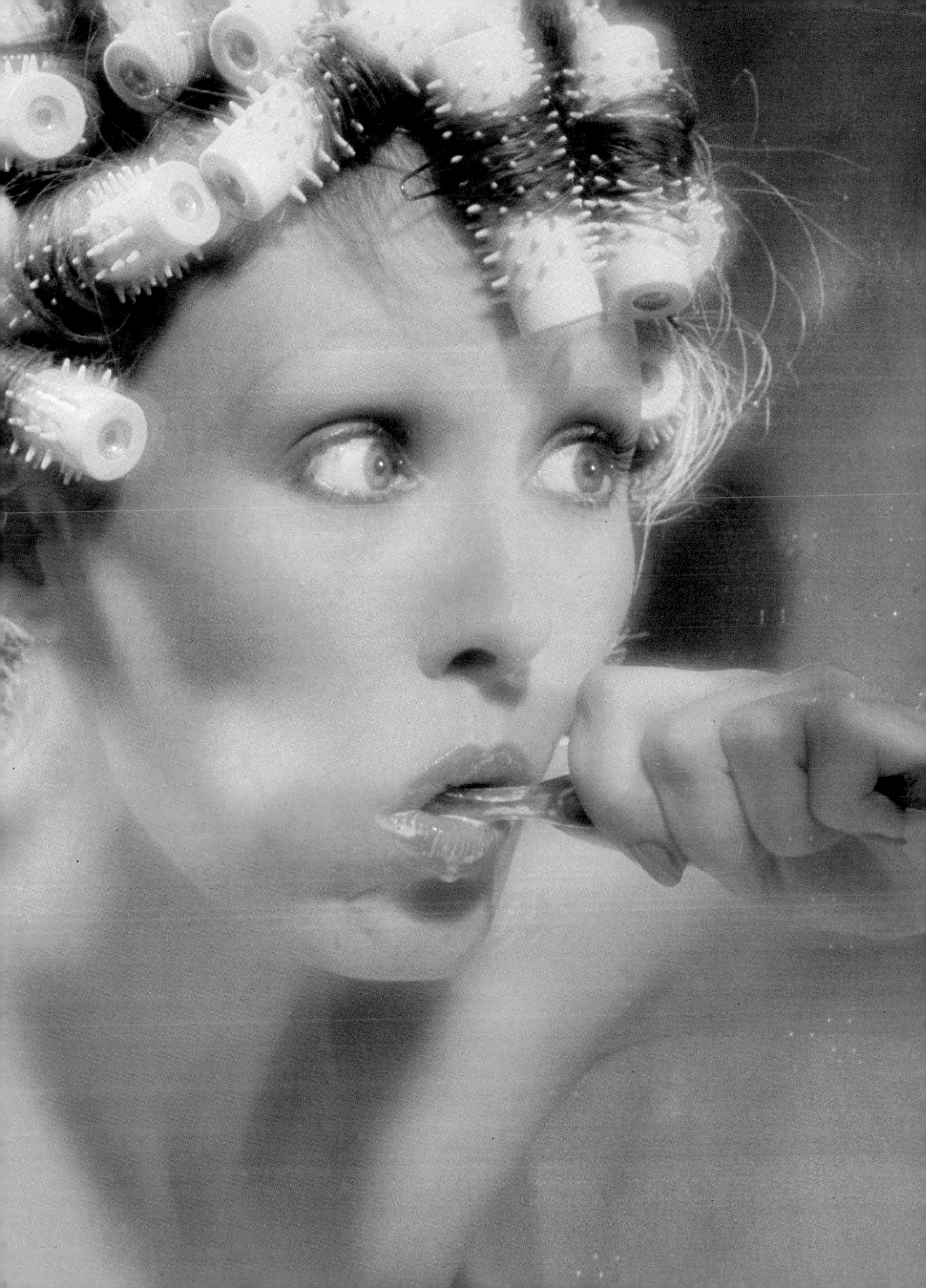

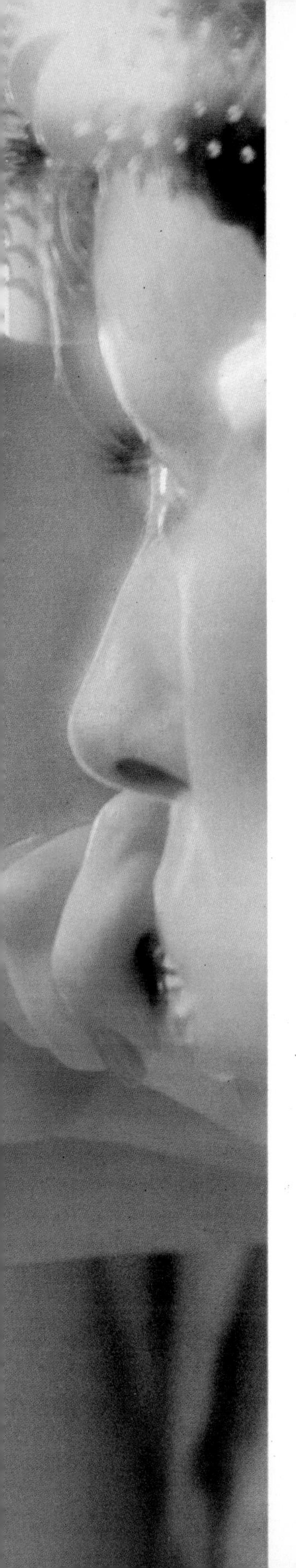

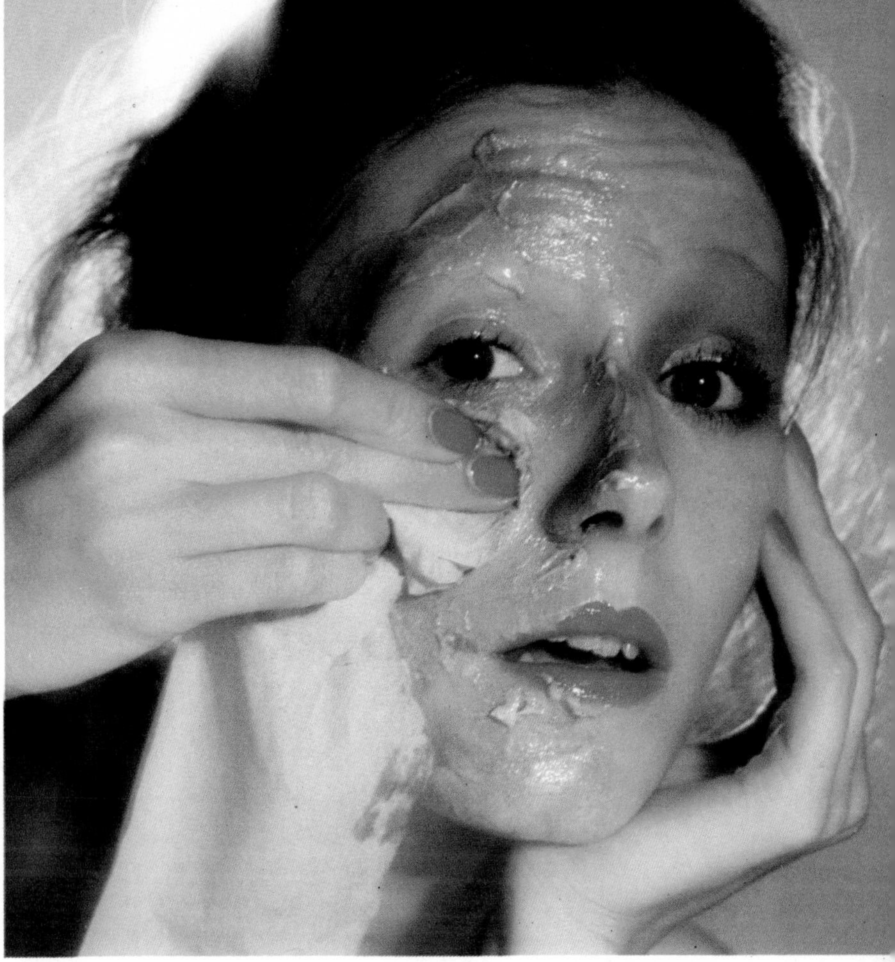

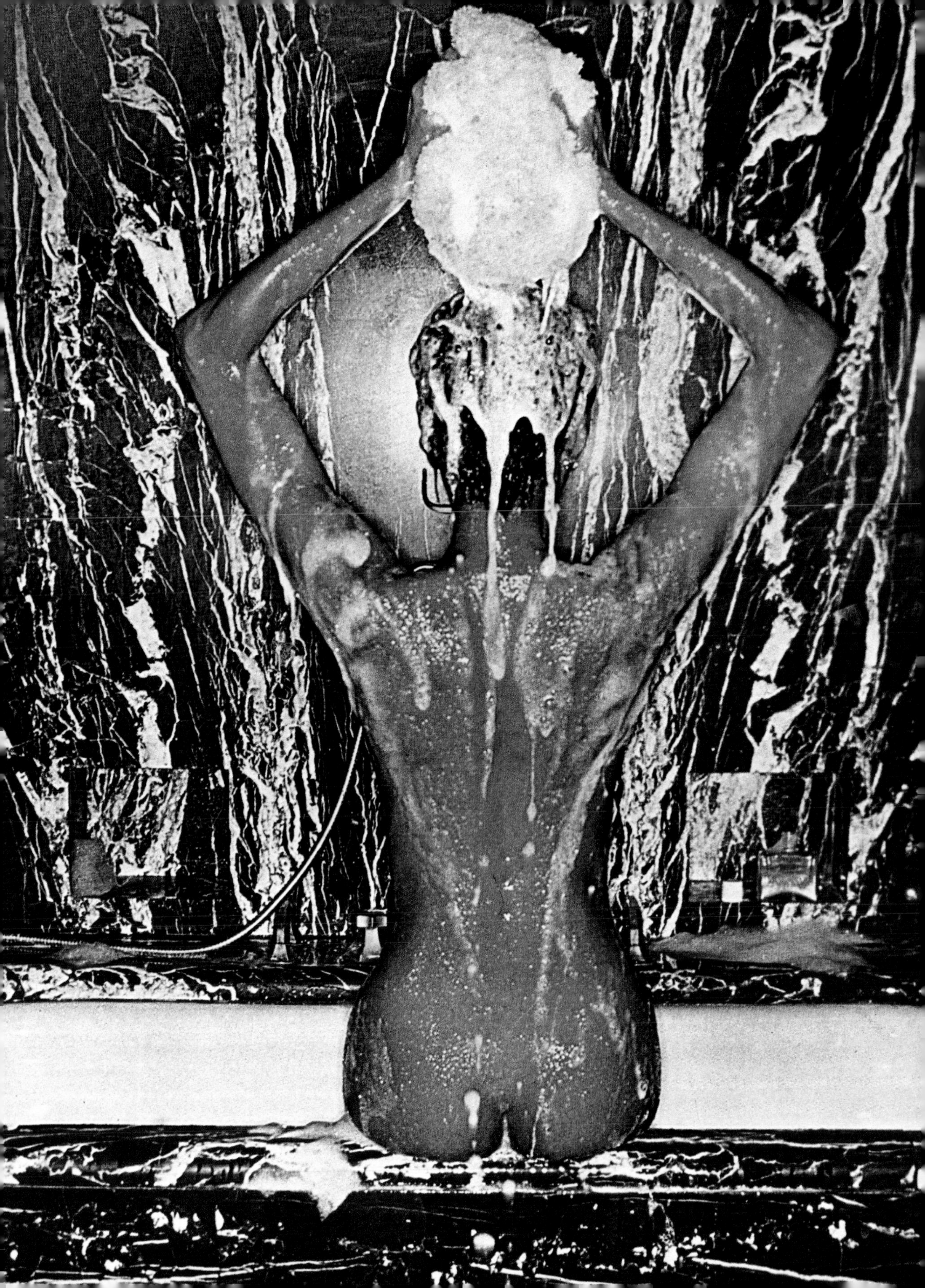

can come through eye strain or incorrect spectacles, or watching too much television.

The basic measurement of good eyesight is that one should be able to see clearly into the distance as well as close up. An optician classifies normal sight as 6/6 which means that you can see at 6 metres (20 feet) what has been precisely gauged to be visible at that distance. For example you should be able to read a car's number plate at 23 metres (80 feet). If your eyesight is 6/8 that means you only see clearly at 6 metres what you should be seeing clearly at 8.

Short sight: Known as myopia. The short sighted eye tends to be longer, so light has further to travel from the eye's own lens to a point on the retina at the back of the eye, which relays the image to the brain. Sometimes the light does not get there, and an unclear picture results.
Long Sight: Known as hypermetropia. The eye is shorter, so the image-carrying light rays go beyond the retina instead of focusing on it. This means that eyes are more comfortable looking into the distance than at close objects.
Astigmatism: This is when part of your vision is blurred, usually because the cornea is misshapen.
Squinting: Usually due to a lazy eye, where the muscle lacks pulling power. When the good eye focuses the other can't, so instead turns inwards, outwards, up or down. Sometimes eyes can harmonize in one direction but not in another. Squints usually show up very early in life and should be corrected before twelve otherwise it may be too late. Sometimes an eye requires a minor operation; exercises often help; or lenses to strengthen the lazy eye.
Colour Blindness: This is not actual blindness, but inability to recognize a few colours only, usually green and red.

INFECTIOUS DISORDERS: Conjunctivitis is inflammation of the thin protective layer over the eye together with a sticky discharge. It usually occurs with an allergy or as a symptom of a nervous disease. It attracts bacteria and sets up an infection, making it possible to infect others too. There are various lotions and ointments which soothe and lubricate the rough areas but the only quick cure is the use of antibiotics.

Blepharitis is inflammation at the roots of the eyelashes, and is inclined to appear if there is a tendency towards dry skin, dandruff or acne. All make-up has some potential allergy problem and unless well cleaned off can produce this sort of inflammation. It is easily treated.

Opposite: Barry Lategan, 1976

AGEING DISORDERS: In old age, the lens of the eye tends to become more opaque and when sight is seriously impaired by this clouding over, it is called a cataract. Cataracts develop slowly and the only treatment when they become severe is surgical removal of the lens which is replaced by strong glasses.

Also with age, pressure within the eye area increases, causing headaches and radiating pain, also coloured haloes around lights. This is known as glaucoma and is often hereditary. Treatment usually comprises keeping open the drainage channels between the iris and lens by contracting the pupil. A small operation may be necessary to increase the channels.

CARE

Conservation of eyesight involves using eyes, not abusing them. Watch for fatigue and if your eyes are constantly tired see a specialist. Try not to read in moving vehicles. Make sure you are living with adequate light: the light should come from behind or above rather than in front. When reading, stop after an hour to give your eyes fifteen minutes' rest.

Vitamin A is important for eyesight and is readily available in vegetables including carrots, celery and tomatoes. Vitamin B-2, vitamin C and vitamin D are also necessary. When there is a lack of B-2, eyes often become bloodshot, itchy and watery.

Eyes need rest and exercise. During the day rest your eyes by simply putting the palms of your hands over them, cutting out the light for five minutes. Another way: sit in front of a picture, look at it. Now gently close your eyes and cover them with the palms. Relax for three minutes or more. You will notice that eyes will see first grey-black, then deep black. Open your eyes and look at the picture again. An additional way to relax tired eyes is to look far into the distance, just gazing.

Eye exercises are simple, quick and efficient. Roll eyes to the right, then to the left in complete circles; 20 times each way. Also look at the tip of your finger, held quite close to the face, then look at a very distant object, then back at your finger. Repeat a few times.

Dark circles and puffiness can be due to lack of sleep or a sluggish kidney. Otherwise it is normal relaxation of tissue which comes with the passing years. Applications of iced water or milk often reduce swollen or puffy eyes. Witch-hazel is helpful – pour a trace over cottonwool pads:

it is best if the witch-hazel is ice cold. Grated potato left under the eyes helps to reduce swelling, as do rosehip tea, fresh figs or strawberries.

For inflamed eyes, squeeze in fresh cucumber juice, or place slices over the eye and leave for 15 minutes. Compresses of an infusion of eyebright or camomile are good natural aids for the eyes.

Bloodshot eyes could be caused by blood vessels congenitally dilated or by some sensitivity. Often alcohol is the cause. Eyedrops are safe but over a long period are not a good idea.

CONTACT LENSES

For aesthetic reasons many women use contact lenses to correct defective sight. Decide with your optician which type most suits your needs.

Corneal lenses, the tiny ones, sometimes only 8 millimetres in diameter, fit only over the cornea. The larger haptic lenses fit over the whole eye, and because of the type of protection they give, are excellent for sports. Hydrophilic lenses, made of extremely soft and flexible plastic, are micro-corneal covering only the iris. These can be worn by those who find the heavier lenses irritating.

Lenses come in many colours. The plastic is patinated. Most people choose light grey to filter the light, or blue or green shades slightly deeper than their own eye to accentuate the colour. The first time you try contact lenses tears will probably stream down your face, but as you get used to the feeling, your vision adjusts. To start with lenses are usually worn for only two hours at a time, twice a day for three days. Then the wearing time is increased by fifteen minutes each session.

The new soft lenses, really flexible flakes of plastic, require less adjustment time. You can wear them for several hours immediately, and finally sleep in them too. Tolerance is no problem, but there is sometimes difficulty in getting exact vision in cases of high astigmatism. They move with the movements of the eye, floating on a cushion of natural eye fluid. They must be expertly fitted and for this a special machine is used to measure the curvature of the eye. There are about fifty-six different kinds of curves and most lenses are made not in one continuous curve, but in a series of three, four or five. If you wear contact lenses, avoid greasy eye make-up because it can work its way into the eyes and even the smallest speck between the lens and the eye can cause blurred vision. Particles of face powder and sparkling eye shadows can cause watering; mascara must be waterproof.

GLASSES

Choosing glasses is not easy. Here are some guidelines:

Always stand in front of a full-length mirror when trying on frames; it is the only way to get the correct sense of proportion.

Make sure glasses fit, sit securely on your nose, don't clamp your head, and that the tops of the frames line up with your eyebrows otherwise you get two sets of parallel lines close together.

Square faces look best in large square or rectangular shapes with the lower corners wider than cheekbones. Round faces need wide but short frames. Long faces need long, deep frames that cover a lot of the face. Short faces are helped by short, narrow, rectangular frames or enormous round ones that sit up on the nose.

Colour is ruled by hair colour, but it is better to keep to neutral tones of beige, browns and greys or light steel rims.

Tinted lenses can be attractive: for indoor wear choose a light tint, darker for sunny or bright artificially lit rooms, while grey is often the best in sunshine.

Eye make-up often needs to be altered when glasses are worn: a little more colour and extra lashes or mascara. Glasses for short sight tend to make the eye appear smaller, so use a darker liner under top lashes for emphasis. Lenses for long sight can magnify eyes, so use light lines and paler colours. Dark frames require a stronger tone of lipstick. Blushing colour should not disappear under frames, so keep it low and use as a contour rather than a highlight.

SUNGLASSES

Tinted glasses are convenient wherever there is a glare and can be very flattering but to wear them consistently is not advisable. The sun is beneficial for it forces the eye into constant activity adjusting from shade to bright light. Good sunglasses help absorb both the infra-red and ultraviolet rays while less expensive ones absorb one or the other or a little of both. Photochromatic lenses are those that change colour depending on the exposure to light – they are very pale in reduced light and darken immediately in the sun.

EARS

Most of us are born with more acute hearing than we ever need and keep it throughout life. If in later years the ability to hear high tones lessens there is nothing to worry about. Constant city and industrial noise can aggravate the ears considerably; loud noises can injure them and affect the general nervous system producing tension.

The ear works this way: sound waves can only exist by a vibration of some material – water or solid matter, but in most cases, air. It is a vibration of the air that we pick up. This is multiplied in pressure many times by the mechanical arrangement of little bones behind the ear drum; then it is taken up within a fluid-filled cavity, which in turn activates the auditory nerves and registers in the brain. It is possible for sound of great intensity to damage this mechanism while some sounds can be beneficial. Music, for instance: no one understands why it can be calming or stimulating or why certain sound patterns can have rejuvenating effects.

Hearing impairment can be congenital, the result of an infectious disease, an obstruction due to dirt, wax, an abscess or congestion, a slight blow on the ear, or a nerve disorder. Over-zealous blowing of the nose can cause damage. Infections of mouth, nose and throat can attack the ear. High levels of cholesterol often coincide with diminishing hearing.

Professional advice should be sought immediately there is any disorder or noticeable change in hearing. More than regular cleaning is not advisable on your own. Even poking around to dislodge impacted wax can be harmful. There is often reluctance to admit to hearing disability yet many surgical and mechanical correction procedures ensure help and minimum inconvenience. In many cases, deafness is due to a hardening of the middle bones; this is called otosclerosis and can almost always be reversed by the manipulation of a tiny bone, the stapes, within the middle ear. Another cause is pressure on the Eustachian tubes which responds well to delicate finger surgery. Finally, artificial eardrums can be inserted.

Modern technology provides amazing miniature units for amplifying hearing. Some are small enough to fit in the ear, others go behind it with a transparent tube leading into the ear's cavity, others are fitted to glasses.

Ear Piercing: Done correctly it is a painless and harmless process. A local anaesthetic should be applied, then the ear lobe punctured by diathermy; afterwards a tiny silk thread is inserted through the hole and acts as a dressing. A few days later, the thread is replaced by a gold ring or rod-and-stud pin which must be worn continually for three months after piercing.

TEETH

It is widely known that teeth need calcium. They are composed of the hardest substance in the body, calcium phosphate. What is not so well known is that a lack of vitamin D restricts the absorption and use of calcium. Vitamin C is also important to strengthen the connective tissue. Fluorine protects teeth and is added to some municipal waters and can be painted on or applied through a toothpaste. Bone meal supplement is said to help fight decay, as it is rich in calcium, phosphorus and fluorine. It is made from finely ground veal and young beef bones and sold as a powder or in tablet form. Apples, celery and carrots clean as well as strengthen teeth. The enemies of good teeth are sugar and white flour. Bacteria thrive on them and decay can start almost at once unless food particles are cleaned away.

The colour of teeth can be deceptive. Very white teeth are not necessarily the healthiest. The whiteness may indicate that they are covered with soft porous enamel, which is thick and transparent. Usually hard enamel is thin and clear showing the yellowish-white dentine underneath. It is impossible to get teeth with this hard enamel coating completely white; all abrasive tooth powders do is to scratch the enamel surface and cause cavities.

DECAY AND DISEASE: Before the age of thirty-five the greatest cause of tooth loss is decay and resulting cavities. After thirty-five the chief culprit is periodontal disease which infects the gums and erodes the supportive tissue and bone structures. Infection can also be carried to other parts of the body and cause trouble. In most cases, periodontal disease can be stopped and prevented. It is a question of controlling plaque, the main cause of both decay and gum disease. Plaque is a mixture of bacteria, saliva and food residue which adheres to the tooth. It is colourless, transparent, invisible. Even very white teeth can be coated with plaque. It settles in the spaces between teeth and around the necks of teeth along the gum line. After twenty-four hours it produces acids which attack the enamel, initiating decay and also providing the perfect environment for the formation of tartar – a rough, hard formation which requires professional treatment for removal.

Unless plaque is removed daily through brushing and flossing it can cause inflammation of the gum tissues, known as gingivitis. The build-up is progressive – gums become inflamed, they bleed, ulcers flare up and the gums begin to recede. At this stage, it can be cured, but if left untreated, it can progress to pyorrhoea (or periodontitis). The teeth become loose as the gums shrink and infection spreads to the underlying bones. This is very serious but surgical procedures by a periodontist may help if the disease is not too far advanced.

Mouth and gums give clear warnings of the disease and the main symptoms are: red, swollen and itchy gums that often bleed, bad breath, pain and pressure between teeth after eating.

HOME-CARE: Normal routine brushing misses 80% of the plaque. If you don't believe it, check by using a disclosing tablet: after you've brushed put one in your mouth and wait until it has dissolved completely. Then look closely in the mirror – the areas where plaque and food debris still remain will show up bright red or purple. There is also a disclosing solution that can be applied to the mouth before brushing. This stains the plaque and so you know where to brush, taking the colour away at the same time. When brushing check these points:

Toothbrushes – should have soft thin bristles with flexible filaments, rounded at the ends, not jagged. Nylon is good because you can change the texture by putting the brush into cold water to make it firmer, into hot to make it softer. A toothbrush should be replaced every three or four months. Electric toothbrushes do not necessarily do a better job. When brushing, angle bristles towards gums, brushing in the direction the tooth grows, downwards for the upper teeth, upwards for the lower teeth, and wiggle the brush around the gum line. A good way is to loosen up plaque first with just the brush, then add toothpaste for polishing. It should take between two and five minutes.

Dental floss – designed to clean between the teeth and under the gums where a toothbrush cannot reach. It should be done once a day, preferably at night and before brushing. It requires a degree of manual dexterity: take a good length, at least a foot (300 mm.), wrap it around the index finger of both hands, winding it from one finger to the other as you need a fresh section, keeping the floss taut. After gently working between teeth, slide it under the gums and scrape the side of the tooth towards the biting surface. Unwaxed floss is usually better.

Watersprays – useful in mouths where bands or extensive fixed bridgework are secured, they clean out debris and help to flush away plaque.

Mouthwashes – dentists warn of overuse of commercial ones, particularly those to freshen breath, as they can disturb the natural flora. An oxidant such as hydrogen peroxide can be used regularly: it kills bacteria and strengthens gums. A good natural mouthwash is a peppermint tea infusion or a mixture of equal proportions of rosemary, anise and mint leaves steeped for half an hour. Parsley and watercress alleviate the bad breath caused by eating over-spiced food.

PROFESSIONAL CARE: Dentistry is now subdivided: a regular dentist does the repair work and cosmetic alterations. The endodontist treats root canal problems. The orthodontist is a dentist who has been trained to consider the good function, balance and alignment of the teeth; he may never do a filling, but his work may eliminate the need for cosmetic dentistry later on. He is concerned with the health of the mouth, gum and bone condition. The hygienist does routine cleaning and scaling: an ultrasonic cleaning device is used with vibrations so fast you don't feel a thing. By gently stroking beneath the gum edge and down the tooth, every particle of plaque is removed.

Everyone should have a clean and a check-up every six months. Cavities should be filled as early as possible but often you cannot see or feel early cavities on your own. Drilling and filling should not hurt at all. Most dentists apply a topical anaesthetic (sometimes a tranquillizing injection beforehand) and then inject a novocain-like liquid into the gum. If enough time is left between the local pain killer and the injection you should not even feel the needle.

Some cavities need root canal work: infection is cleaned out and the area sterilized, then filled with silver or rubber-like materials. Sometimes a post is inserted in the root so a porcelain cap can be attached on the top. There are many filling preparations so like natural enamel that they no longer show. Silver amalgams are still used for back teeth for resistance reasons and there is nothing better than gold for a really big filling.

COSMETIC DENTISTRY: A denture is an unsatisfactory substitute for teeth and cosmetic dentistry can radically change what nature or neglect created. Permanent crowns and bridges look like natural teeth, including the slight imperfections and variations of colour. Porcelain is usually more effective than plastic and is fused onto a strengthening metal, normally a mixture of an amalgam and gold.

Having a tooth capped means first grinding it down to a pointed peg and a temporary plastic jacket being cemented over it. An impression is made, and the permanent crown is cemented in place on the following visit. If teeth are missing, a fixed bridge can be made, attached to neighbouring teeth which either have to be capped or pinned with metal points to base the bridge. The life of the crown or bridgework cannot be guaranteed as the tendency of the gum is to recede as you get older, necessitating additional work at a later date. A minimum of four to five years can be expected, ten is reasonable, and many caps have been known to last much longer.

An alternative to capping a chipped, cracked or broken tooth is to adhere a special malleable resin to the damaged spot; this blends in with the colour and texture of the natural tooth. These resins are also used as a protective coating for eroded areas near the gum line.

Sometimes removable bridges need to be constructed and these have precision attachments as fine as jewellery. They don't look like false teeth and only need to be taken out for cleaning.

Implants are not always one hundred per cent successful. Natural ones, such as resetting a tooth knocked out but still intact in itself, last only about five years as the jawbone usually invades the weakened root area and kills the tooth. Artificial implants involve securing a steel base or post to the jawbone, then capping it with porcelain or plastic. Individual reaction determines their lasting power.

Another cosmetic technique is contouring where teeth are shaped to give the illusion of regularity without altering the basic structure. Bonding is the process that puts a white veneer over teeth to mask any discoloration and pitting. It also helps to prevent decay.

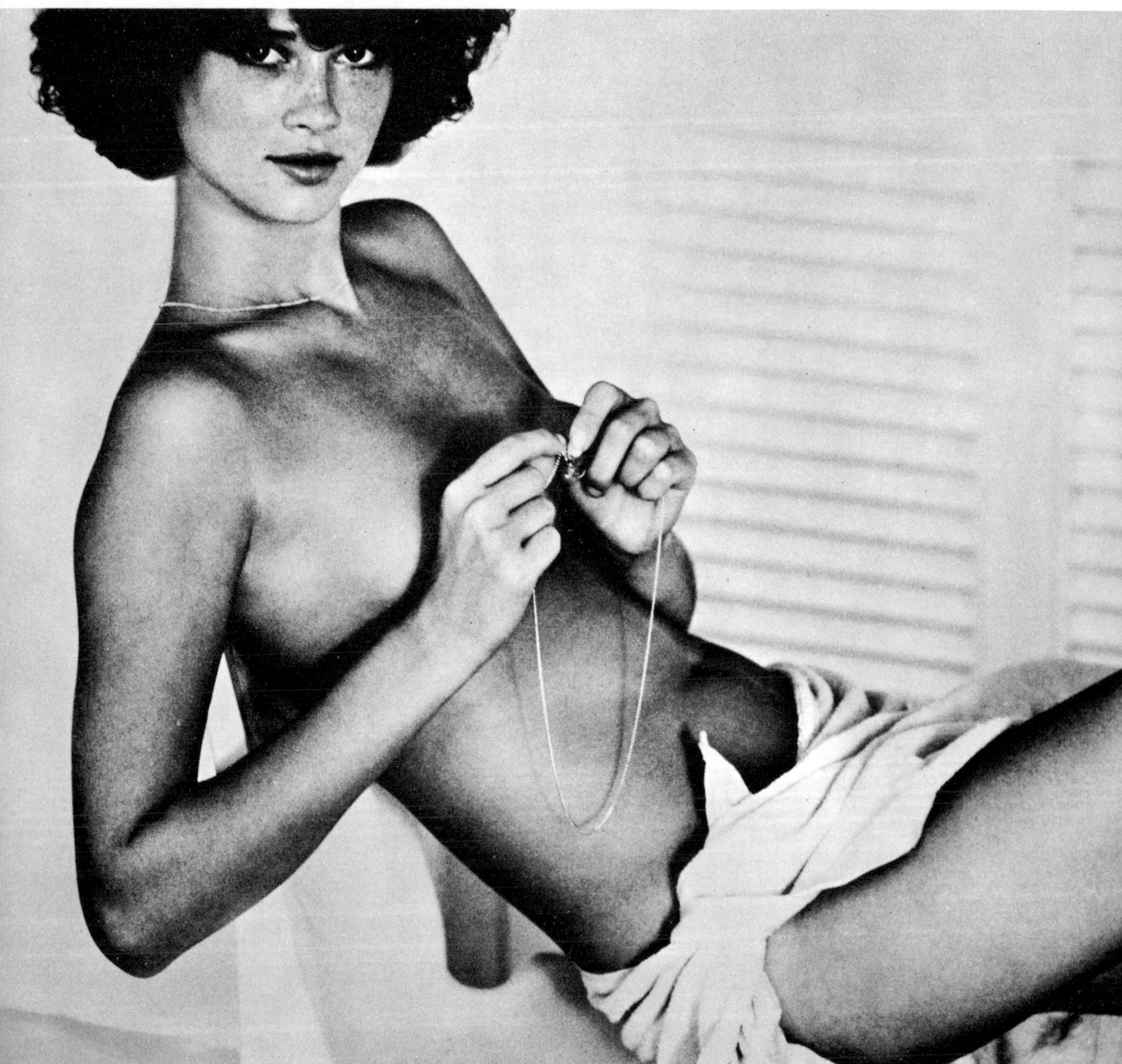

MCCABE

8

LIMBS

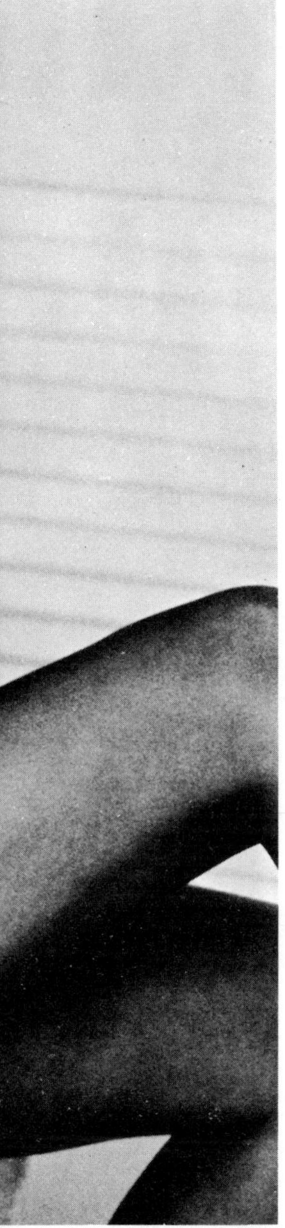

ARMS

Changing the shape of arms is very difficult. Though slender arms are desirable, skinny ones are not – but to put flesh on the arm is almost impossible unless combined with an overall weight increase. There is a tendency for the upper arm to be flabby, particularly noticeable as one gets older, and this is usually due to poor muscle tone. Also upper arms can get a mottled look because of sluggish circulation. Daily exercises can help both conditions – see below for illustrated details. If upper-arm flab is really excessive and hangs down, in some cases it can be corrected by plastic surgery. This is often necessary when considerable weight loss results in loose skin, as there is no other way to eliminate it.

Arms need moisturizing and massaging just like any other part of the body. When applying lotion, use the entire palm with strong upward motions that start at the wrist and go all the way to the shoulder. Don't forget the elbows and try not to lean on them as this causes a rough and bumpy surface – rub the lotion in with circular movements. If elbows are badly ingrained with dirt, use a deep cleansing cream or rub with lemon; if rough, try first kneading in an oatmeal-and-water paste, which is also a marvellous cleanser. All arms have hair; unless it is particularly heavy, it is best to leave it. If it is very dark, bleach first before thinking of removal. If it really bothers you, never shave – use other methods of depilation.

ARM EXERCISES

Four good exercises to help improve muscle tone and circulation of the upper arm. They should be done daily; a little constant exercise produces better results than a lot once a week. It is not necessary to do all, choose just two, if you prefer.

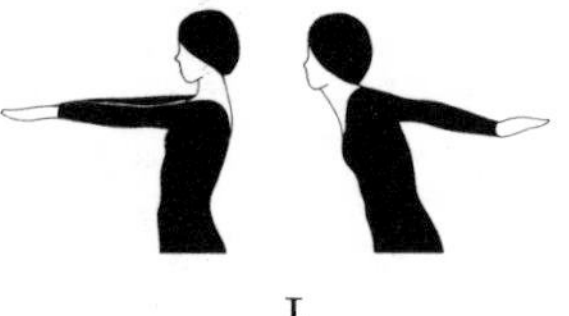

1

1. *Arm circle:* Stand with feet a little apart, stretch both arms out in front, holding them at shoulder level with palms turned down. Swing arms backwards trying to keep them high all the time, and at the back push hard until fingertips touch. Repeat a minimum of 6 times.

2. *Shoulder bounce:* Stand, feet apart, raise arms straight out at sides to shoulder height, palms facing front. Clench fists. Draw fists to touch shoulders above bosom, imagining you have a force resisting this movement. Push hard as though you were squeezing the sides of the bust together. Bounce fists twice in this position; extend arms slowly to starting position. Repeat a minimum of 6 times.

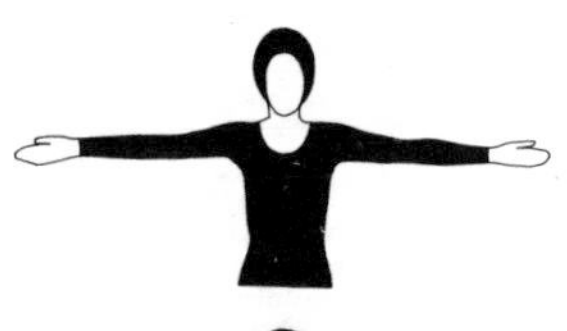

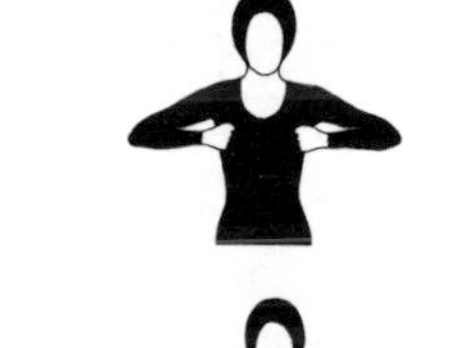

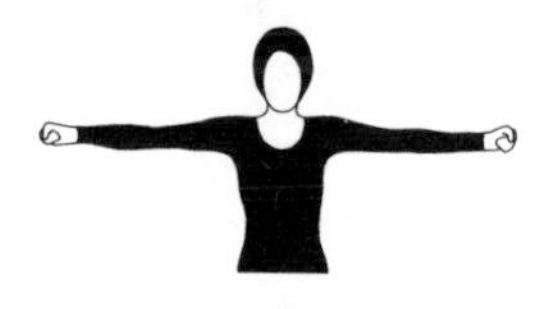

2

3. *Weight lift:* Use a weight of about 3 lbs – dumb-bell, weight-sack, book – grasp firmly in hand and raise arm above the head, keeping it straight with elbow close to head; keep back straight too. Bend elbow and lower weight backwards to touch back of opposite shoulder. Raise arm up again. Repeat 10 times for each arm, slowly, firmly. Work up to 20 times.

4. This is an isometric exercise, where action presents resistance to movement. Stand in a doorway, feet a little apart; make fists of hands and raise arms in a triangular position to rest fists against door-frame – palms facing forwards. Breathe in deeply and try to push out the door-frame. Push, counting to 3, relax. Start with 3 pushes and work up to 5.

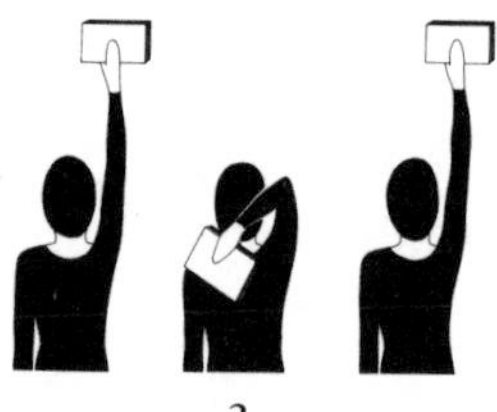

3

HANDS

There are twenty-eight bones in the hand and the wrist, all finely balanced to give remarkable mobility. The skin on the back of the hand is fine and soft, with numerous sebaceous glands (those that produce oily sebum to protect the skin) and sweat gland openings. The palm of the hand is coarser and tougher: well supplied with sweat glands, but unlike most other parts of the body, it has no sebaceous glands. This means that it is one of the dryest parts of the body.

A hand can show age faster than any other area – a face can be lifted, a hand can not. Liquid silicone has been tried for 'plumping up' hands, but its transient properties proved dangerous. Therefore, prevention through care is essential. First, water is fatal to hands; detergents and household cleaning agents are destructive. Exposure to elements – sun, cold, wet, sea, earth – takes its toll. Protection and care are a daily concern.

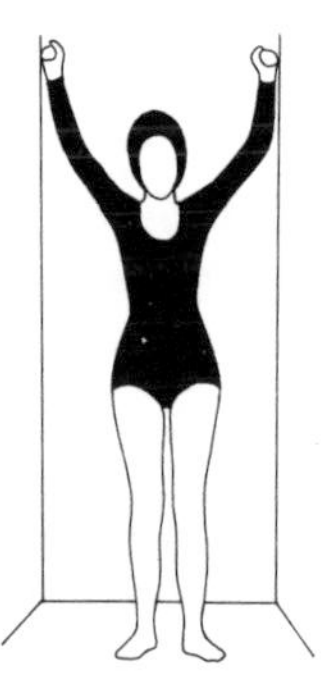

4

Some points to remember:

Wear rubber gloves for all wet work; cotton-lined are the best to absorb excess moisture. Wear heavy fabric gloves for gardening, cotton gloves for housework, gloves outdoors when it is cold or raining – or snowing.

Every time your hands get wet, dry them well and smooth on hand lotion.

Wash hands thoroughly several times a day with a mild soap, run clean water over them before patting dry, cream; at least once daily scrub fingers and nails with a firm brush.

A smooth pumice stone used with soap and water removes stains and rough skin.

Once a week massage (twice if time) with a rich lubricating cream; begin at finger tips and work firmly down each finger, then over the palms and backs; a good time to do this is before going to bed.

When you can, wear cotton gloves overnight – put on over a layer of hand cream or petroleum jelly.

First aid treatment: a sheath of warm paraffin wax which opens pores, removes toxins, and cleanses.

A lemon will clean and bleach fingers; cream afterwards, as the juice is drying.

A masque – the same as the one you use on your face – will cleanse and tone hands.

Warmed oil – preferably olive or almond – is the best handbath for dryness; soak once a week for half an hour – marvellous for nails too.

Rinsing in a mild vinegar-water solution after washing will protect hands against drying, chapping, and other irritations.

There are certain conditions that need special care:

Brown spots: The development of these so-called 'age-spots' can be retarded and in many cases prevented by the use of a suncream. Existing spots can be partially bleached out with a de-pigmenting cream, or hidden with a waterproof cover-up make-up (good for hiding veins too); dermatologists can professionally lighten these spots and remove scaly bumps by therapies including cryotherapy and electrodesication.

Chilblains: Usually due to lack of finger activity and inadequate protection from the cold and damp. Exercise to stimulate circulation, massage fingers frequently and check you have enough calcium in your diet. Wear warm gloves.

Rough skin and cracks: Caused by cold weather, hard work and handling drying things. Remove dirt from cracks with lemon, then rub olive oil into cracks with absorbent cotton. Wash hands in warm soapy water, rinse with clear water. Follow with a massage using a really rich emollient hand cream. Do this daily. If cracks are bad, you must not allow air to get to them: seal by covering with adhesive tape or plaster, and only remove for cleansing and creaming. Even the most stubborn cracks will vanish this way.

Swollen knuckles: Could be due to a rheumatic or arthritic condition, in which case check your diet and see your doctor; can also be aggravated by over-exertion. Important to do finger and hand exercises and give hands a daily massage.

Tobacco and fruit stains: The most reliable stain removers are peroxide or lemon juice. Pressure is needed to remove the more stubborn marks, so use a pumice stone. Afterwards cream well, as both peroxide and lemon juice are very drying.

1

HAND AND FINGER EXERCISES

Exercises for hands to make them more flexible and graceful – and to aid circulation.

1. *Fist fling:* Clench the fist tightly, hold a second, throw open the fingers, forward and as wide as possible. Both hands at the same time, repeat 6 times.

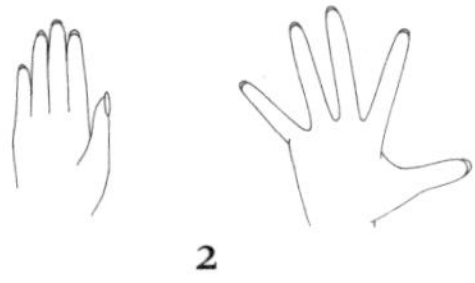

2

2. *Finger spread:* Put hands straight in front of you, palms down, fingers pressed tightly against each other; thrust fingers apart, opening to as wide a separation as possible. Repeat 6 times.

3. *Hand circles:* Be sure hands are limp and relaxed, then rotate them from the wrist in circles, first in one direction, then another – 10 in each direction.

4. *Vertical lift:* Holding hands gracefully, palms down, lift up slowly from the wrist, then move down. Keep the hand very relaxed, but not absolutely limp; 10 times.

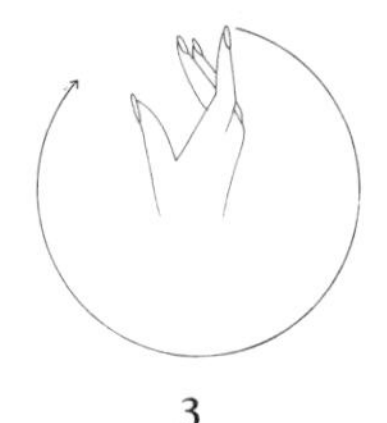

3

NAILS

Nails are horny extensions of the skin. The visible nail, that hard plate, is only about half. The other half is the matrix, invisible except for the uppermost tip which we recognize as the half-moon or lunula. The rest of the matrix is oval, rather like the nail itself, and extends down to the first joint. This is where the nail is formed, where the body turns protein plus a few trace elements into fingernails. Nails are composed of horizontal layers of keratin and how strong or brittle your nails are is partly a

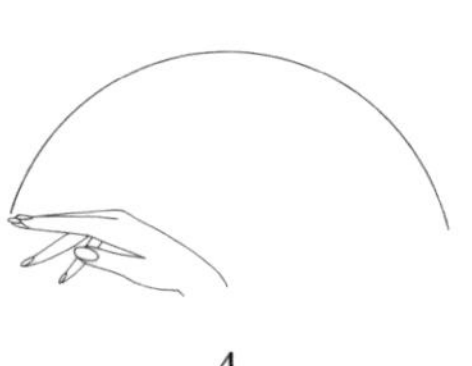

4

matter of inheritance, but nutrition is also important. A protein-high diet rich in iron, calcium, potassium, vitamin B, and iodine will help keep nails healthy. Foods such as yoghourt, celery, carrots, soya, eggs, and seafood are particularly good. Nails are good indicators of circulation: if you put pressure on the nail, watch how quickly the blood returns.

What causes irregularities? From time to time we all get a few ruts, bumps, and marks. Horizontal ridges, regular on all nails, denote a past illness – though if only on one nail, it means you've given it some rough treatment and possibly damaged the cuticle by using a sharp instrument. Good nail care will eliminate most horizontal ridges. Vertical lines tend to be hereditary and the older you get, the more they show; sometimes they indicate dryness. White spots can be a sign of disease or stress or caused by air pockets forming in the nail as it grows in which case they eventually grow out. Yellowing of the nails comes from smoking or medicines or because of nail polish pigment – that is why it is important to apply a base coat. Lack of care causes split or broken nails.

Nails grow at the rate of a quarter of an inch a month, so a new nail takes about four months to reach the tip from the cuticle. If you start helping your nails now, you can soon see the results. Nail growth varies with the individual: fastest in youth, decreasing with age. Pregnancy increases nail growth, so does warm weather, any activity of the fingers (like typing, piano-playing), and massage of the fingers towards the tips. Middle fingers grow fastest, and nails on the right hand (if you are right-handed), which indicates the greater the activity, the faster the growth.

Nails become brittle if they are exposed to extreme cold, too much sun, chlorine or cleaning chemicals. They become soft if you use too much soap and water. Cutting with scissors encourages splits and fractures. Nail polish is not harmful, it protects and strengthens as well as beautifies. A few women are allergic to nail enamel; for them there are formulas free of irritants. Nail polish remover, however, is very drying. To use neat acetone is false economy; even an oily remover should be used sparingly just once a week when you manicure. It is better to touch up polish when there's a chip rather than remove it every time. Cutting the cuticle is generally bad since it protects the nail base from infection – cuts in the cuticle, if too deep, can cause infection.

Basic rules for nail care:

Shape by filing with an emery board, safer and easier than a metal file.

File to an oval; filing to a point is asking for breakage. Don't file too deeply down the sides.

Keep cuticles soft by keeping them well moisturized; after applying hand lotion, gently push back softened cuticles with a towel or tissue as often as you can.

Problem nails need special care, but if you stick to the following guide lines, you may be amazed at the good results:

Keep hands out of water as much as possible; wear gloves; cream-clean hands instead of washing them several times a day.

Use cuticle cream at bedtime; get it to the root of the nail using an orange stick to gently lift the cuticle and put the cream underneath.

Once a week soak nails in olive oil, leave some on; wear gloves in bed.

When manicuring, use warm oil instead of soapy water, but go over nails again with remover before applying enamel or it will slither off.

Before applying polish, buff nails with paste or powder polish; this stimulates circulation and provides a smooth base for the enamel.

Avoid using metal manicure instruments: use emery boards for filing, orange sticks for lifting cuticles and cleansing nail tips.

Paint nails with white iodine before applying polish.

Try the gelatine cure – three level teaspoonfuls in cold fruit juice or dissolved in a cup of hot consommé; taken every day this should improve nails after two months. There is one snag: sometimes when the treatment is discontinued, nails once again become brittle, flake or break.

MANICURE

An expert, professional manicure is not difficult, and done slowly, methodically, and regularly, will result in good-looking, immaculate nails. You need one every week to keep nail shape and cuticles in trim. A professional manicurist spends about half an hour on the job – you will need longer, about forty-five minutes, and if you do it with your legs resting and raised your feet will benefit too.

Equipment:

Basics – towel, absorbent cotton, bristle nail brush, dish of warm soapy water (no detergent, but a shampoo, or a bath product).

Tools – emery board, nail clippers, cuticle clippers, orange sticks, nail buffer.

Creams – hand lotion, cuticle-remover cream or oil, cuticle massage cream or any rich emollient cream, buffing paste – tinted or clear.

Nail Cosmetics – oily polish remover, white nail pencil, base coat, nail enamel, top sealer, nail patch paper and fixative.

Procedure:

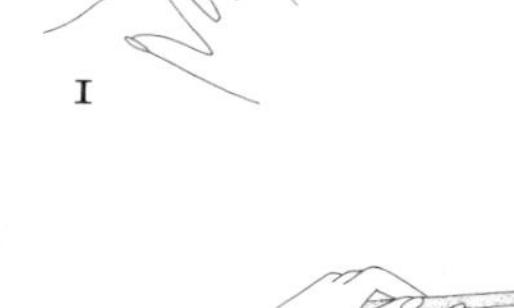

1

1. Remove old nail varnish: wet cotton with oily remover and press it against nail for a second to pre-soften polish, wipe off slowly. A quick swish over is not enough; this press-then-wipe method cleans the varnish from under the cuticles as well.

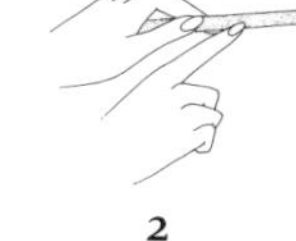

2

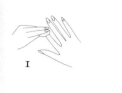

2. Shape nails into an oval with an emery board, working with long strokes from side to centre. Don't saw, and never cut nails with scissors. If nail is damaged or much too long, use nail clippers to trim it straight across then smooth edge with emery board, leaving tip and sides straight if nail is short. The nail will grow out stronger in this squarish shape and can be rounded later. If nails are brittle, keep them short – just slightly longer than the finger is still long enough for elegance. Don't file too low at the corners; this weakens growth.

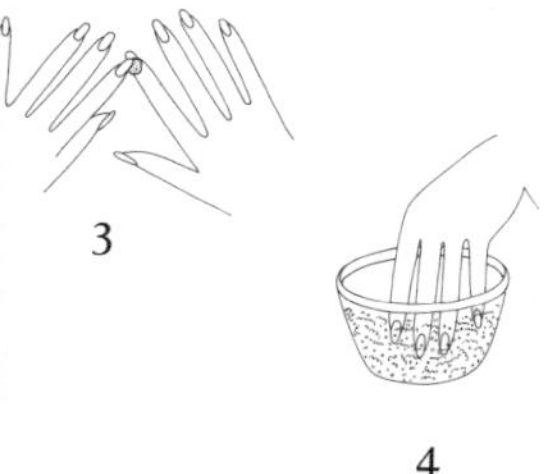

3

4

3. Massage nails with cuticle massage cream or any rich emollient; this stimulates nail base and helps loosen dry skin.

4. Soak nails in warm soapy water for ten minutes; if grimy and stained scrub gently with a bristle nail brush. After soaking, dry each nail in turn gently with a soft towel.

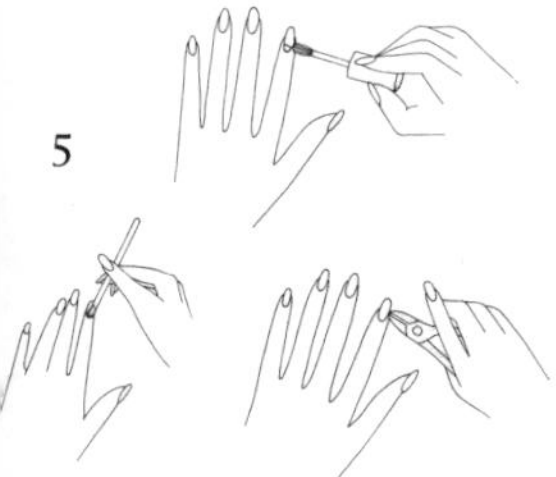

5

5. a) Apply cuticle remover or oil around the cuticle.

b) With an orange stick wrapped in cotton wool and kept moist by dipping in the soapy water, push back and carefully lift the cuticle away from the nail. Very gently; if pressure is too great, the matrix of the nail may be dented and the new nail will grow in ridges.

c) If there are still loose pieces of dead skin or cuticle, clip neatly with cuticle shears. Do not clip the entire cuticle; too much trimming should be avoided, as it makes the cuticle tough and encourages it to grow back stronger. If stains have got under, or down the side of, the nail, dip cotton-wrapped orange stick into peroxide and rub them away.

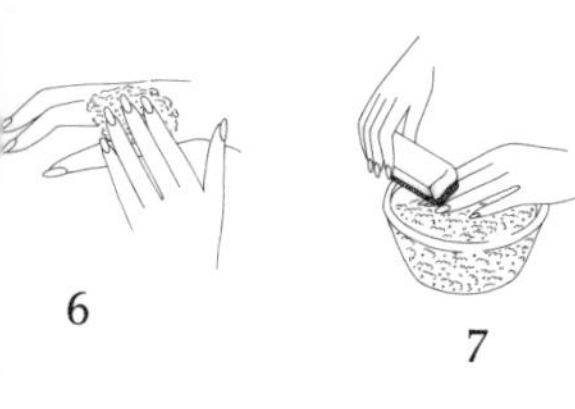

6

7

6. Apply hand lotion and massage hands and fingers; during massage give the fingers a good pull from their joints.

7. Dip fingertips back into the water and wash and scrub away the left-over bits of skin. Remove all traces of grease from the nail area.

8. If tips of nails need whitening, run a white nail pencil under them.

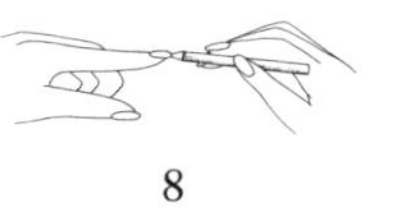

8

9. If you are going to buff your nails, or if you have splits or breaks that need mending (for details see below), now's the time to do it. Buffing is one of the best treatments for nails, either as a pre-polish reviver to stir up blood circulation, or as a polish in itself. Dab buffing paste on nails and buff gently in one direction only with a nail buffer or a soft chamois

cloth. Continue for about one minute a nail. For a pink shine, use a tinted paste. If you are buffing for circulation before applying polish don't use the cream.

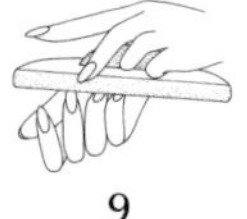
9

10. Apply varnish. With all applications try to do it in three straight strong strokes: one down the middle, one either side. A base coat gives a smoother surface and prevents colour pigment from discolouring the nail. The enamel strengthens as well as colours; the number of coats is up to you – two is a minimum, while top manicurists recommend four. The top coat or sealer helps protect the nail and guards against chipping. In addition to covering the surface of the nail, brush across the top edge and behind it. Colour tricks with polish: minimize the look of large hands by polishing the entire nail; cover all the nail if it is short or small; lengthen short fingers and make wide nails appear narrower by applying polish down the centre only, leaving sides bare; pale shades are best on short nails or stubby hands; dark shades give hands a delicate look; apricot, golden reds, and pink flatter a tan.

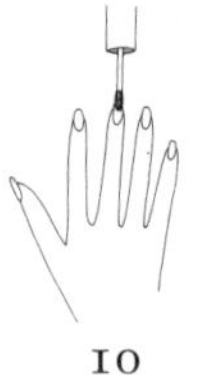
10

11. For a neat finish, run an orange stick tipped with cotton and dampened with polish remover along the outside edge of the cuticle and finger tip, to remove any smudges of polish.

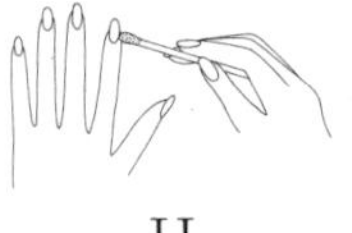
11

Patching:
If a nail splits or tears, it is often not necessary to clip it down – sometimes if the rip is deep, it can be both painful and ugly, as well as inviting infection. It can be temporarily patched until it grows out. There's a knack to doing this and it takes time to learn, but you can make a patch smooth enough to be invisible under any nail enamel:

1. With cotton dampened in remover, take away all traces of polish, oil or cream from nail.
2. Tear off a patch of nail paper – slightly larger than the area to be covered. Don't cut, the ragged edge blends more easily with the nail surface and resists peeling off.
3. Brush over patch with the fixative; lift it with tweezers or brush onto the nail. The jagged edge should face the base of the nail, and there must be a flap-over long enough to fold under the nail tip.
4. Mould the patch to the nail with a cotton-wrapped orange stick dipped in remover. Tuck extension under nail tip; be sure edges blend on the surface and excess glue is removed; check to see there are no air bubbles between patch and nail.
5. Cover first with base coat, then layers of polish and finally sealer. A patch should last through two polish changes, if you treat it with care.

Protective Patching:
The same principle can be applied to problem nails to protect them during regrowth. On each nail apply a tissue patch at the top – a jagged edge at the bottom to mould onto the surface of the nail, an extension at the top to tuck under the tip. You might need a little extra glue under the tip to secure the paper. Cover with base coat, polish layers and sealer.

False Nails:
Only to be used in an emergency. There are two kinds – those you glue on, and those you build up with a kind of cosmetic cement. They can look very effective, but they are drying, not good for the nails, and can be detrimental to new growth.

LEGS

The length and basic shape of the leg is hereditary and cannot be altered . . . fat and cellulite are accumulated, and can be prevented or controlled. Most things that go wrong happen after maturity or because of complete neglect in the teenage years.

The leg is about one-third of body weight, but the ankle has to bear the entire weight of the body and is one of the strongest hinge joints we have. The knee-joint is the largest and has to support the largest, heaviest, strongest bone in the body: the thigh. The look of the thigh depends on the upper and lower sections of muscles and flesh which cover the bone. It is in this area that trouble starts, partly because most of us don't use it enough, and partly because it has a particularly thick layer of adipose tissue, just waiting to be filled out with stored-up fat. Only regular exercise and diet control can prevent, correct and maintain shape. What's wrong with most legs is simply that they are too fat above the knee. Swollen legs are another matter, for they retain too much fluid.

Legs by nature are rather dry – there are not enough active oil glands in the limbs to keep them smooth and gleaming. It is important to lubricate them with a body lotion or cream after every bath; more often in the summer when they are bare and drier because of exposure to sun and sea.

Legs grow hair. Though in some cultures it may be considered erotic to keep it on, from a beauty point of view, it is better off.

CELLULITE

Cellulite is ugly and it tends to accumulate on thighs, around the knees, on hips and buttocks. It is the result of abuse more than age. It can affect women of normal weight, indeed even thin women are often troubled by cellulite. It takes time to appear and a long time to repair. It is caused by bad circulation and retention of fluid, the latter being the reason why the skin looks puffy, dimpled and soggy. It is also a sign of lack of exercise and a diet too full of the sugar and starch carbohydrates. Some doctors believe it is caused by an excessive secretion of oestradiol (female hormone) and it would seem logical that there could be a counter-balancing treatment. But at present cellulite is helped only by physical means – self care and salon treatment. Try the following with daily regularity – the only way to get good results:

Diet: Cut back on fats, sugars and starches; concentrate on high protein meats, green leafy vegetables, salads and fruit. Eat plenty of cucumber, first and foremost a diuretic food which helps to firm tissues. Every day eat cucumber salad – finely sliced complete with skin, a little olive oil, garlic, lemon juice and parsley (to counteract the smell of garlic).

Exercise: Walking and swimming are ideal, so is bicycling whether the real thing or simulating the movement by lying on your back supporting hips with hands and cycling in the air. Walk around the house doing the goose-step – you'll feel the inner thigh muscle working hard to keep the leg in a straight line.

Applications: Anti-cellulite creams can be massaged into the skin (see below for method) but it is usually the movement more than the cream that aids the area. Ivy is an ingredient in many creams and when used on its own it has a noticeable effect on cellulite. Ground ivy can be crushed and rubbed into the skin or applied as a poultice. You can make a solution by steeping ivy in cold water for twenty-four hours and using it as a wash to bathe the dimpled areas repeatedly.

Friction: The idea is to improve circulation, stepping up the metabolism of the fat cells. Pinch flesh through a towel; slap area alternately with hot and cold sponges or cloths; rub with a loofah or a friction glove made of string, nylon, or rubber nodules; put rough kitchen salt on the glove and vibrate the flesh.

Massage: You must be careful not to over-massage and be too rough with your flesh; use an oil, emollient or cellulite cream, and always be sure movements go up in the direction of the heart, never down. Don't just rub; using both hands wring and twist the flab as though you were squeezing out water; then with fists, iron the flesh upwards. For legs, grasp one ankle with both hands, wring and twist up to knee. For inner thighs, knead, then iron out. For buttocks, stand sideways about four inches away from a wall; turning slightly hit first one side then the other.

Water: Any force of water against the flesh is good – a jet in a swimming pool, a strong shower faucet; contrasts of hot and cold water help – take a cold shower followed by a hot bath, or force alternate hot and cold blasts from the hand-shower on special areas; nightly warm baths with Epsom salts are recommended.

Treatments: Beauty specialists offer individual methods to get rid of cellulite – wax, mud, steam, water, electrical and enzyme treatments, usually followed by a massage. Aromatherapy also claims to have good results with cellulite. See also page 289.

THICK ANKLES

Some people have naturally fleshy or sturdy ankles and no amount of attention or exercise can alter them. In these cases the flesh, though ample, is usually firm. However, if flesh is flabby, it is caused by fluid retention on the same principle as the formation of cellulite, and the same rules apply for getting rid of it – diet, exercise, massage, treatments.

SWOLLEN ANKLES

The sort of swelling that is usually temporary and abnormal: to test, press a finger on the swollen area. If it leaves a dimple that slowly disappears, then it is a transient condition. Gravity causes the most simple form: blood and body fluids fighting against gravity to return to the heart from the lower body extremities. When you have been on your feet all day, some of the body fluid can seep into the tissue around the ankles and puff them up. If you are barefoot or wear open sandals the feet swell instead. This can be dealt with easily by resting the feet, raising them higher than the head, to help the fluid back into circulation and upwards. The swelling will go down but it can take more than an hour. The swelling caused by varicose veins is similar; this too can be helped by raising the feet, and support stockings are of value.

Another cause of ankle swelling – and one of the most common – is the shift in hormone balance which occurs in the premenstrual period and in pregnancy. Many women in their thirties and forties complain of swollen ankles the week before their period begins. Artificial increases in hormone levels cause fluid retention and for this reason some women are unable to tolerate birth control pills. Older women who take hormone pills may have the same trouble. To counteract swelling it is essential to minimize fluid retention. First, control salt intake; it is the high hormone level that causes the kidneys to hold salt in the body and retention of salt always causes retention of water. Second, eat foods that are diuretic;

green vegetables, fruits, and herbal teas all have diuretic properties – cucumber and artichoke are of particular value. Third, bathing the feet and ankles in Epsom salts can help, also ivy compresses.

SPIDER VEINS

Little clusters of veins can gather on thighs, behind knees and around the ankles. They may look unattractive but usually have no serious effect. Sometimes thread veins are controlled by hormones, which is why they can appear during pregnancy. You may get them if you take the Pill and other causes include alcoholism and cirrhosis of the liver, but in such cases they are accompanied by other symptoms. Tight girdles, garters, and boots don't cause vein trouble but it is not healthy to wear them all the time, nor constantly to have legs encased in synthetic fibre tights; legs need to breathe. Thread veins are really a cosmetic problem and can be concealed by leg make-up applied in upward strokes. They can be treated by injections of a chemical and although the veins will fade and usually disappear, bruise marks may show for a while. Surface veins can be prevented from spreading by an electrical treatment that coagulates the blood. The time required to clear up blemishes of this type depends on how long you have had them; a series of treatments is usually needed, and the blue-purple veins are easier to eliminate than the reddish spider ones.

VARICOSE VEINS

This is an ugly and potentially dangerous condition. Varicose veins are caused by malfunction of the blood vessels in the legs, and are very common among Western peoples. Great pressure is put on the leg veins, as they have to defy gravity when they take the blood up to the heart. Some veins cannot stand the strain. Veins are long, elastic-walled tubes with a one-way flow of blood controlled by valves. Sometimes the vein walls become flabby or the valves don't work well and instead of closing to prevent backflow, they relax, sag, and let some of the blood seep back where it promptly meets blood going in the other direction. This makes the elastic wall bulge and in time there is a permanent knotty bulge with twisted bluish veins. The causes of valvular inefficiency are not known exactly, but there is a hereditary factor. Overweight puts pressure on the veins, and in pregnancy hormones relax muscular strands in the vessel.

The varicose vein cannot cure itself. The condition is usually progressive and should be treated in the early stages, for it can get so bad that there are medical complications of thrombosis, eczema and ulceration. The most serious type of varicose vein is the post-thrombotic. It usually appears as a group of small veins around the ankles that cause swelling and produce brown pigmentation marks. If not treated, they can lead to ulceration.

Varicose veins can be treated by surgery or injection. The two methods are completely different and it is a personal and medical decision as to which is preferable. The most commonly affected vein is the great saphenous which travels from the foot up the inside of the leg to the groin: the short saphenous may be affected and this shows at the back of the leg. Surgery is successful in 95 per cent of cases. The operation is called 'stripping' and involves removing the whole vein from the leg. It is literally pulled out by a special instrument; incisions are made in two, sometimes four, places. Many surgeons prefer stripping in a downward direction as there is less risk of nerve damage in the ankle area. It is usually necessary to be in hospital for a week. A careful operation means that this particular vein will never cause trouble again but other veins may need treatment later on.

Injections are used for all types of veins, but it is not just a matter of injection. Treatment consists of injections plus bandaging plus exercise plus patience, and the whole procedure involves a minimum of six weeks before legs are cured. A sclerosing fluid is injected into the vein; this acts as an irritant, roughens the surface walls and encourages them to close up. Legs are then tightly bandaged from thigh to ankle. The fluid injected is of far less importance than careful diagnosis and the technique of compression bandaging. The injection simply initiates a chain of events that results in the vein emptying itself and fusing the two surfaces. It is most important that the bandages are not disturbed; you cannot take a bath, only shower with plastic bags protecting the bandages. It is essential to walk a minimum of a mile each day (some doctors say two miles). The injections and bandaging take less than an hour, but the subsequent care is considerable. The method has a high proportion of success; some brown pigmentation marks are often visible after the veins have fibrosed up but these can be covered by make-up.

Prevention, of course, is better than anything. If there is a family history of vulnerable veins, you should rest your legs often, wear support stockings, avoid standing for too long, and walk as much as you can every day. Watch your diet; obesity puts great strain on legs, and even a slim woman is less likely to develop varicose veins if she eats plenty of protein and cuts down on sugar and starches.

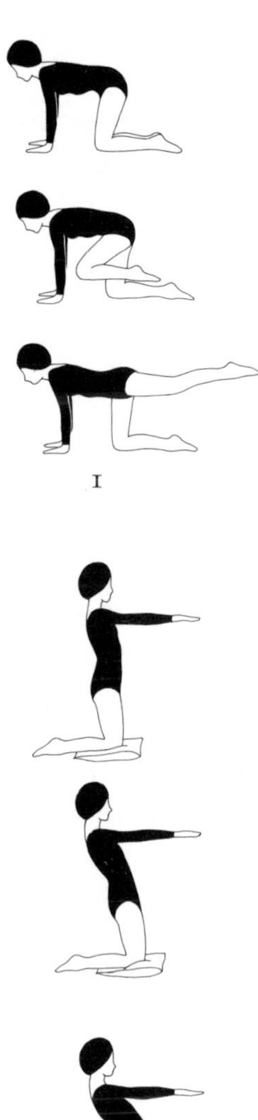
1

2

SCORCHED LEGS

Scorch marks are caused by sitting too near the fire. Once the skin has been damaged, it takes time for the marks to disappear. This is because the damage is usually below the top layer of skin which has to flake off before the scarred cells come to the surface – and they in turn flake off in the growth cycle. To help bleach the discoloration, try diluted peroxide in water. Keep legs moist by thoroughly creaming after bathing, particularly around the shin bone where there is a minimum of flesh.

LEG EXERCISES

To keep legs in good shape and condition requires daily exercise. Here are four basic movements designed to trim and firm them. Do each a few times at first, and work up to twenty minutes for the group. This is the sort of attention legs ideally require; not only will shape improve, but health benefits by keeping circulation at an invigorating level.

1. *All-fours stretch:* (for thighs and buttocks). Position yourself on hands and knees with back straight, arms rigid; bend left knee forward and up to chest, then extend back, stretching in line with buttocks. Do 10 times without touching floor. Repeat with other leg.

2. *Angled kneeling:* (for thighs and legs). Kneel on floor with back straight, arms at shoulder level; keeping body in a straight line with bottom tucked under and hips forward, slowly lean back as far as possible – without straining thighs, without collapsing. As thighs become stronger, you'll be able to go further back. Return to vertical position. Repeat 8 times.

3. *Knee bends:* (legs and thighs). Stand with feet a little apart, palms on thighs; raise toes, then bend knees pushing them outwards and lower the body to a crouching position, straighten legs, lower heels. Repeat at first 10 times and gradually work up to as many as possible.

4. *Knee bounce:* (for knees and calves). Sit on floor with legs spread in a wide V; bend knees slightly, drawing heels in towards you; stretch legs and bounce backs of knees on floor twice; bring legs together, straight in front, bounce knees on floor twice. Repeat 10 times.

FEET

Feet make our vertical posture possible. Much of the strength comes from the big toe, which is attached to a muscle centred across the shin; weight is absorbed by the arch. The true point of balance is in the ball of

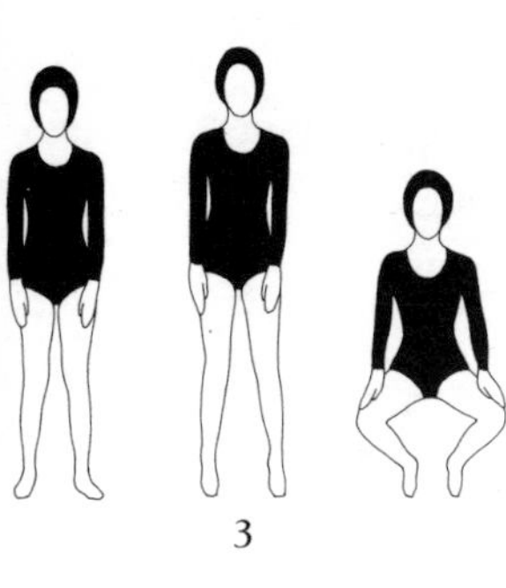

3

the foot, the exact position is individual. The way you place your feet and balance your body determines your standing and walking posture. This ideal point of balance can be found by standing barefoot, feet straight ahead about eight inches apart. Relax, hold arms loosely at sides, then keeping heels on the floor, sway gently. If you do not tense your body, it will steady itself at the correct balancing point for you. Concentrate on the spot, remember its exact position on the foot and from that moment on be conscious of using it. You'll be surprised how much lighter you feel.

In the structure of the foot the order of importance is: muscles, bones, then skin, for it is in this order that feet deteriorate. There are twenty-six small, delicate bones in each foot, the highest concentration of bone in the body. There are also three to four times as many ligaments and muscles which bind the bones into place and give spring and elasticity to the foot. The arch, which has to bear the weight and provide the grace, is strictly not one arch but three, two being in the length of the foot and one across it.

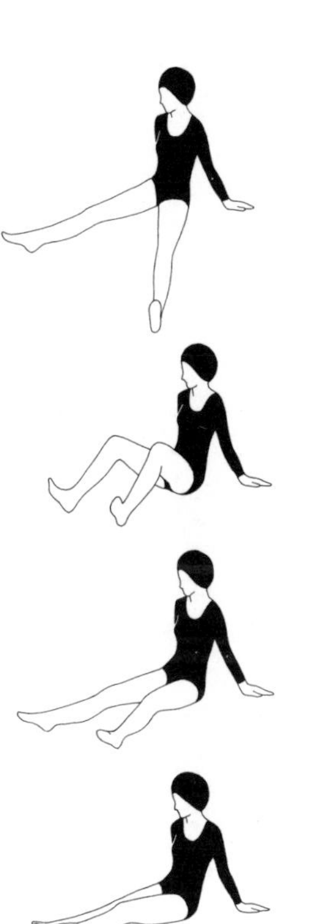

4

The structure of the foot is very similar to that of the hand, but the toes lack the mobility of thumb and fingers. However, feet should not be so inactive and inert as they generally are. Feet with toes that are practically never used are feet with poor circulation and subsequent problems. Feet that are never exercised permit muscles to slacken so that they can no longer take the weight of the body, nor bind or support the bones as they should. This means that the bones, because they take too much wear and tear, get out of alignment, arches drop, bunions form and the skin gets rubbed so corns and callouses appear.

Ninety per cent of foot trouble is caused by wearing a shoe that is too small, too narrow, too pointed or too high. Limited width causes corns and bunions to build up in defence against pressure; any heel over two inches upsets the shock-absorbing function of the arch, causes headaches and backaches, and adversely affects leg muscles and posture.

Alternate heel heights during the day and from day to day. The lower the heel, the better the legs are exercised naturally, but as each heel height exercises muscles that others don't, vary them. Avoid wearing shoes that have no support, but wear sandals in warm weather – the thong type with low or no heels that permit the feet, particularly the toes, to straighten out without restriction.

Make sure shoes really fit. There should be a good pinch of leather between the outer and inner side of the shoe across the ball of the foot (usually the widest part), and no less than a quarter of an inch of space between the end of the big toe and the tip of the shoe. Never buy shoes with the idea of breaking them in. The best time to buy them is in the afternoon; feet are at their smallest in the morning and a shoe that might be fine at nine, is murder at four. Think of shoes like gloves and take them off when you get home.

Footcare: Daily attention goes a long way towards getting feet in better shape and they respond very readily to such consideration:

Scrub feet daily with a stiff bristle brush, toe by toe, arch, sole, heel.

Pumice any callouses or hard spots.

Massage feet often with a hand or body lotion, working around each toe, particularly the heel area.

Push back cuticles when you cream, just as you would for finger nails.

Powder feet, this helps absorb moisture.

Pamper feet with cologne before putting on shoes or stockings.

Give yourself a pedicure every ten days.

For dry sandpaper heels and soles try an overnight treatment of petroleum jelly rubbed well in then sealed in with cotton socks.

Protect sensitive areas by wrapping or covering with absorbent cotton.

For tired feet, give them an Epsom salts bath – two tablespoons of salt to a quart of lukewarm water; then immerse in cool water, rub with alcohol, moisturize with a cream, prop them up for twenty minutes.

Another tired feet remedy – plunge them into hot water softened with bath salts or oil, then put them into very cold water adding a little astringent.

A few drops of lavender oil in a tepid footbath will relieve fatigue.

Lemon juice softens skin and helps tired feet.

For sweaty feet, dab twice a day with surgical spirit, then powder – particularly in hot weather.

A foot soother: stir one teaspoon of malt vinegar into a small carton of natural yoghourt (enough for three applications but keep in fridge); brush on mixture then rub over feet, between toes; leave on for five minutes and rinse away with warm water; the vinegar works on the dead skin and rough patches, the yoghourt softens hard skin and cools it.

Blisters are helped by sprinkling on cornflour.

Go barefoot whenever possible – on sand, grass, carpets; feet need air and freedom.

Check stockings: if they are too tight or too short they can lead to foot problems in the same way as shoes do.

Feet need vitamin D to help maintain bones – and the sun is a good source.

Feet that hurt should be taken to a chiropodist for treatment; even a simple corn should be professionally attended to.

CORNS

Corns are formed because of pressure or friction from footwear. They are really the foot's protection, with the body trying to form a thickened layer of skin to buffer and pad the foot. They are built up of hard dead skin, cone-shaped, with the point facing inwards and known as the eye. When this presses on a nerve, it can be very painful. Corns usually appear on the joints of toes; quite common is a hammer toe, where the second toe (often the longest) becomes bent at its two joints and forms corns over the bends. Corns also appear on the under surface of the foot, caused by unevenness of the sole of the shoe. When corns are between toes, they are moist and are known as soft corns.

The way to get rid of corns is to have them professionally removed. In the meantime, relief may be obtained by bathing your feet in hot salt water for a quarter of an hour, then wearing a ring of felt around the corn to free it from pressure. It is unwise to use a knife, scissors or razor blade to reduce the corn yourself; you could set up an infection.

BUNIONS

A bunion is found over the joint at the base of the big toe; it is a thickening of the skin at the head of the metatarsal bone and forms a painful lump at the side of the foot. It is started in many ways – short shoes, narrow shoes, tight stockings. Particularly significant is the slackening of muscles around the centre of the foot and lack of activity in the big toe joint, which consequently becomes stiff and rigid. At the first sign of a bunion, see a specialist, do foot and toe movements and wear a pad of lint or rubber for protection. If the joint becomes really angled with the built-up bunion, surgery may be the only answer, because although the bunion is hardened skin to an extent, it is basically bone growth. An incision is made along the joint of the big toe to a point just beyond the widest point of the bunion. The part of the bone forming the bunion is removed. The operation requires a week in hospital and the immediate after-effects can be painful, particularly at first attempts to walk. Stitches are removed after two weeks but it is six weeks before normal shoes can be worn.

CALLOUSES

Caused by friction from badly fitting shoes, a callous is an area of flattened hard skin. It is less painful than a corn because it has no pointed root, but it can cause a very unpleasant burning sensation. It is better to have it removed by an expert, but you can help by rubbing the area with a pumice stone or friction pad, afterwards creaming well.

VERRUCAS

These are warts, caused by a virus picked up by bare feet. Because they grow inwards, they can be painful. Sometimes they appear singly, sometimes in clusters. If the spot is relieved by a hollow ring of felt, the infection will often clear up. Otherwise go to a chiropodist who will get rid of the virus as well as removing the verruca. There are four methods of removal: acid pastes or liquids, an electrical treatment, freezing, or surgery if the wart goes very deep.

ATHLETE'S FOOT

This is a fungal infection, so-called because at one time only athletes ran the risk of catching it by going barefoot in gyms and swimming pools. It thrives in warm, damp skin, spreads easily and is highly contagious. A kind of ringworm, it can appear between toes and on the soles of the feet. Symptoms include an itchy rash, splitting and peeling of the skin between the toes, and blisters under the toes.

Prevention is not easy: wash feet after walking around a pool, drying them thoroughly, particularly between the toes. Keep feet as dry as possible at all times, and free them from moisture-holding stockings and shoes. There are a number of preparations in both liquid and powder form for dealing with this problem, but should it persist, get professional help. Treatment is effective within two weeks.

NAIL INFECTION

The most common foot infection is one that attacks the nails. It is called onychomicosis and is caused by a fungus that makes the nail discolour and thicken to such a degree that it is impossible to cut or clip it. It is not necessarily painful, but looks dreadful, and can cause a corn or sore if it presses against an adjoining toe. The big toe nail is most affected. The fungus is infectious and flourishes in warm, damp conditions. Treatment consists of paring and filing away the thickened nail so that a liquid can be painted on the soft surface underneath to kill the fungus. This may have to be done over some weeks, but it only takes a few minutes. Sometimes the whole nail must grow out before it is completely healthy again.

INGROWING TOE NAIL

This can be terribly painful as the sides of the nail are forced into the skin. It is caused either by incorrectly cutting the nail (down the sides instead of straight across) or by wearing shoes that are too tight or shallow. At the beginning seek expert advice; the longer it is left or mismanaged, the more difficult to cure. Some toe nails remain problems for life simply because they were not taken in hand early enough. Feet can be poisoned easily, so don't risk inflammation or the chance of dye from stockings or shoes getting into the bloodstream via a nail cutting into the flesh.

FOOT AND TOE EXERCISES

Feet get little opportunity to exercise freely; here are four exercises that should be a daily routine – to be done barefoot:

1. *Joint stretch:* Stand and take weight on one foot, raise heel of the other foot and bend the toe joints at right angles to the rest of the sole; hold to the count of 2; then balance the foot on tip toe, to the count of 2; return to bent position and finally to floor. Repeat 6 times for each foot.

2. *Muscle toner:* Standing on a book or a step, let toes hang over the edge; then bend them firmly downwards, hold to count of 2; pull them strongly upwards, hold to count of 2. Repeat 10 times.

3. *Toe control:* Sit or lie with legs straight in front, hold feet up and try to spread out toes as you would fingers; then try to work each toe up and down individually. Repeat 10 times. (At first you will find it almost impossible to do this exercise, and it helps at the beginning to hold four toes and let the free one work individually. Start doing it in the bath, when foot circulation is usually at its peak.)

4. *Foot circles:* Sit or lie with legs stretched out in front, knees braced. Make wide circles outward, arching the foot. Do 10 times. Repeat, making inward circles. (Particularly good for strengthening and trimming the ankles, as well as helping to improve the shape of the foot.)

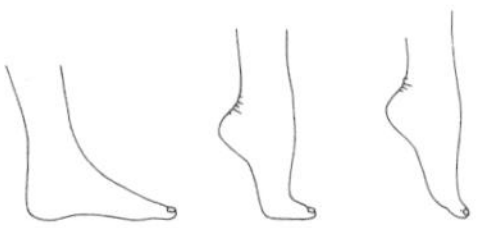

1 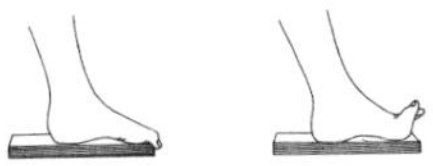 2 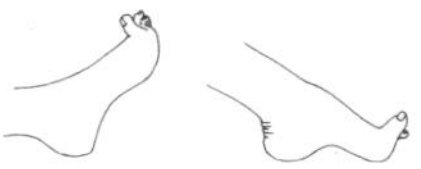 3 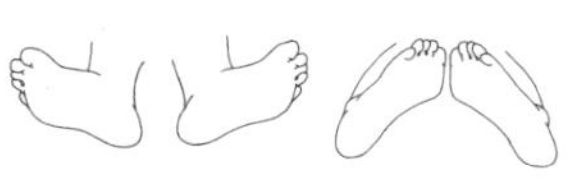 4

PEDICURE

You need a pedicure every ten days and it takes about forty-five minutes.

Equipment:

Basics – towel, absorbent cotton, bristle nail brush, pumice stone or friction block, large bowl of soapy water (bath oil or foam is preferable).

Tools – emery board, nail clippers, cuticle clippers, orange sticks, nail buffer, foot scraper.

Creams – hand or body lotion, cuticle-remover cream or oil, buffing paste, tinted or clear.

Nail cosmetics – oily polish remover, base coat, nail enamel, top sealer.

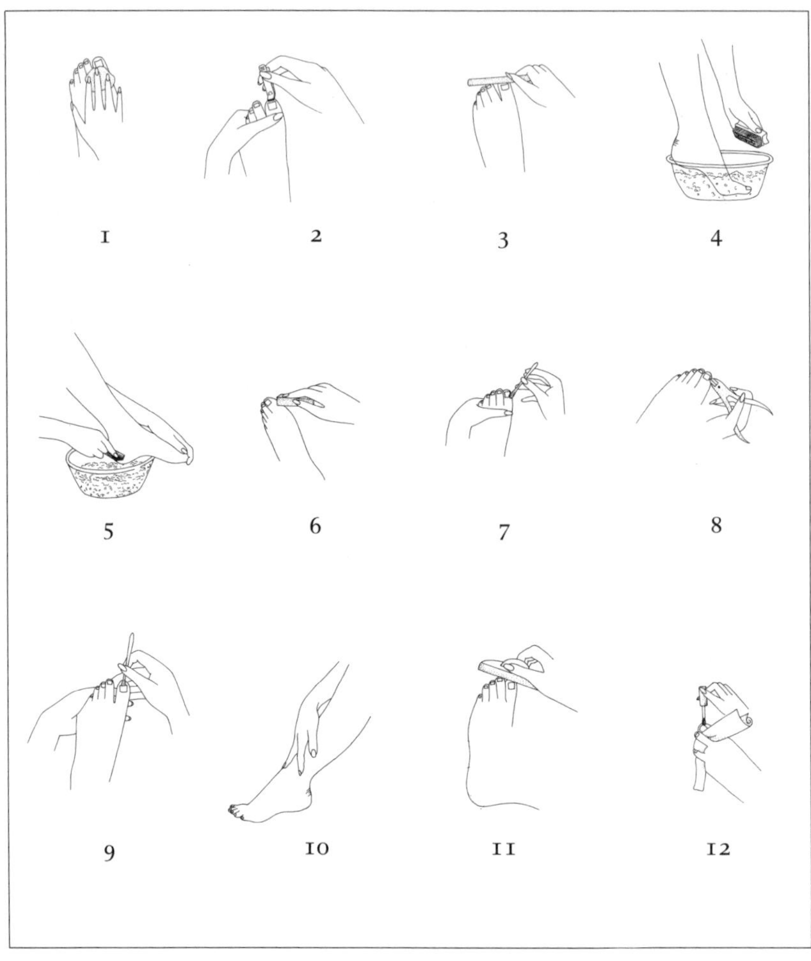

Procedure:

1. Remove old varnish by pressing cotton soaked in oily remover against nail, then wiping off.
2. Clip nails straight across, neat and square, using nail clippers, never scissors. It is particularly important to keep toe nails straight even if long, to prevent the possibility of an ingrowing nail.
3. File nails smooth but not to a shape; keep straight and square line; no sawing back and forth.
4. Soak feet in sudsy water for a good ten minutes; scrub feet with a bristle brush – across the toes, the heel, the underside of the foot.
5. Use a pumice stone or friction pad on the really dry rough spots, on any calloused area too. If there is a lot of flaky dry skin, this can be scraped away with a bladed foot-scraper, but be careful to use this gently. It's easy to nick the skin – short swift movements are the best. Put feet back in the water to brush away remaining shreds of skin.
6. Clean under the nails and down the sides with a cotton-wrapped orange stick dipped in the suds. If nails are stained, dip stick into peroxide and try to rub away. Stains, however, may be due to infection, not dirt.
7. Apply cuticle-remover cream or oil around the cuticles, massage gently and with an orange stick-plus-cotton push gently back.
8. If there are stubborn strands of skin – they often appear at the side of the big toe – that do not break away with the cuticle cream and massaging, clip with cuticle shears to neaten edge. Don't clip the entire cuticle, only the straggly ends.
9. Check toe joints to see if hard skin is beginning to build up, if so gently file down with a pumice stone or a sandpaper stick.
10. After dipping again in the water to get rid of the last bit of skin or dirt, towel dry, then massage in body lotion – over the foot and lower leg with firm upward strokes; massage each toe individually.
11. Buff nails to aid circulation – in one direction only otherwise the nail becomes too heated. One minute a nail is adequate. If you are not going to use polish afterwards, a tinted paste gives a coloured sheen – just cream it on before buffing.
12. Apply polish as for manicure but before doing so, separate toes with wads of cotton or a strip of tissue. This prevents polish smudging from one toe to another. After base coat, apply two colour coats, then a sealer. Clean away any smudge marks with a cotton-tipped orange stick dipped in polish remover.

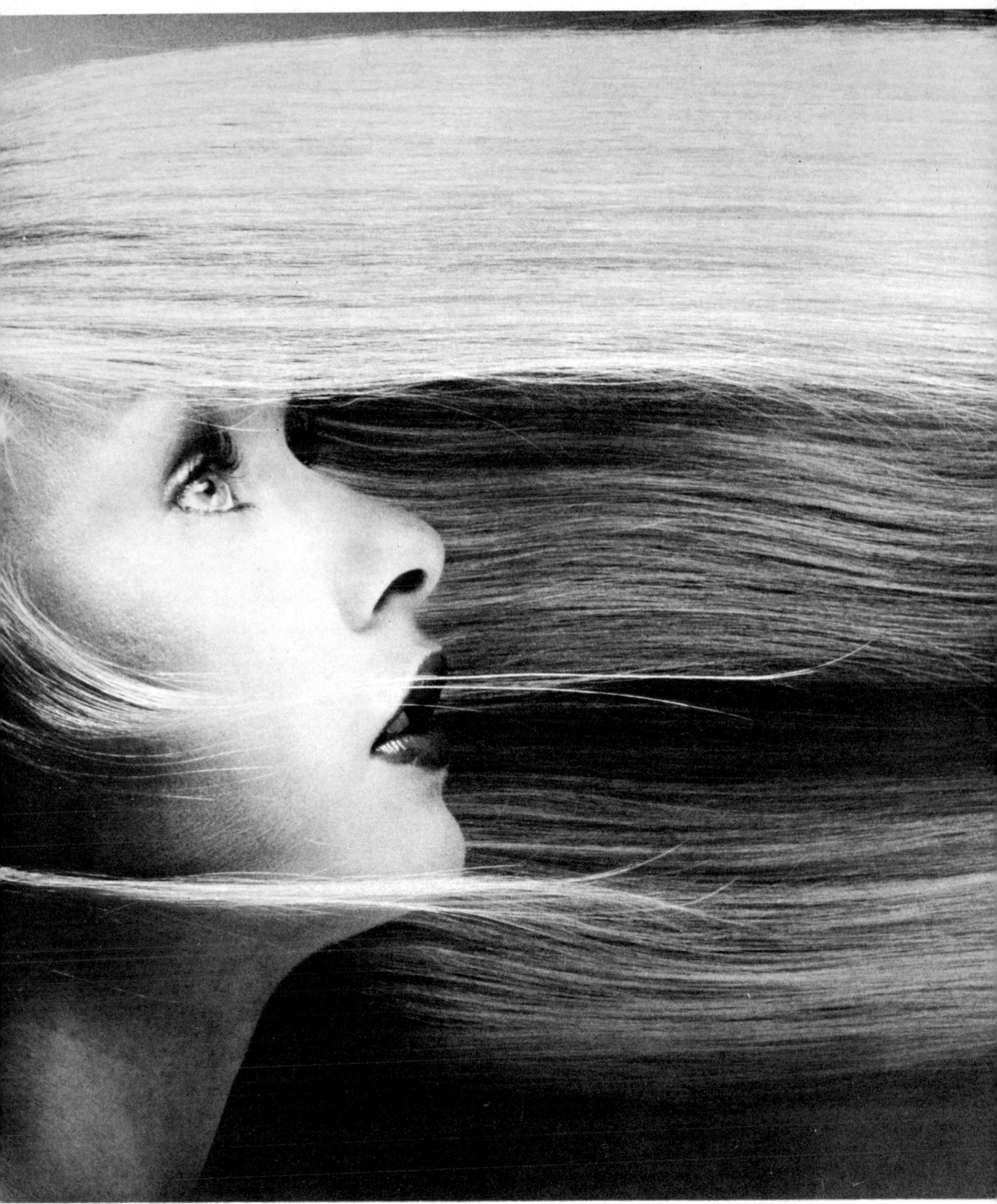

PATRICK HUNT

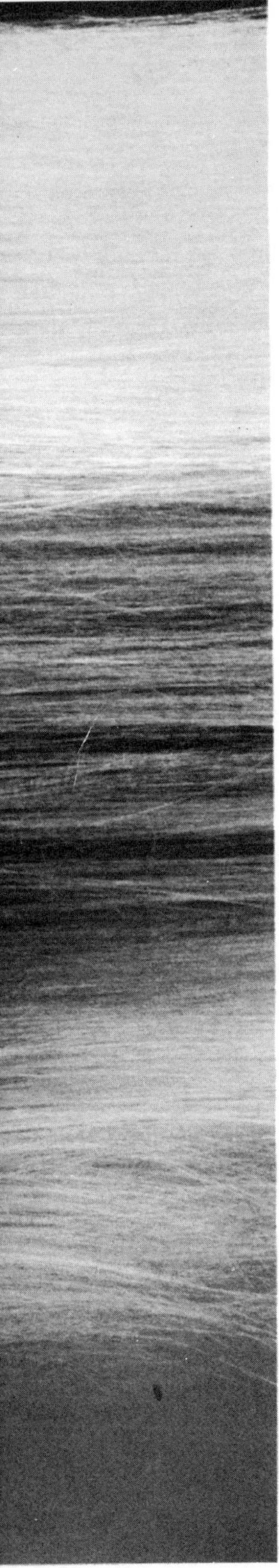

9

HAIR

More time, thought, energy and money are spent on hair than on any other aspect of body-beauty. And yet we don't see nearly enough good-looking heads around. Health and beauty are of equal importance and there is no possibility – as in the case of skin and make-up – of covering up lack of one with the other. Texture, condition, type, colour and shape have to be taken into consideration simultaneously. Hair that bounces, shines and has a look of vitality and control is the result of a healthy working body together with a programme of correct care.

ELEMENTS

Hair is a complex cellular structure and varies from one person to another. The structural form is basically the same: each strand, no matter how fine it may look, consists of three layers. The outer layer, or cuticle, is made up of overlapping scales which protect the inner layers. The next layer, or cortex, is made up of long thin cells and is the most important for it gives the hair its elastic resilience and contains the pigment which provides the colouring. The innermost layer, or medulla, is spongy tissue and the cells sometimes contain granules of colour pigment.

The part of the hair that you can see above the skin is the shaft, and the part that lies beneath the scalp is the root. The root is not a single entity, for it is enclosed in a sac known as the hair follicle, and at the base of this is a tiny nodule called the papilla, which is really the store house for nourishment of the hair strand. When you pull hair out 'by the roots', although there is a tiny globule of white at the end of it, you leave behind the papilla which will eventually manufacture and nurture a new hair. This is why plucking is never a permanent way to get rid of unwanted hair, and why hair loss through abuse and breakage can eventually be replaced.

Interlinked to the follicles are sacs containing sebum which lubricates the hair and gives it gloss and suppleness. An underactive or blocked sebaceous gland means dry hair, an overactive one means oily hair.

Each strand of hair grows out straight or curly depending on the inner structure of the root. If the root is smooth, the hair comes out as a perfect cylinder and is straight. If the root is distorted, the hair shaft is more oval, at times quite flat, and emerges as waves or curls. Whatever the texture, you usually have between 90,000 and 140,000 individual hairs on your head. Blondes, because their hair is finer, have the most; then dark-haired people, whilst redheads have the least though their hair is the thickest and therefore appears the most abundant. The life-span of a single hair can vary from a few months to several years. Each strand has its own cycle of growth, then a period of rest which ends in its falling out and being replaced by a new hair. This process is evenly distributed at different stages throughout the head and it is perfectly normal to lose a certain number of hairs every day.

On the average, hair grows at the rate of half an inch (13 mm.) a month, though this slows down as we get older. It grows faster during warm weather, and faster at night. The reason why some women can grow hair to their waists is because they have the combination of a quick growth rate and a relatively long life-span for each hair. It usually happens when you are young and in good health. Nothing can make hair grow faster and most hair, after reaching a length of ten inches (255 mm.), slows down to half the normal rate of growth. It is not true that cutting will encourage the hair to grow. It may seem to simply because, having got rid of split and impoverished ends, the illusion is created of thicker, healthier hair.

Hair colour is determined by three pigments – black, red and yellow. Black and dark brown hair are concentrations of black; red begins to show up in brown hair; light brown hair contains traces of yellow; red hair is mostly red pigment with black or yellow shadings; blonde hair is yellow with traces of red. Hair doesn't really turn grey, but loses its colour. The middle section of the hair shaft stops producing pigment and fills up with colourless air bubbles, but because the white hairs are intermixed with the coloured ones, the general effect is grey. The age at which hair turns grey is usually hereditary. It cannot turn grey overnight but it can lose its colour quickly due to an illness or emotional shock.

We are inclined to forget that healthy hair is part of a healthy body, and directly affected by physical metabolism and emotional balance. Its texture may be determined by genes but its strength and condition are determined by what it is fed. A high-protein diet with lots of fresh fruit and vegetables is good for hair. Foods containing vitamins of the B complex are essential. Important too are vitamins A and C. Of the minerals, iron, iodine and copper are the most beneficial, and lack of iodine can be most detrimental. A supplement of brewers' yeast tablets is recommended for anyone with a hair problem. In some cases, if premature greyness has been caused by a nutritional deficiency, it can be helped by massive doses of vitamin B.

TYPES AND TREATMENTS

Beautiful hair is immaculately clean and glossy, and the result of a planned programme of care. To work out a routine, it is important to know your hair type. Is it dry, oily or balanced? Has it been tinted, bleached, permed or straightened? That is all you need to know. Texture, thickness and curling ability influence styling and shape, but not basic care. The wonderful washability of hair is one of its main assets, and all hair needs frequent washing. Once a week is average for normal or dry hair, but if you are exposed to city grime or pollution, do it every five days. Oily hair usually requires washing every two or three days. The rule is: wash when hair looks or feels dirty. Some hair requires special rinsing. All hair needs pampering from time to time with a deep conditioning treatment. Check the chart overleaf to work out your general pattern of care, then check for details of each procedure.

THE ROUTINE

The ritual of washing hair was probably the first beauty routine you learned – but it's worth checking to see if you are getting the most out of it. The modern rule is: wash often, wash lightly, use shampoo sparingly; in this way enough lubrication stays in the hair, and the natural fungicides and antiseptics are not removed – they are useful for they protect the scalp from infection. Here are the steps to a perfect wash:

1. Brush hair gently to remove dead hairs and particles of skin that cling to the hair and scalp.
2. Massage scalp with gentle kneading motions; use pads of fingers and do it gently; this helps loosen more dead particles.
3. Deep conditioning treatment is given now, when needed.
4. Wet hair very thoroughly with warm water, lots of it – using a shower

spray is the easiest method. Work a small quantity of shampoo into a mild froth. Rinse hair with warm water. If necessary work in a second limited portion of shampoo – but it shouldn't be necessary.

5. Rinse hair thoroughly until it is squeaky clean. This may take three or four rinsings; let the final one be of cool or cold water to close the pores.

6. Use instant conditioner or cream rinse now if you need one; rinse away if instructions say so.

7. Mop hair with a soft towel to absorb a lot of the wetness; don't rub, simply blot dry.

8. Comb gently into shape for setting or drying; never brush hair when it is wet.

FORM	DRY	OILY	BALANCED
Natural hair not tinted, bleached, permed or straightened	Shampoo for dry hair Cream rinse Deep conditioning treatment every 3 weeks	Shampoo for oily hair Astringent rinse Deep conditioning treatment once a month Dry shampoo when needed	Mild shampoo Natural rinse, avoid very creamy ones Deep conditioning treatment once a month
Tinted, permed or straightened hair; hair overexposed to sun or chlorine; problem split ends	Shampoo for tinted or dry hair Cream rinse Instant conditioner once a week Deep conditioning treatment every 3 weeks	Shampoo for tinted or dry hair Instant conditioner every 2 weeks Deep conditioning treatment once a month Dry shampoo when needed	Shampoo for tinted hair or mild one Instant conditioner every 2 weeks Deep conditioning treatment once a month
Bleached or lightened hair – or hair bleached then coloured with a light shade	Shampoo for lightened hair Cream rinse Instant conditioner once a week Deep conditioning treatment every 3 weeks	Shampoo for lightened hair Instant conditioner once a week Deep conditioning treatment once a month Dry shampoo when needed	Shampoo for lightened hair Instant conditioner once a week Deep conditioning treatment once a month

BRUSHING AND MASSAGING

Daily brushing stimulates circulation and gives new body and fullness to the hair. Brushing before a shampoo is essential and the first step in the cleansing routine. Invest in a first class brush. Natural bristles are the best, but if you choose nylon be sure the ends are rounded. Always keep your brush spotlessly clean, otherwise you'll brush dirt back into the hair. A quick dip of the brush in a mild solution of ammonia and water quickly lifts the grime, then swish around in warm soapy water, rinse and dry upside down. Use two brushes if you prefer, one in each hand.

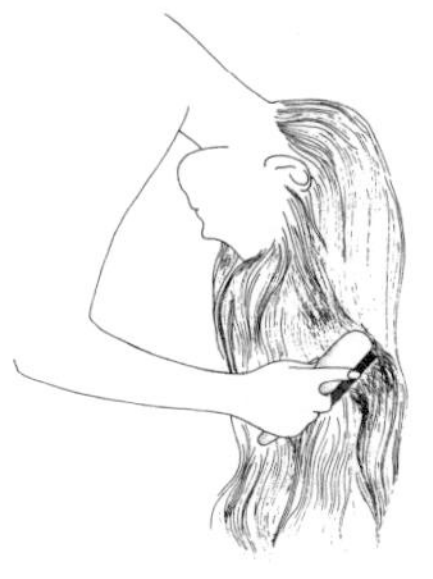

Hair should be brushed firmly but not over zealously – it responds better to a gentle treatment than to an attack. Every time you brush your hair you are going to lose some hairs. It's quite normal; hairfall is estimated at between forty and a hundred hairs a day. Hair should be brushed inside out: stand or sit, bending head forward and down, so that your hair is hanging in front of your face. Start with the brush at the nape of the neck and close to the scalp – though not scraping it – and make long lifting strokes away from the head. If hair is snarled, divide it into sections and work your way piece by piece towards the forehead. Stand up and throw your head back, and when the hair has settled back and down, use your brush to smooth it lightly. If you are not going to shampoo, put a piece of silk over the brush to polish the hair.

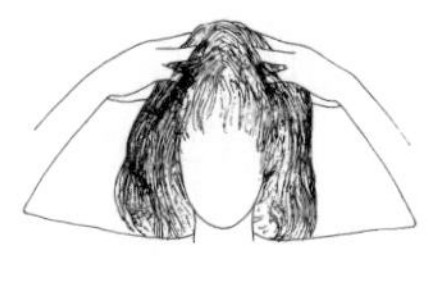

Massaging helps to improve circulation and loosen tense muscles. Do it before a shampoo and whenever you can spare a few moments. Start at the back of the head with fingers rotating slowly and gently; don't scratch, don't push with palms. Work your way in circular movements up the sides, over the crown and to the rim of the forehead. The scalp should move even with the slightest pressure.

SHAMPOOING

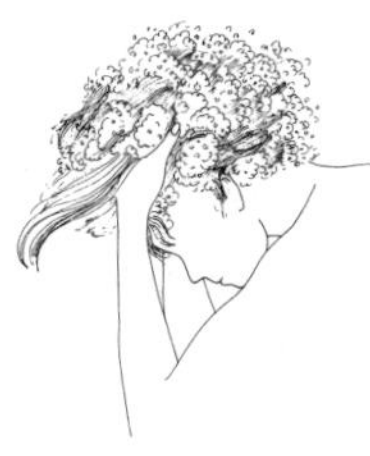

Careless shampooing can be harmful, either because it is the wrong type of shampoo for your hair, or because it is wrongly used. After wetting the hair thoroughly with warm water, use just a teaspoon of shampoo for a mild lathering. No hard rubbing; the hairline can be cleaned with a soft nailbrush, while the ends of long hair should be treated as you would treat fabric. Only if the hair is very dirty should two soapings be necessary. Modern detergent shampoos are very concentrated and if over-used stimulate the oil glands to greater activity.

Commercial shampoos are basically divided into two categories – soap shampoos and detergent ones. Read the labels which provide information as to whether the shampoo is for dry, oily or balanced (normal) hair; whether for tinted or bleached hair; whether enriched and with what; whether medicated or hypo-allergenic, whether based on natural sources or not. Tests have shown that some of the protein molecules from enriched protein shampoos are absorbed by the hair shaft and feed the hair; the remaining molecules coat the strand temporarily and are washed away with the next shampoo. They can make hair more manageable and slightly thicker. Many products make a reference on the label to pH, which means a measure of the acidity or alkalinity. Hair is surrounded by a liquid mantle of moisture (from the atmosphere, perspiration etc.) and it should be slightly acidic. However, certain alterations to hair – including colouring and perming – frequently leave an alkaline residue which makes the hair less resilient and can cause breakage and splitting. So the pH content of a shampoo (or a rinse, or conditioner) can be significant if you need to restore or maintain the natural acid-alkaline balance of the hair. A scale of numbers is used to define the acidity or alkalinity of any solution: 7 is neutral, 7 down to 0 are acidic, 7 up to 14 are alkaline. Most shampoos range from 6 to 8.

To find the right shampoo is a matter of experiment. Judge by seeing how effectively it cleans your hair, how your hair feels and behaves.

There are several shampoos you can make yourself:

Simple Soap Shampoo: For really delicate hair there's nothing better than soap; buy old-fashioned green cream soap and dissolve 4 oz. (120 g.) in a pint (6 dl.) of warm water – it may take a few days to coagulate evenly. Use in small quantities.

Herbal Shampoo: Add a strong infusion of herbs – rosemary or thyme – to a Castile shampoo.

Egg Yolk Shampoo: Beat 2 egg yolks into a cup of warm water; massage into scalp and hair for 5 minutes; leave to saturate for 10 minutes. Rinse off – no other shampooing before or afterwards is necessary.

Egg and Brandy Shampoo: Beat 2 egg yolks into ½ cup brandy and ½ cup warm water; massage into hair, leave to absorb for 10 minutes. Rinse.

Camomile and Egg Shampoo: Make a strong infusion of camomile flowers; for oily or balanced hair add an egg white, beaten to a froth; for dry hair add a beaten egg yolk. This shampoo is for light hair only. For dark hair use the same recipe, but substitute an infusion of sage or rosemary in place of the camomile.

Oily Hair Wash: Beat 4 whole eggs, massage through hair; leave for 15 minutes; wash off well with water; then rinse with a mixture of a cup of rum with a cup of rose water.

DRY SHAMPOOING

If pressed for time or in case of illness, a dry shampoo can be useful. Most come in powder form and the most common error is to use too much. Shake a little into the hair, gently rub in and around, then brush it out, using upward strokes away from the head. It takes about five minutes, and it helps to put a piece of gauze over the brush to absorb dirt and oil. Hair can also be dry cleaned with eau de cologne: cover brush with a piece of gauze or cheesecloth, sprinkle it with eau de cologne and brush through the hair. A natural dry shampoo is powdered orris root: sprinkle a minimum amount in the hair, brush for 5 minutes.

RINSING

Hair that has not been properly rinsed might just as well not have been washed at all. A water rinse is essential after every type of shampoo. Rinse, rinse, rinse – three, four or more times until every particle of soap has gone. The slightest residue of soap will leave hair dull and sticky enough to attract dirt immediately. The final rinse should be cool water, cold if you can stand it, particularly for oily heads as it closes the pores tight. Dark hair can have a little vinegar added to the last rinse; light hair benefits from the addition of lemon juice to the final water. These both help to restore the acid covering of the hair and remove the last vestiges of soap. Natural rinses with special effects are:

To add sheen to hair: boil parsley in water for 20 minutes, strain and use as a final rinse.

To add lustre to dark hair: pour a pint (6 dl.) of water over 2 tablespoons of rosemary, steep for 30 minutes, strain, add to final rinse.

To improve natural hair colouring: simmer a handful of nettles in a pint (6 dl.) of water until soft; strain, add to final rinse. It also gives the hair body.

To restore light tones to blonde hair: simmer a cup of dried camomile flowers in a pint (6 dl.) of water, after 30 minutes strain and use as a final rinse; catch the liquid in a basin and repeat the rinsing several times.

To lighten hair: simmer 4 tablespoons of ground rhubarb root in $1\frac{1}{2}$ pints (9 dl.) water for 30 minutes, steep for several hours, strain; rinse through hair several times.

There are also cream rinses which act like fabric softeners. They make the hair silky and easy to comb after shampooing, reducing the pulling and tangling that causes breakage and split ends. They add sheen and also help control the hair by minimizing static electricity. It is important to control the quantity used, otherwise the hair becomes too slithery. They should not be used on oily hair.

Here's a natural recipe that adds sheen and softness: pour 1 pint (6 dl.) of boiling water over 2 tablespoons of rosemary (for dark hair) or camomile (for light hair), steep for 30 minutes, strain; add 3 oz. (90 g.) oil of sweet almonds and 20 drops of lavender essence.

CONDITIONING

Regular conditioning is a protective measure for all hair. It is essential for hair that shows signs of dryness, dullness or breakage. It is necessary to counteract the alteration treatments of tinting, dyeing, perming, straightening and bleaching. The purpose of conditioning is to restore hair to its natural condition, to make it manageable, to prevent breakage, to reduce split ends and to smooth out rough straw-like texture.

There are two types of conditioner – instant and deep. An instant conditioner is usually an enriched liquid (more likely than not containing protein) that is combed through freshly washed hair. It softens, adds resilience and bounce. Some have to be lightly rinsed away; others stay on to also serve as a setting lotion.

Deep conditioning involves products or home treatments rich in creams and oils. They are massaged into the hair and left on for anything from 10 to 30 minutes in order to allow the rich ingredients to penetrate the hair shaft. They are extremely valuable for dry hair and hair that has been abused or damaged. They are sometimes applied before the shampoo and sometimes afterwards – read instructions carefully. If hair is in very bad condition, a weekly deep conditioning is recommended until there is an obvious improvement. Usually a treatment every three weeks is adequate to preserve and maintain it.

Deep conditioning treatments can be made from household items:

Hot Oil Treatment – warm 2 tablespoons of olive oil, gently massage into every part of the scalp. Wring out a towel in hot water and wind it turban-style around the head. As it cools, repeat the process 2 or 3 times to ensure total saturation. Afterwards shampoo hair and rinse thoroughly. Good for brittle, dry hair.

Procedure

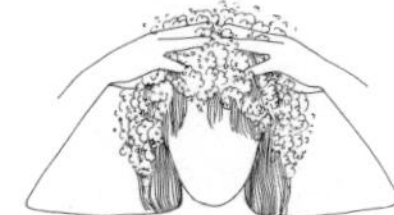

1. Shampoo hair and rinse until absolutely clean – till it squeaks.

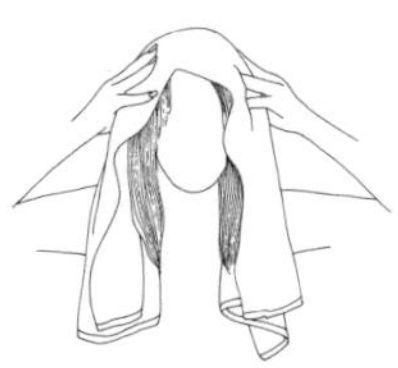

2. Blot dry with a towel, gently comb until smooth without tangles.

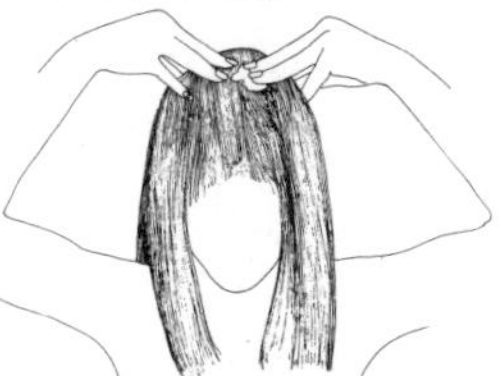

3. Section the hair and apply treatment product; massage into scalp.

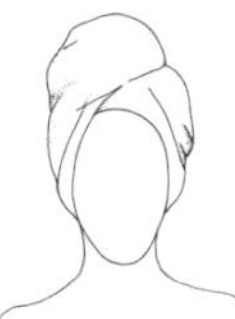

4. Dip towel in hot water, wring out, wrap around head; leave 15 to 30 minutes.

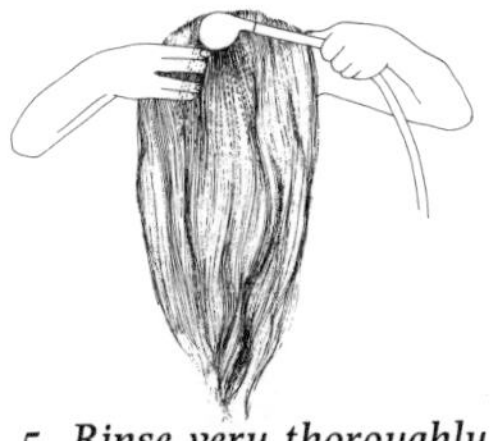

5. Rinse very thoroughly, 3 or more rinses preferably with shower.

Castor Oil Treatment – warm ½ cup of castor oil, massage into scalp and gently comb it through hair; wind a steaming hot towel around the head; wait 30 minutes before shampooing. Good for fragile hair.

Olive Oil and Honey Treatment – stir together ½ cup of green olive oil and 1 cup of liquid honey; shake vigorously; allow mixture to steep for a day or two. Massage into scalp, comb through, but don't let teeth scrape the scalp. Cover with a plastic bag, make airtight to permit the heat of the head to aid penetration. Leave for 30 minutes. Then shampoo and rinse. Keeps dark hair shining and lustrous.

Protein Treatment – beat 2 eggs, continue beating and slowly add 1 tablespoon of olive oil, 1 tablespoon glycerine and 1 teaspoon cider vinegar. Apply after initial shampoo and rinse; leave on for 15–30 minutes. Rinse well. A restorer for all types of hair.

Cocoa Butter Treatment – in the top of a double boiler, melt ½ cup safflower oil, 1 tablespoon cocoa butter and 1 tablespoon anhydrous lanolin; when completely dissolved and blended, take off heat and beat. Then take 3 tablespoons of the mixture and add 1 tablespoon of water, mix thoroughly. Massage into hair, leave on for 15–30 minutes. Then shampoo, rinse. Gives new life and lustre to dark hair.

Salad Dressing Treatment – beat together 1 egg, 1 tablespoon vinegar, 2 tablespoons vegetable oil just before using. Massage well into scalp and comb evenly through hair; leave on for 15 minutes. Shampoo and rinse. Helps to moisturize the scalp and provide lubrication for dry hair.

PROBLEMS

If hair is treated well it is easy to keep in good condition. It is by nature both elastic and plastic: elastic because it can be stretched and pulled around without breaking; plastic because it can be moulded temporarily or permanently into any shape you please. Yet resilient as it is problems crop up time and time again. Home treatment is often effective but any persistent or serious disorder should be treated by a trichologist.

ENVIRONMENT

It is not only air pollution that is bad for the hair. Day in day out, whatever the climate, hair is constantly exposed to heat, humidity, wind, cold, sun, water, central heating or air-conditioning.

Industrial pollution – particles of soot, grime and smog attach themselves to the hair, particularly if it is oily or sprayed. This makes hair dirtier and it is thought that it can affect the colour of tinted or bleached hair.

Sun – a little is good for the hair, but too much can be its worst enemy. It dries out hair, often causing breakage and split ends. It lightens natural-coloured hair, but seriously changes the shade of tinted or lightened hair, making it dull or brassy – it always brings out the reddish tints. If exposed to a lot of sun, keep the head covered and have a deep conditioning treatment every three or four weeks. Hair often acclimatizes to sun so that women from the tropics find their hair deteriorates in a northern climate and of course the reverse is also true.

Heat – intensifies the natural condition of hair: if it is dry it will become drier, if it is oily, oilier. It usually makes hair dirtier due to the head perspiring and dirt adhering to the moisture. Normal balanced hair will need washing more frequently and deep conditioning once a month. Dry hair will require an instant conditioner after every wash and a deep one every three weeks. Oily hair requires more shampooing than usual, and a long conditioning treatment every three or four weeks.

Humidity – adversely affects all hair. Curly hair becomes curlier, straight hair, straighter and even balanced hair will lose its shape more quickly. Choose simple styles and a stronger setting lotion. A deep-conditioner for all types of hair is a great help.

Water – rainwater is harmless – unless in polluted areas – but sea and swimming pool water can harm. The chlorine in pools dries and bleaches normal and tinted hair; it is always better to wear a cap, and if you can't, wash hair immediately on coming out of the water, adding an instant conditioner if possible. Sea water dries and bleaches hair, often because the hair is also exposed to the sun and the salt content accelerates both the drying and the bleaching processes. Always rinse hair in fresh water after swimming in the sea, again adding an instant conditioner if your hair is naturally dry or chemically altered.

DANDRUFF

The most common of all scalp disorders. It forms noticeable white flakes near the roots of the hair and is really dead tissue from the scalp and not in itself an infection although it can lead to one. It is an unhealthy condition and early and mild cases should be dealt with by a vigilant programme of home care. A very irritated scalp should be treated by a trichologist. Hard brushing, combing or scratching can precipitate a condition called seborrhoea by removing partially attached scales leaving exposed sore areas in which bacteria flourish. There are two forms of this condition: dry and oily. In the dry type, the scales are constantly visible; it is not only unsightly but can lead to eye trouble. The oily type is common in adolescence and is often accompanied by acne.

The causes of dandruff are many but difficult to pinpoint. Not enough fresh air in the hair is one reason, so is sleeping in rollers, never brushing the hair, fatigue, emotional upset and climatic conditions – people who live in cold areas tend to have more dandruff than those living in tropical climates. Doctors suggest hereditary factors and hormone imbalance – but nothing has been proved.

If you suffer from dandruff first look to your diet. Too much sugar and starch can lead to acidity and skin eruptions while a diet too high in fats can stimulate overactive oil glands and aggravate the condition. Stick to lean meats, vegetables, salads and fresh fruit.

It is essential to keep the scalp clean. Dandruffy heads need constant washing with a medicated shampoo, and this applies to dry as well as oily hair. A teaspoon of antiseptic in the rinsing water is helpful. A treatment is to make a liquid of 1 part apple juice to 3 parts water – to be rubbed into the scalp 2 or 3 times a week.

ABUSE

Tinting, bleaching, perming and straightening all damage hair to some extent, but the two treatments that cause the most trouble are bleaching and straightening. Strong bleaching should be avoided: it can weaken the hair and the scalp. If you are dark don't bleach year after year but try to be content to lighten it just a few tones. Straightening can stretch the hair dangerously: it is far worse than permanent waving. Other things that destroy hair are: constant use of brush rollers, heated rollers, hot irons, pulling the hair when blowing dry, elastic bands and any constant restriction.

Damaged hair results in broken strands, split ends and dryness. The way to counter-balance these problems is constant use of a conditioning treatment. The only remedy for split ends is to have them cut off, if not they will continue to split up the entire hair shaft. Even long hair should be cut regularly so that the ends are healthy. Some hairdressers singe the strands to remove split ends: a section of hair is twisted tightly so that the broken or split ends pop out and are carefully singed off with a flame. It is a time-consuming job, and only for an expert.

HAIR FALLOUT

Alopecia areata can mean loss of hair in patches or a diffused hair fall all over the head. It is causing concern because an increasing number of women are beginning to lose their hair. As women assume more responsibilities and tensions, it is thought that they are also producing more of the male hormone androgen. The normal ratio of hormones in a woman's body is eight parts oestrogen (female hormone) to one part androgen. The oestrogen affects skin texture and hair resilience. If the balance is disturbed, trichologists believe that regrowth of hair is affected.

Traditionally women have often suffered excessive hair loss a few months after giving birth because after a very high oestrogen level during pregnancy a sudden reduction adversely affects hair. The Pill keeps female hormone levels high and it has been found that women who stop taking it are often subject to the same post-natal symptoms of hair loss.

Anxiety, worry, lack of sleep and bad teeth all contribute to alopecia areata. Mistreatment through indiscriminate colouring or heating can go further than breakage and produce permanent hair loss.

Pulling the hair tightly back into a pony tail can cause inflammation on the scalp's surface or below the outer layer. This disturbs normal growth and the intolerable strain on the hair when repeatedly stretched can make it give up growing at all. The papilla sometimes shrinks and dries up and either a straggly hair emerges or there's stoppage.

Hair loss can often be reversed by finding the source of trouble. Extreme and sudden loss is a medical problem not an aesthetic one. An examination of the body and not just the head, is necessary including a thyroid test, kidney, calcium, enzyme and liver studies. The latest test is to establish if the body is manufacturing enough oestrogen.

UNWANTED HAIR

Everyone has body hair and except in a few cultures it is considered attractive to get rid of it. Dark-haired women usually have more of a problem than fair, because the hair shows more and is coarser. Haphazard hair growth is normal in every woman past puberty. Hormonal changes are a prime influence which is why growth becomes more profuse after the menopause and sometimes during pregnancy. There are many hair-removing methods and the choice depends on personal preference and place of removal:

Abrasion: Use a pumice stone or sandpapery glove. First cut hairs level with the skin, lather with soap and water, then rub away hairs using circular movements. For arms and legs.

Bleaching: For dark hair that is only a soft down. If you use a commercially prepared bleaching preparation, follow instructions carefully. You can make one yourself by mixing 30 per cent peroxide with a little ammonia and water. It is wise to make a skin-patch test 24 hours before the first bleaching. Swab on where needed; hair must be completely stripped of colour, not just to its reddish tones, and this may require two bleachings – done 24 hours apart. For facial hair, forearms and body.

Depilation: The application of chemical depilatories in powder, gel, cream or spray form. They soften and dissolve the hair shaft but do not disturb the root, therefore do not prevent regrowth. They take from 10 to 15 minutes to work on some areas and longer if you have previously shaved. Use of depilatories over a period of time tends to weaken hair growth so new hair is slower to appear and often less noticeable. If you are using one for the first time, make a trial test on a small patch of hair. For legs, arms, underarms – avoid using on the face unless definitely specified for such application.

Electrolysis: This is the only technique that offers reasonable assurance of permanent removal of superfluous hair. A fine wire needle – of platinum or stainless steel – is introduced into the opening of the hair follicle. An electric current of low voltage, lasting up to 40 seconds, is transmitted down the needle to destroy the papilla. The hair shaft is automatically loosened for instant removal. When it is done properly there is a slight burning sensation, though the intensity of feeling varies from person to person. Some women can sleep through a treatment, others find it really hurts. There are no ensuing scars and the hair from that particular papilla should never grow again. The operator needs skill, patience and good eyesight – plus good co-ordination. It takes time because only a certain number of hairs can be removed during one session. Multiple treatments are usually necessary. The alternative to destroying the papilla is to use the same electronic treatment to cauterize the blood vessel and hence stop growth; this is called diathermy. Electrolysis is expensive, but for those with a chronic problem it is worth it. For facial hair primarily, where the area to treat is quite small and doesn't take long, provided you haven't used other methods before. It is often used for hairs around the nipple.

Shaving: The quickest, easiest and cheapest method – and it does not cause hair to grow faster, coarser or darker. What happens is only that the new hair from the shaved pore emerges blunt-cut rather than tapered, so it seems – and indeed feels – more bristly. Use a safety or an electric razor. Watch out for, and try to prevent, dryness and nicking or scraping the skin. The nicks are prevented by always using a clean, sharp blade; for dryness use a special shaving soap or cream which lubricates the skin and stops moisture evaporating. Never shave dry. Wiping a blade can dull its shaving edge, so to clean loosen razor and rinse with hot water, shake, drain. Shave legs upward in long even strokes. Regrowth is rapid because the root is neither removed or damaged but this is a normal rate of growth. For legs and underarms. Don't shave the face, forearms or sensitive body areas. Pubic hair that extends to the upper thighs can be eliminated this way.

Tweezing: Plucking with tweezers is the only practical way to get rid of isolated hairs on the face and chest; it is the one method for trimming eyebrows too. Before tweezing, swab area with an astringent-soaked cotton pad to remove any oily covering and help you to grip the smallest hairs. Re-plucking is required after two to twelve weeks.

For scattered facial hairs – but don't pluck if hair is coming from a mole or wart, check with a dermatologist first. For hairs around the nipples, pluck in the direction of growth while holding skin taut with the other hand. It can hurt.

Waxing: One of the oldest methods of temporary hair removal – a thin layer of melted wax is applied to the skin, allowed to cool, then quickly stripped off tearing the hair out with it but not destroying the roots. The hairs are pulled out from just below the surface of the skin (though the papilla is left intact) which means new hairs are only visible after quite some time, even months. There is no regrowth stubble and in time waxing retards and weakens regrowth. It can hurt enormously depending on the part of the body and your pain endurance level. It can be done in a salon or with a commercial product at home. A home-made recipe is to mix 5 tablespoons of sugar into 5 tablespoons of water, add the juice of half a lemon; cook slowly or in a double boiler, stirring and waiting until it turns a caramel colour. Pour onto a plate and work into little balls. Press the ball firmly onto the skin, hold, pull it up sharply extracting excess hair with it. It takes a long, long time.

THE FACE

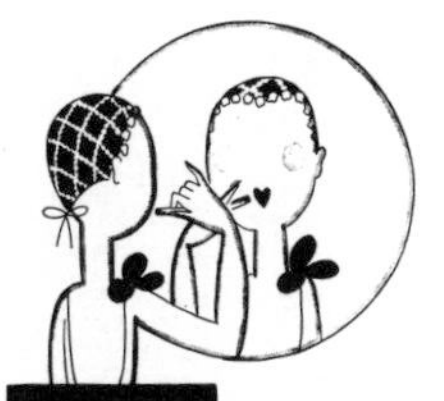
Groundwork

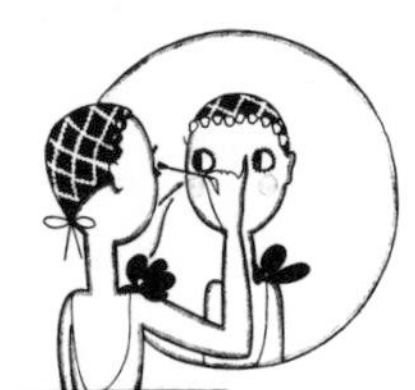
Chiaroscuro

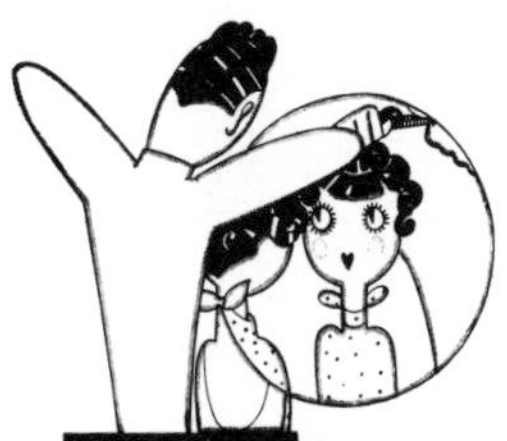
Expert Assistance

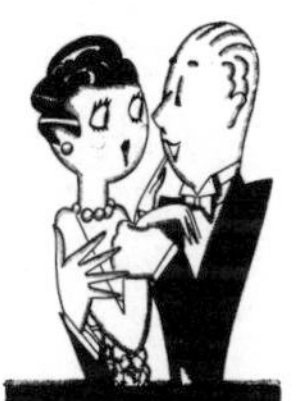
The Kill

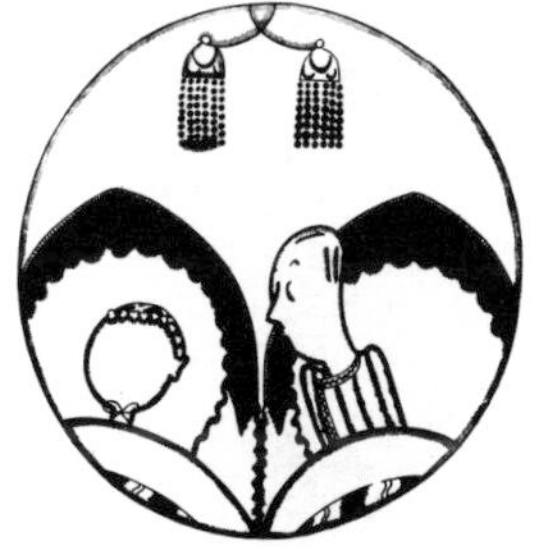
Disillusion

An Artistic Adventure
With A Catastrophic Climax
Drawn by Fish

In 1921 Vogue *said: 'The face that can render a song without words has a lasting charm, for expression is the better part of beauty, being much more than skin deep.' Obvious make-up was in 'disrepute' and cosmetics designed to 'reproduce natural tints to perfection'. But by the end of the decade beauty meant more than 'a pink and white doll's face' and it could 'cost as much in upkeep as a Rolls Royce'. In the 1930s the movies were 'the most perfect visual medium for the exploitation of fashion and beauty'. Everyone wanted Joan Crawford's bow-tie mouth, Dietrich's plucked eyebrows, Vivien Leigh's gypsy colouring.* Vogue *said: 'It is your job to spend gallantly, dress decoratively, be groomed immaculately – in short to be a sight for sore eyes.' Cyclax promised to transform 'jaded Lady into glamorous Jade' and Tattoo lipstick offered 'soft, inviting, youthful lips . . . luscious alluring colour that does not smear but stays on . . . through cocktails, cigarettes . . . everything!' With the war cosmetics disappeared from the counters but ladies were reassured: 'Four fundamental cosmetics you need are unrestricted – sleep, diet, exercise, rest for 20 minutes a day after lunch.' But in 1947 Dior's New Look gave women a new outlook on beauty and 'natural' make-up was considered rather 'mawkish'. Skin care was all important in the 1950s with the 'famous three' steps – cleansing, stimulating and nourishing. With a 'Magic Iron' you could make 'fine lines disappear . . . crepiness give way to smoothness . . . and formant tissues wake up to fresh activity'. With Helena Rubinstein's Estrogenci Oil you could even make 'time stand still'. Eyes became 'doe eyes' and eye make-up even more important than lipstick.* Vogue *suggested: 'Eyes made mysterious with eyebrow pencil and a dusky shadow, and strip eyelashes of nylon.' The 1960s saw the beginning of the back to nature trend while the cosmetic industry still promised 'miracles' . . . 'revelation in nail polish chemistry' . . . 'revolutionary creams and preparations'. The London Look of the mid-1960s was copied throughout the world and Jean Shrimpton's was the look; Elizabeth Taylor the last of the world-famous movie stars. With the 1970s your face, like fashion could be as you like it . . . spectacular like Bianca Jagger . . . naturally sophisticated like Twiggy . . . naturally beautiful like Marisa Berenson. A last suggestion: 'Try looking like a lady.'*

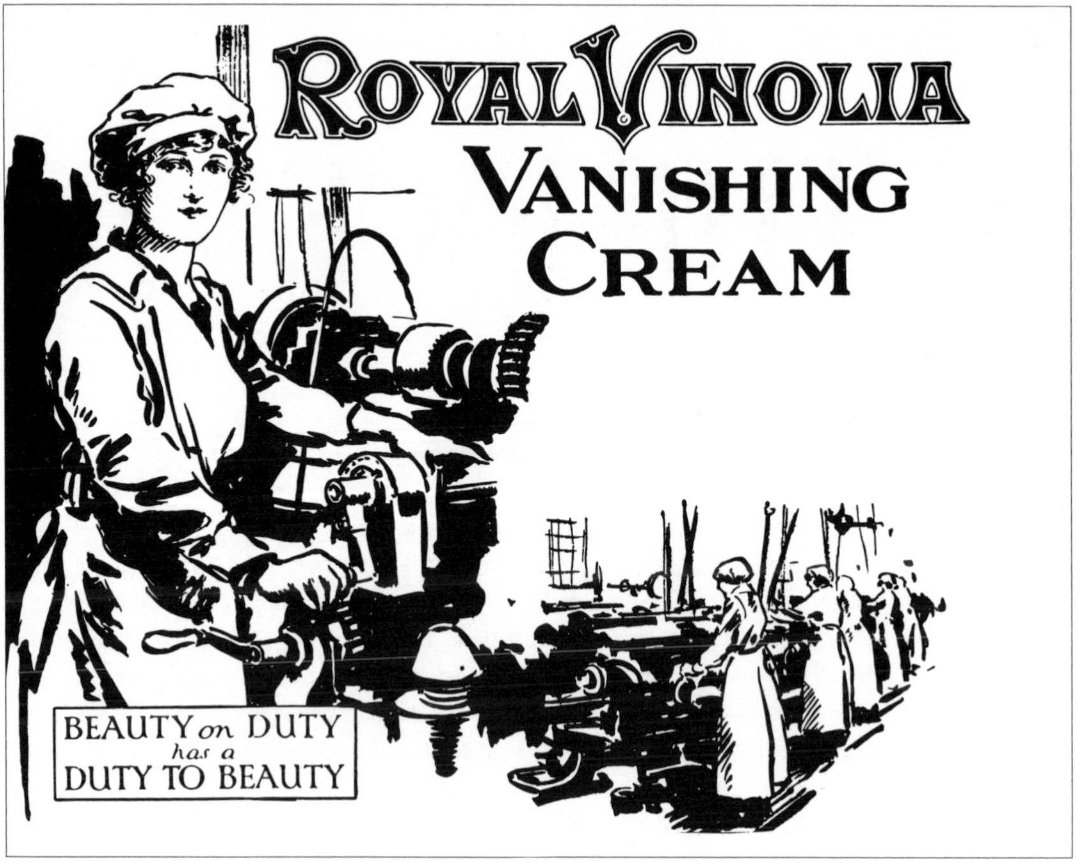

ROYAL VINOLIA
VANISHING CREAM

BEAUTY on DUTY
has a
DUTY TO BEAUTY

1918

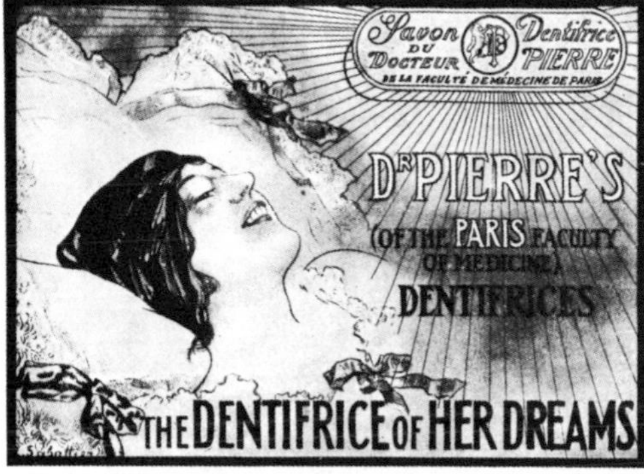

Savon du Docteur Dentifrice Pierre
DE LA FACULTÉ DE MÉDECINE DE PARIS
DR PIERRE'S
(OF THE PARIS FACULTY OF MEDICINE)
DENTIFRICES
THE DENTIFRICE OF HER DREAMS

1919

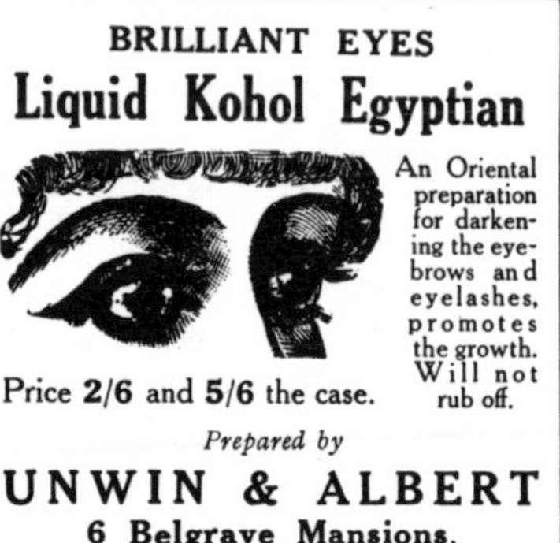

BRILLIANT EYES
Liquid Kohol Egyptian
An Oriental preparation for darkening the eyebrows and eyelashes, promotes the growth. Will not rub off.
Price 2/6 and 5/6 the case.
Prepared by
UNWIN & ALBERT
6 Belgrave Mansions,
LONDON S.W.

1916

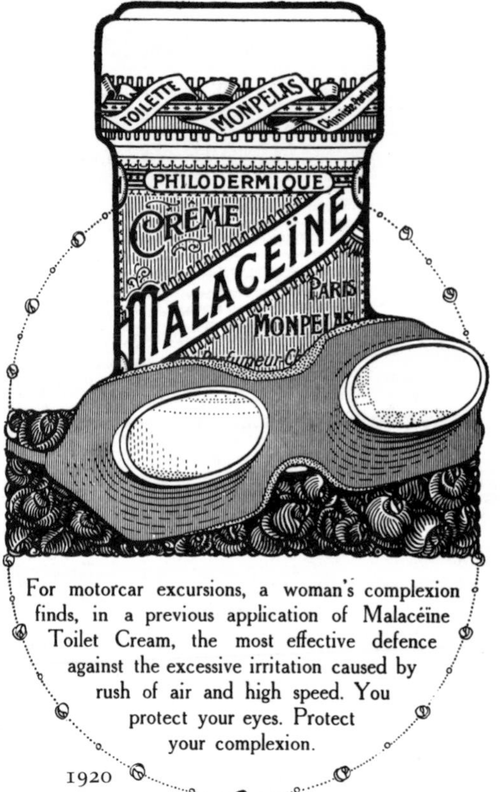

TOILETTE MONPELAS
PHILODERMIQUE
CRÊME
MALACEÏNE
PARIS
MONPELAS
For motorcar excursions, a woman's complexion finds, in a previous application of Malacéïne Toilet Cream, the most effective defence against the excessive irritation caused by rush of air and high speed. You protect your eyes. Protect your complexion.

1920

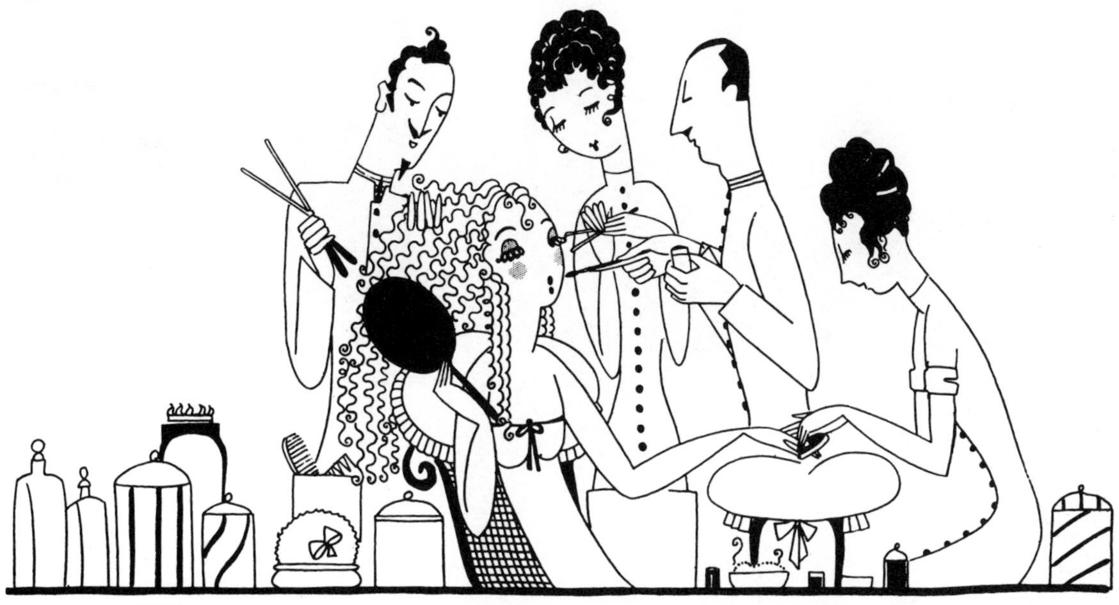

FISH 1923

'A woman who is a beauty has no need – and no time – to be anything else. Courage, patience and perseverance must be among her virtues, but the end justifies the means. Success in her chosen career brings everything that is most dear to the heart of woman – a jealous husband, envious women friends and admiring grand-grandchildren. Besides which she gives pleasure to connoisseurs and employment to many amiable and deserving people.'

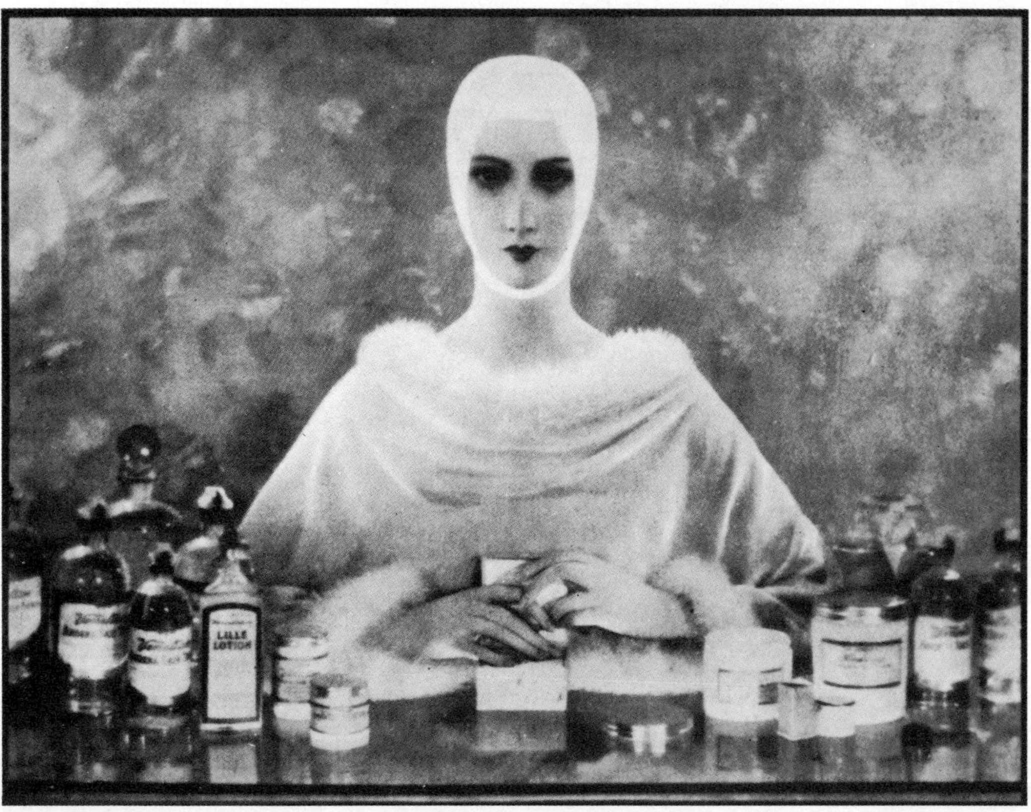

DE MEYER 1932

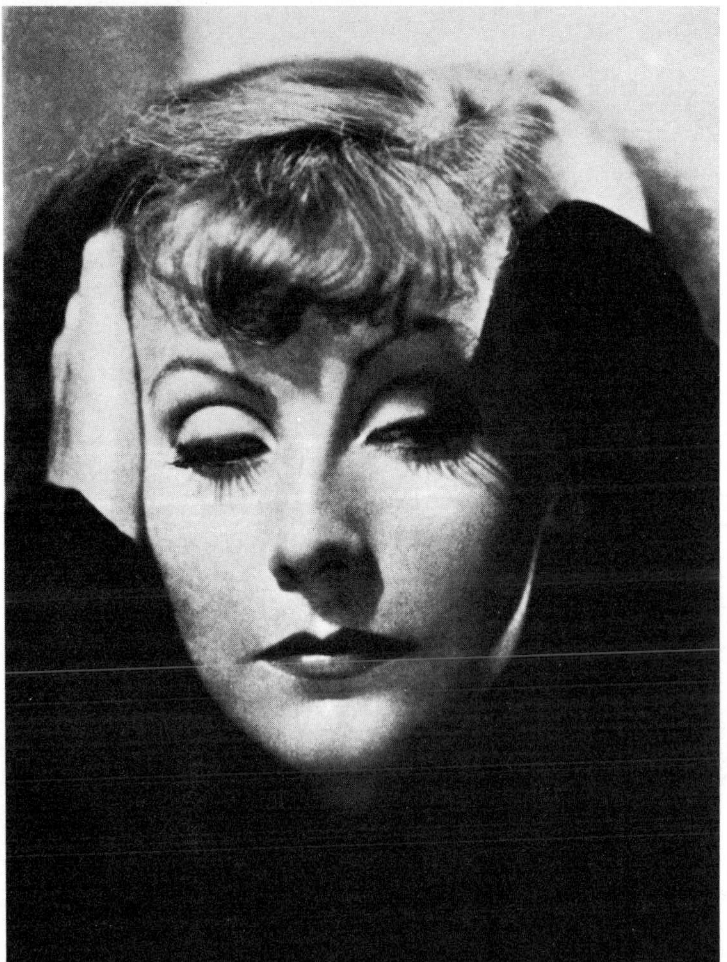

Garbo STEICHEN

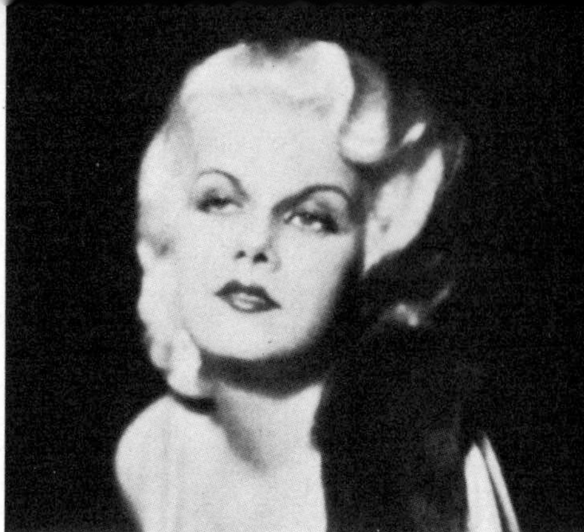

Jean Harlow

'Anthropologists of the future, when bending their beards over cinema archives, will unearth a perplexing phenomenon. They will discover that whereas early in the twentieth century the female citizens of Hollywood were various in type, about 1931–32 they suddenly all began to look alike. The chief points of this resemblance are blondish hair, worn untidily in a long bob, narrow eyebrows arching skywards, and incredibly long eyelashes. These are augmented by a sullen lower lip and a gaunt look which will doubtless cause the inference that all actresses at this era were the victims of an unpleasant internal disorder. Of course, this is not true. What has really happened is demonstrated in the photographs (below). The upper row depicts them in the sunny days of their pre-Nordic innocency. Then came Garbo. Below are shown the ensuing metamorphoses.'

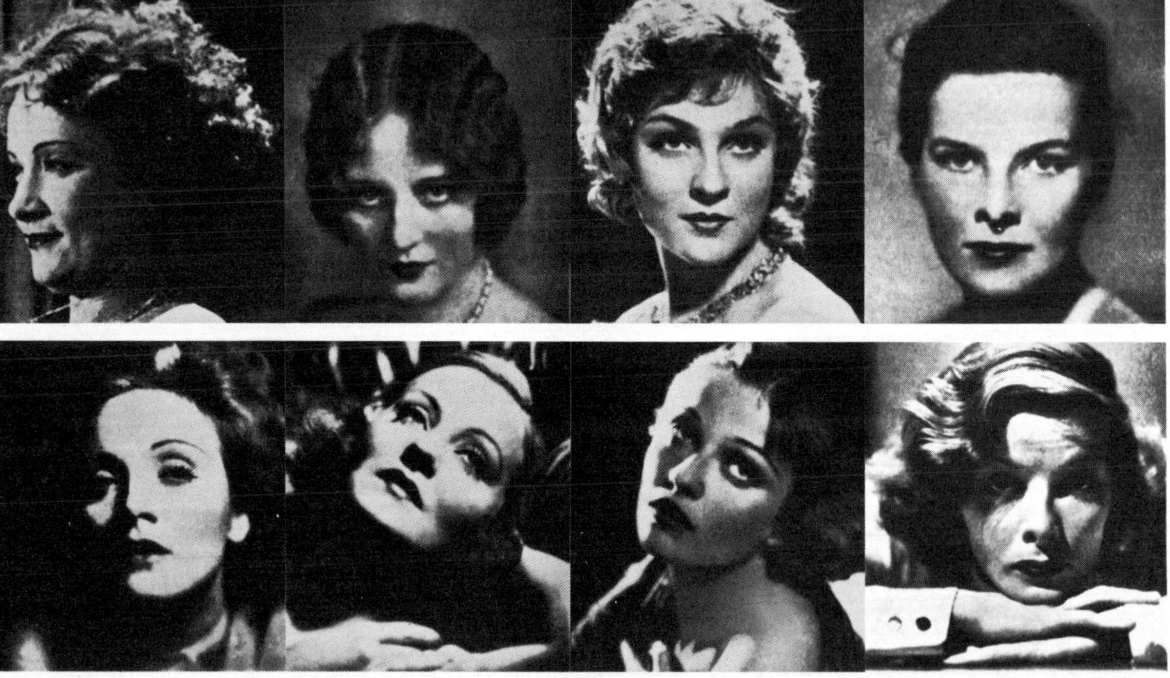

Marlene Dietrich Tallulah Bankhead Anna Sten Katharine Hepburn

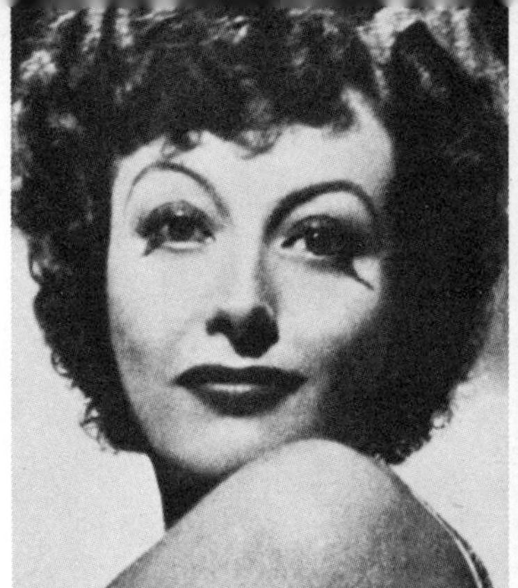
Joan Crawford

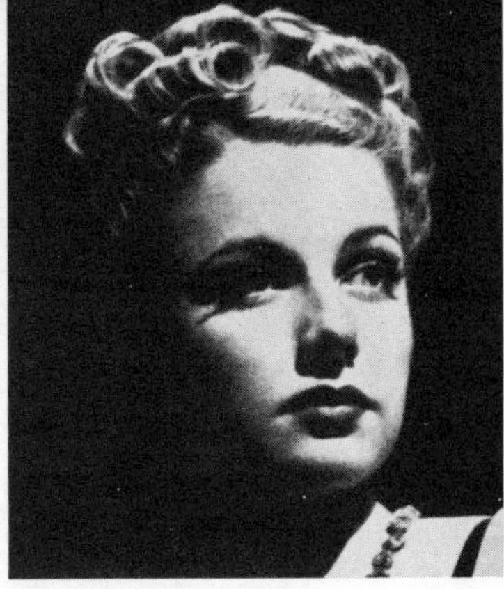
Ann Sheridan

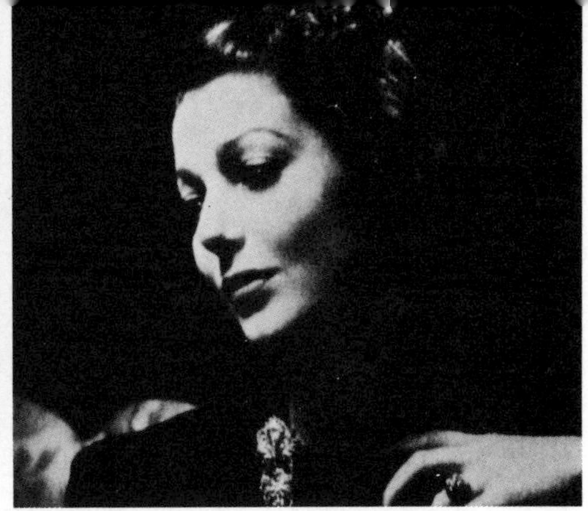
Loretta Young

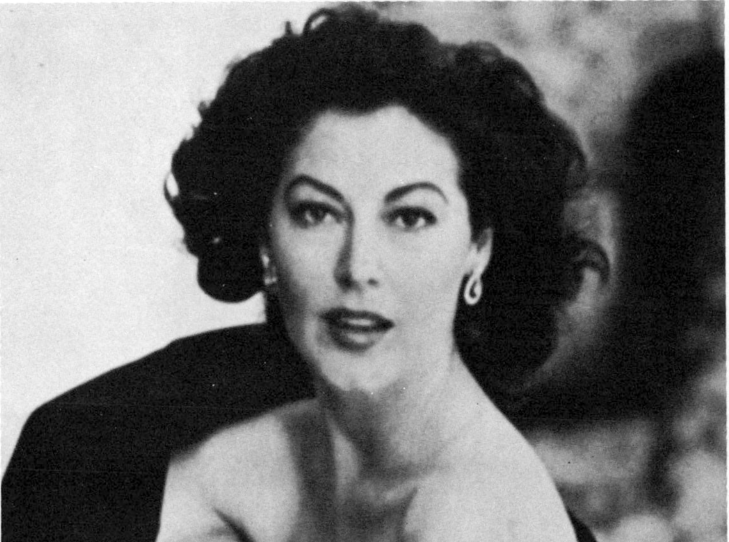
Ava Gardner

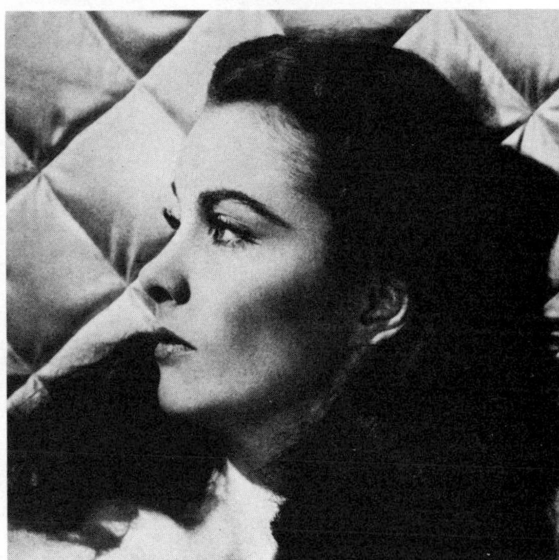
Vivien Leigh

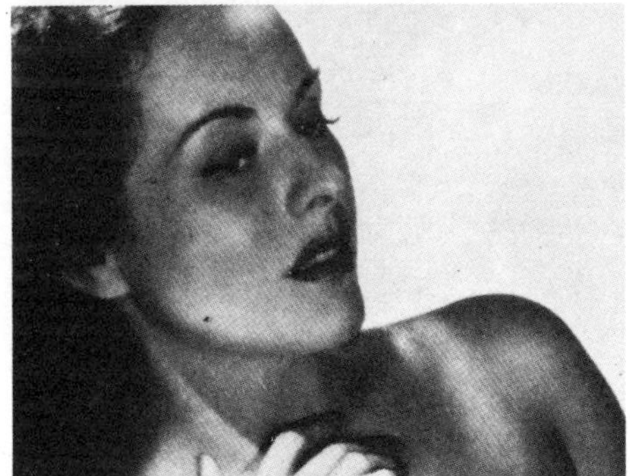
Paulette Goddard

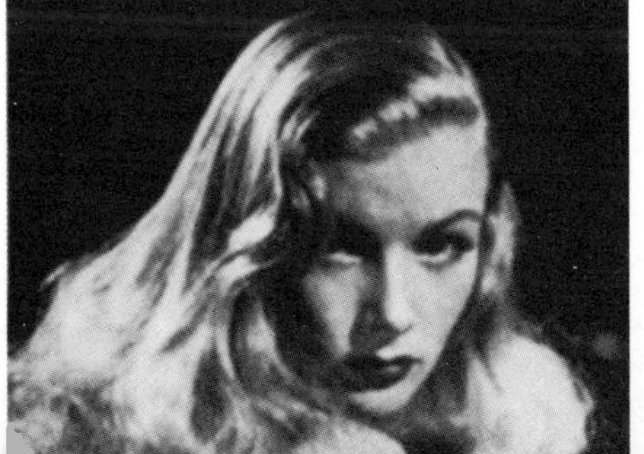
Veronica Lake

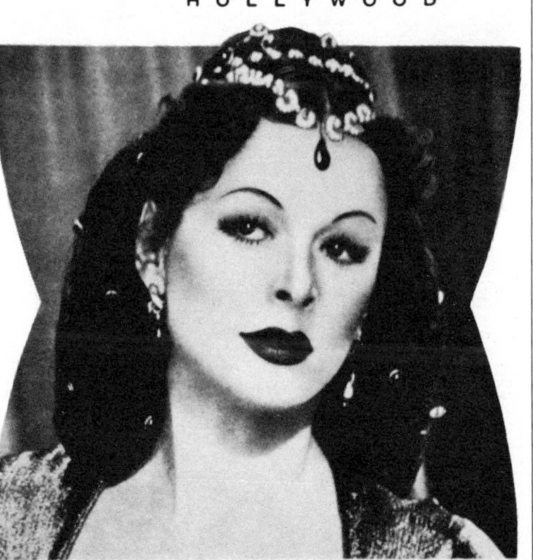

Hedy Lamarr

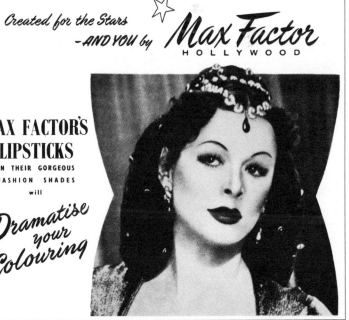

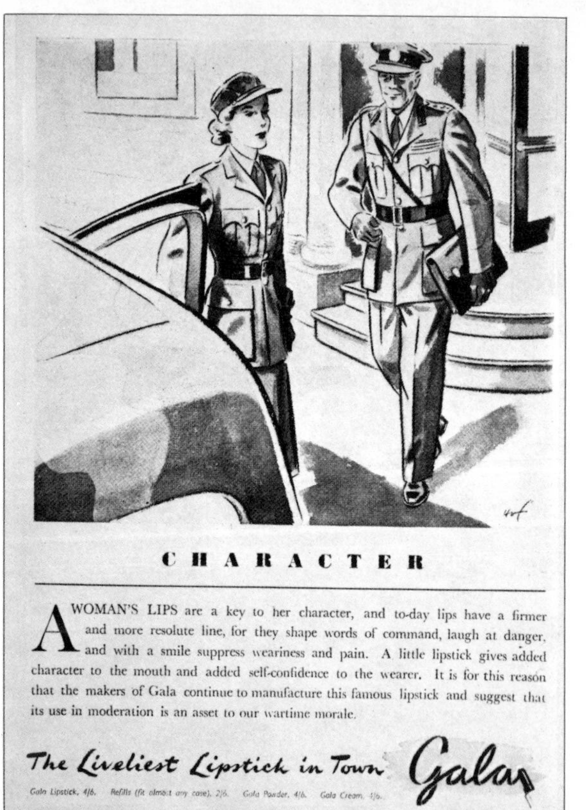

CHARACTER
A WOMAN'S LIPS are a key to her character, and to-day lips have a firmer and more resolute line, for they shape words of command, laugh at danger, and with a smile suppress weariness and pain. A little lipstick gives added character to the mouth and added self-confidence to the wearer. It is for this reason that the makers of Gala continue to manufacture this famous lipstick and suggest that its use in moderation is an asset to our wartime morale.
The Liveliest Lipstick in Town
Gala
Gala Lipstick, 4/6. Refills (fit almost any case), 2/6. Gala Powder, 4/6. Gala Cream, 4/6.

1943

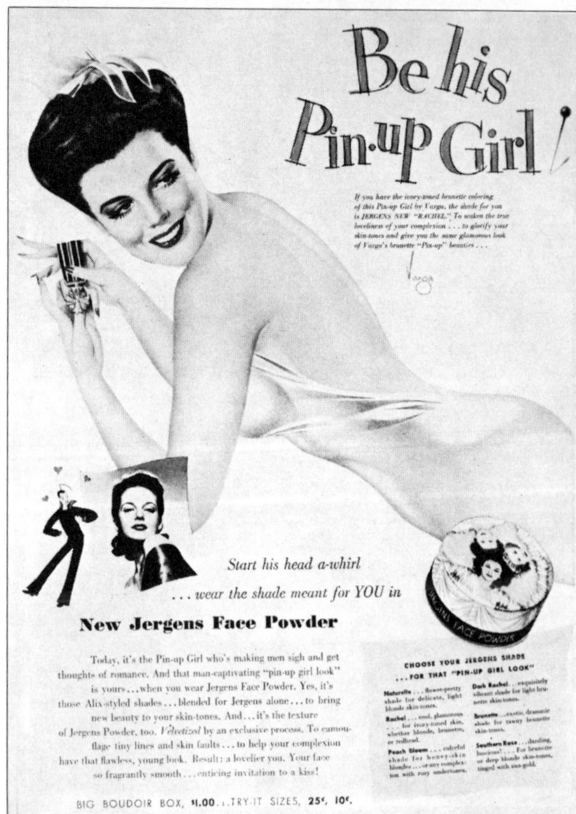

Be his Pin-up Girl!
If you have the ivory-toned brunette coloring of this Pin-up Girl by Vargo, the shade for you is JERGENS NEW "RACHEL." To waken the true loveliness of your complexion . . . to glorify your skin-tones and give you the same glamorous look of Vargo's brunette "Pin-up" beauties . . .
Start his head a-whirl
. . . wear the shade meant for YOU in
New Jergens Face Powder
Today, it's the Pin-up Girl who's making men sigh and get thoughts of romance. And that man-captivating "pin-up girl look" is yours . . . when you wear Jergens Face Powder. Yes, it's those Alix-styled shades . . . blended for Jergens alone . . . to bring new beauty to your skin-tones. And . . . it's the texture of Jergens Powder, too. Velvetized by an exclusive process. To camouflage tiny lines and skin faults . . . to help your complexion have that flawless, young look. Result: a lovelier you. Your face so fragrantly smooth . . . enticing invitation to a kiss!
CHOOSE YOUR JERGENS SHADE
. . . FOR THAT "PIN-UP GIRL LOOK"
Naturelle
Rachel
Peach Bloom
Dark Rachel
Brunette
Southern Rose
JERGENS FACE POWDER
BIG BOUDOIR BOX, $1.00 . . . TRY-IT SIZES, 25¢, 10¢.

1943

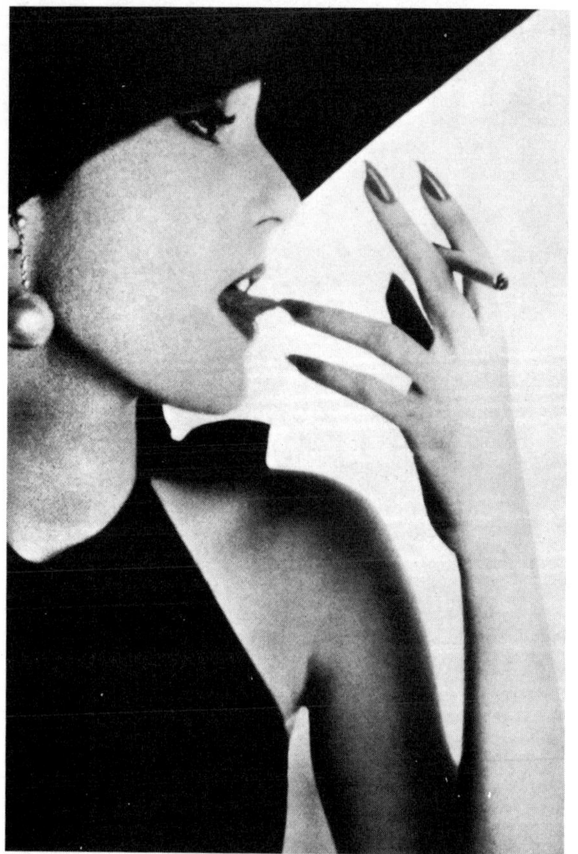

PENN 1951

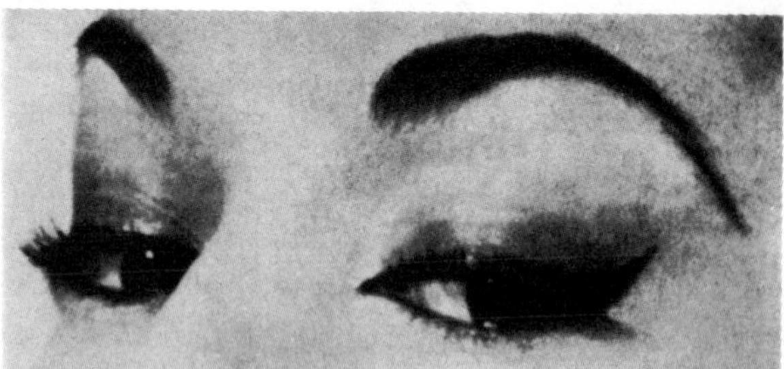

BLUMENFELD 1950

'The 1950 look is the "doe-eyed" look introduced by Piguet in Paris. It could become, we think, as generally and excitingly new as the use of lipstick was in the twenties.'

'With summer and the prevalence of black and white comes a new silhouette-sharpness of make-up. The eyes, lips and nails – often the only colour in the ensemble – are emphasised with bold strokes. Strengthen the browline, sharpen the outline of your lips. This is the moment to use your eye and lip liners, your battery of brushes, and – new too this season – to file your longer nails to an accentuated point, as those of the girl in the picture.'

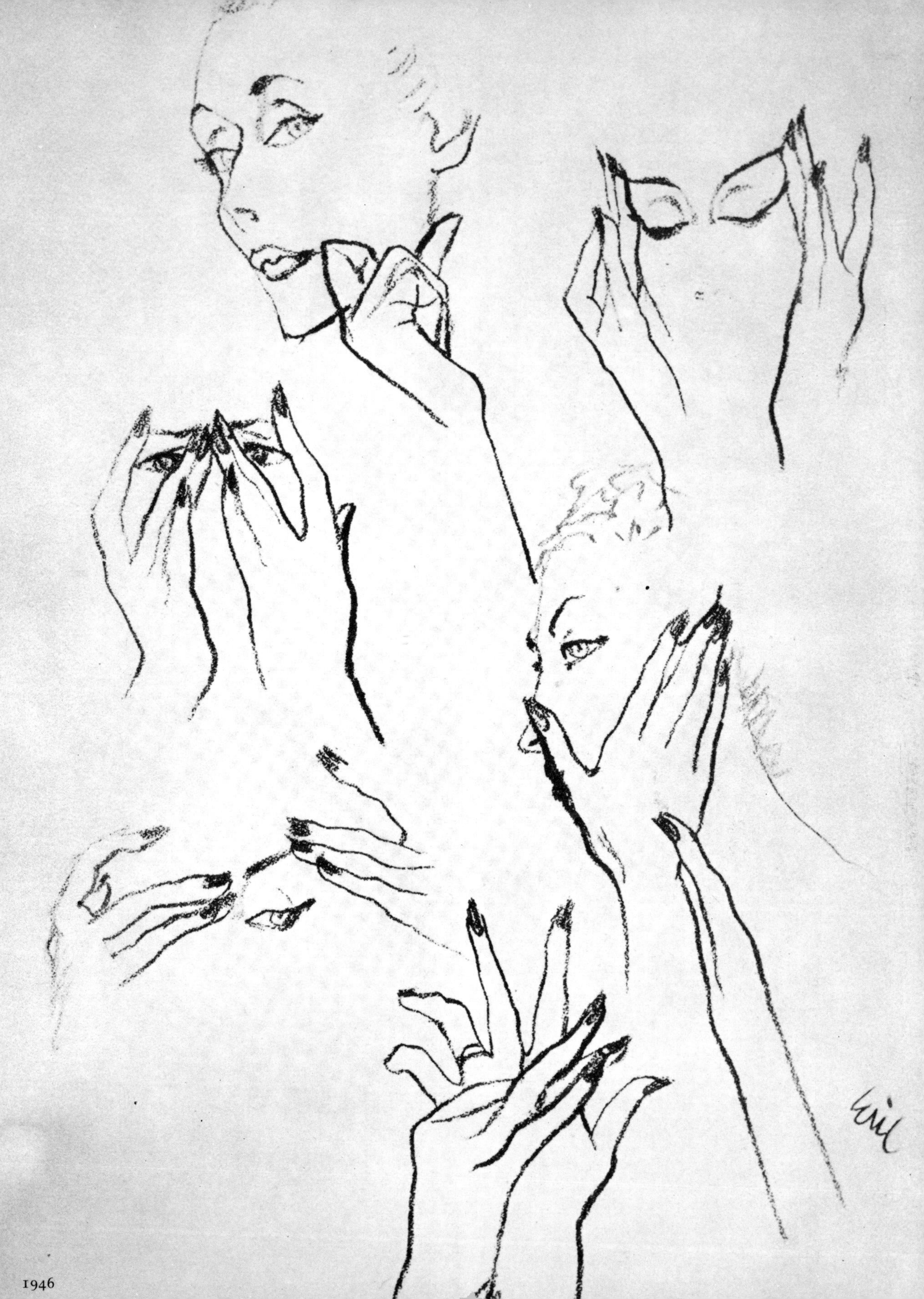

1946

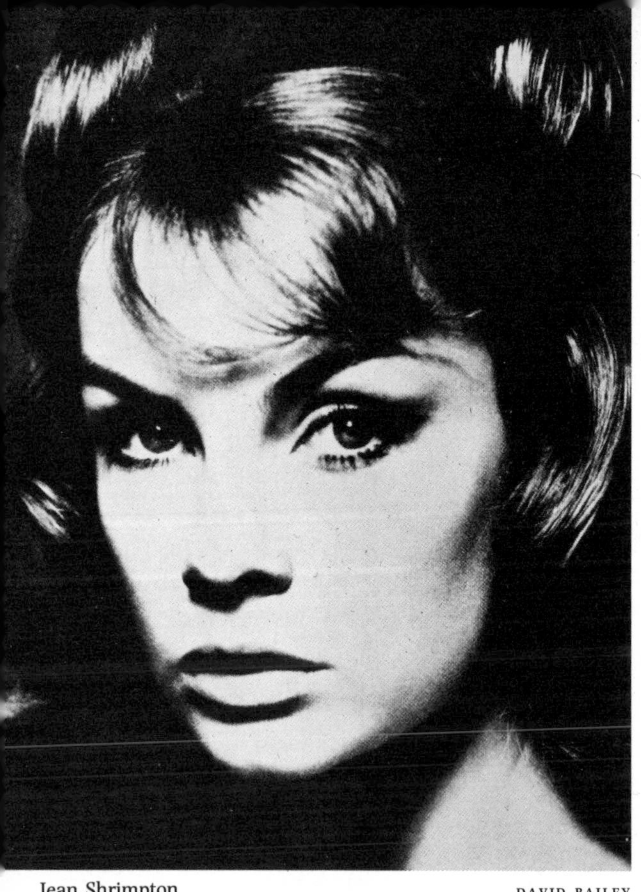

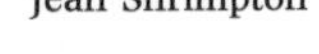
Jean Shrimpton 
DAVID BAILEY

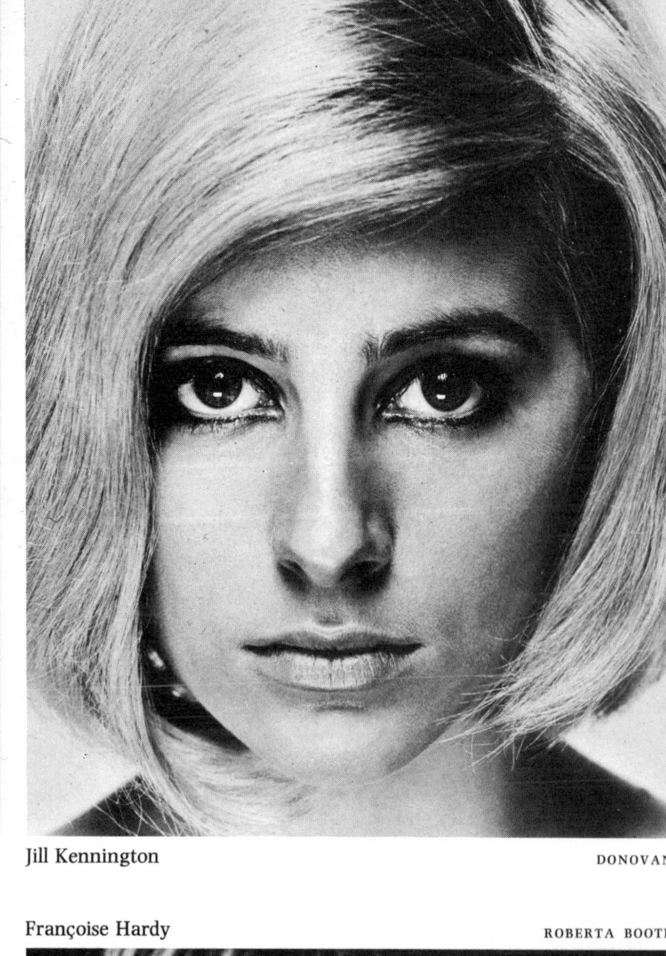

Jill Kennington DONOVAN

Twiggy NORMAN PARKINSON

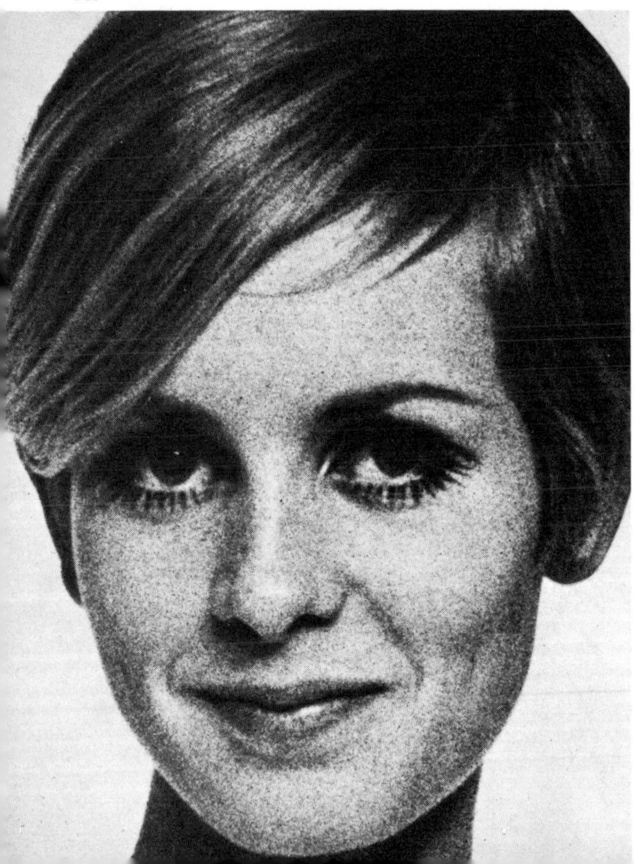

Françoise Hardy ROBERTA BOOTH

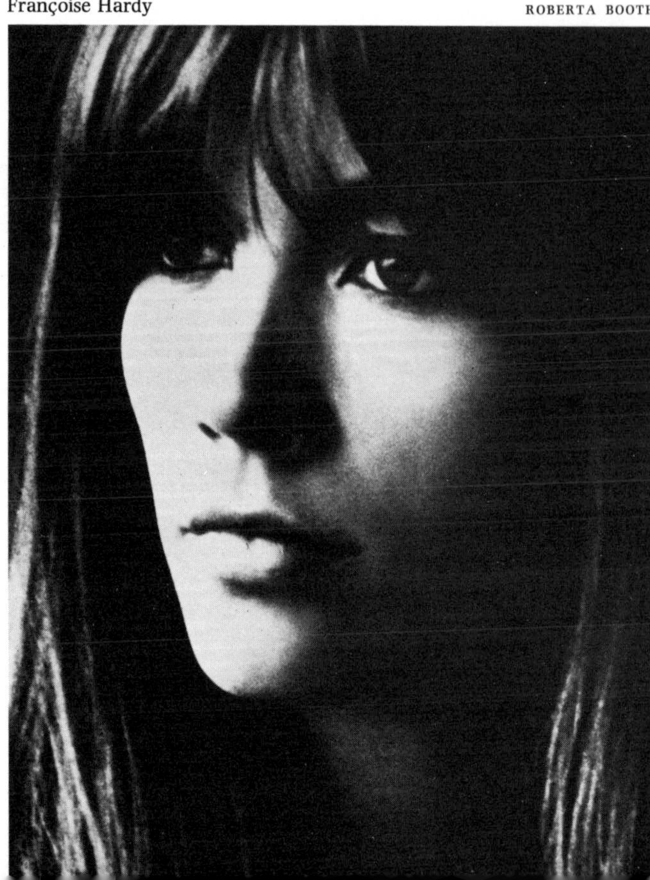

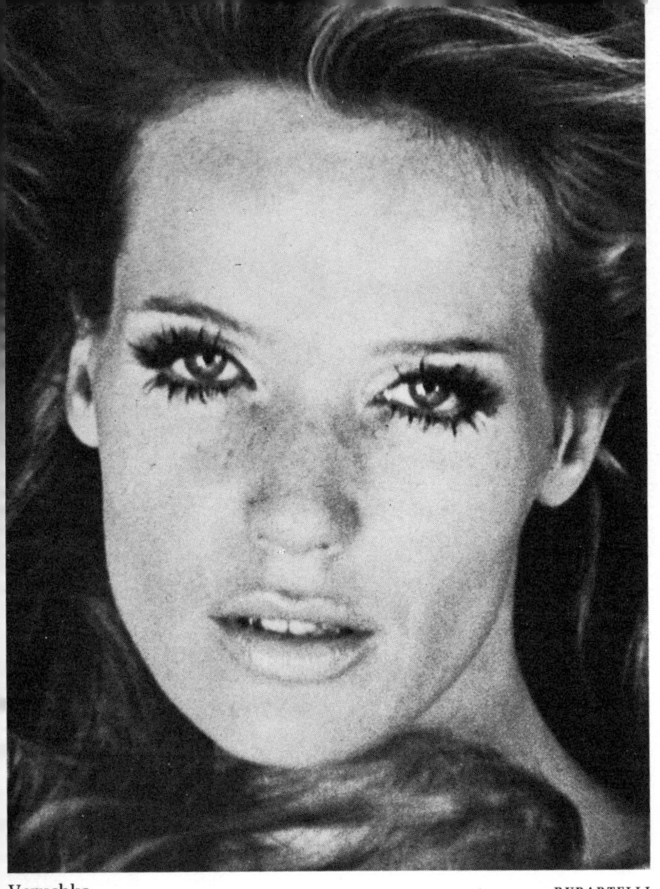

Verushka RUBARTELLI

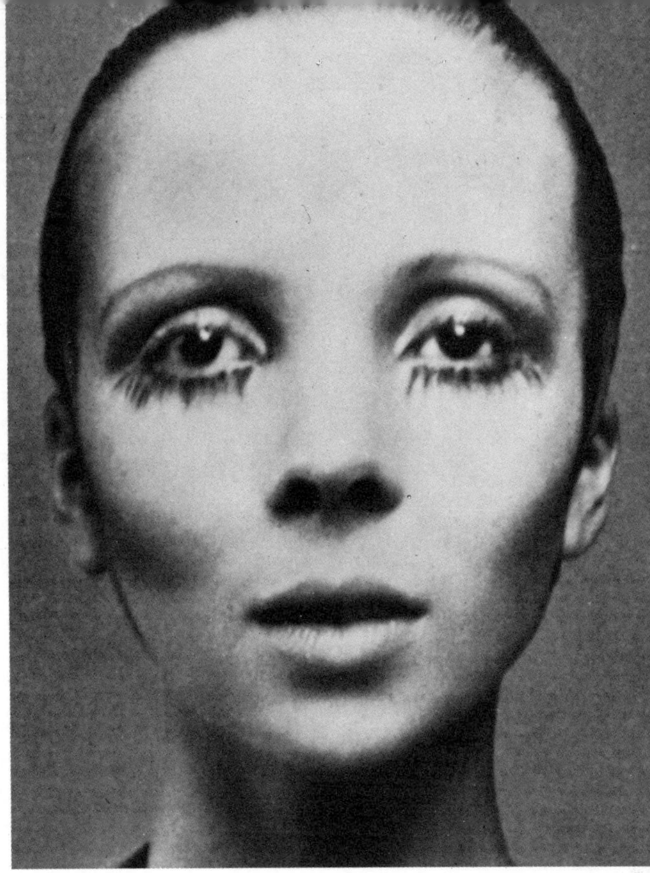

Penelope Tree AVEDON

Karen Graham KOURKEN PAKCHANIAN

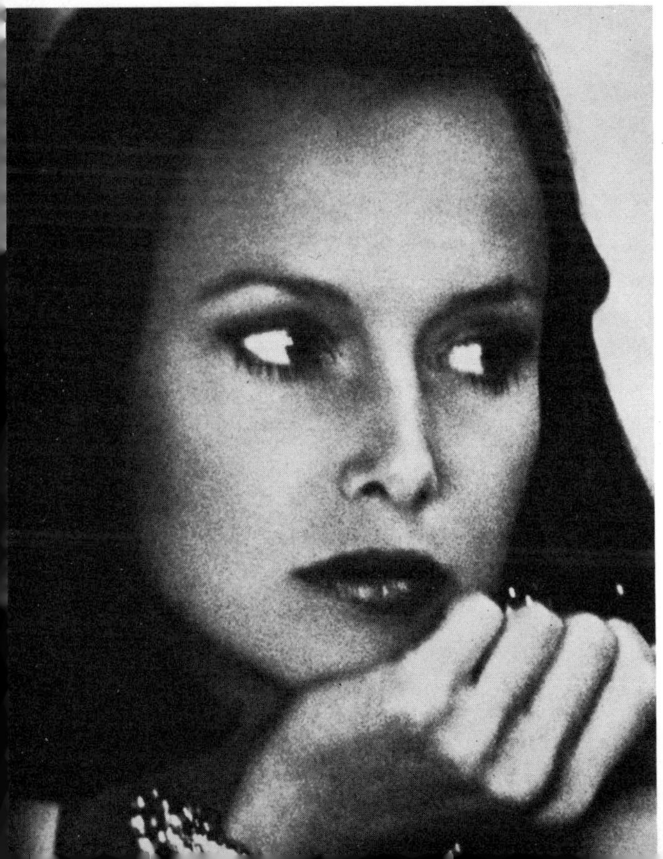

Maudie James DAVID BAILEY

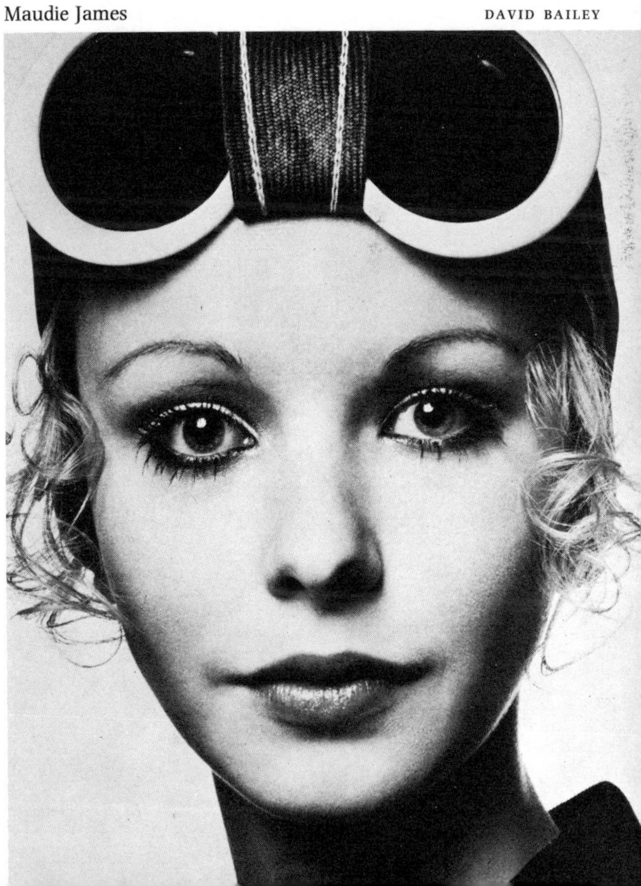

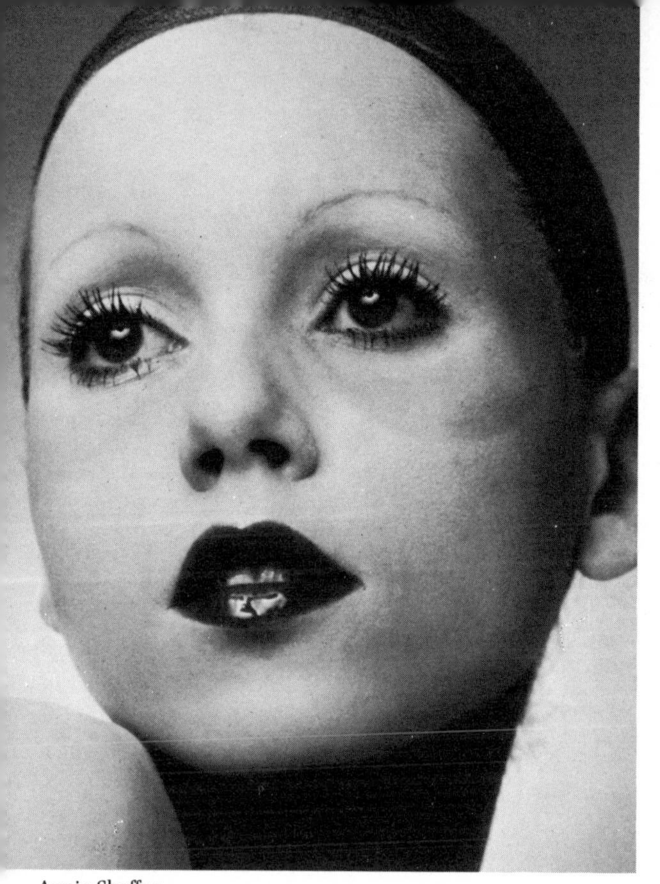

Annie Shaffus ARROWSMITH

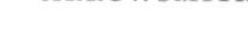

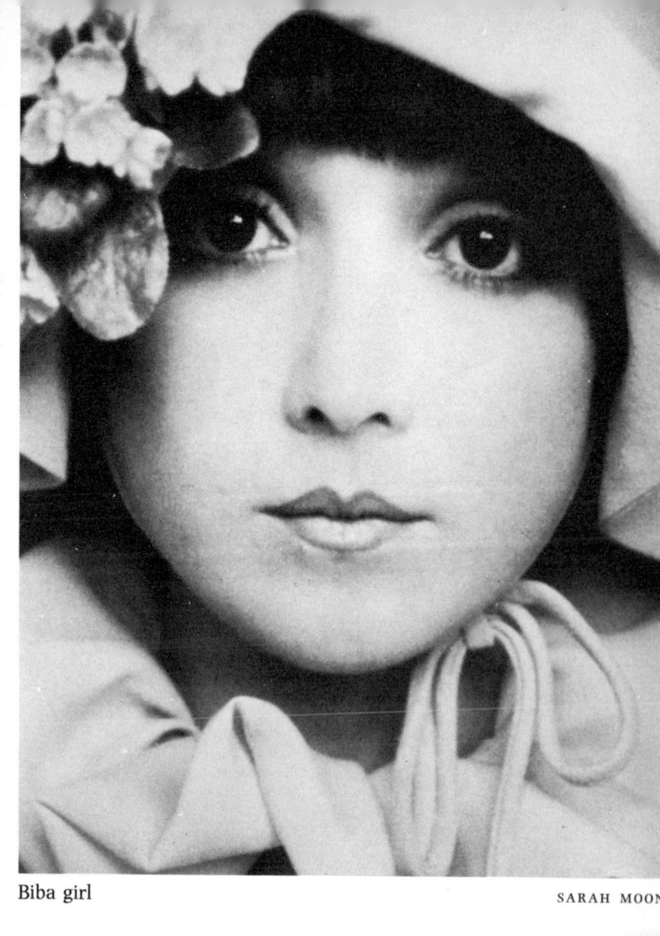

Biba girl SARAH MOON

Grace Coddington BARRY LATEGAN

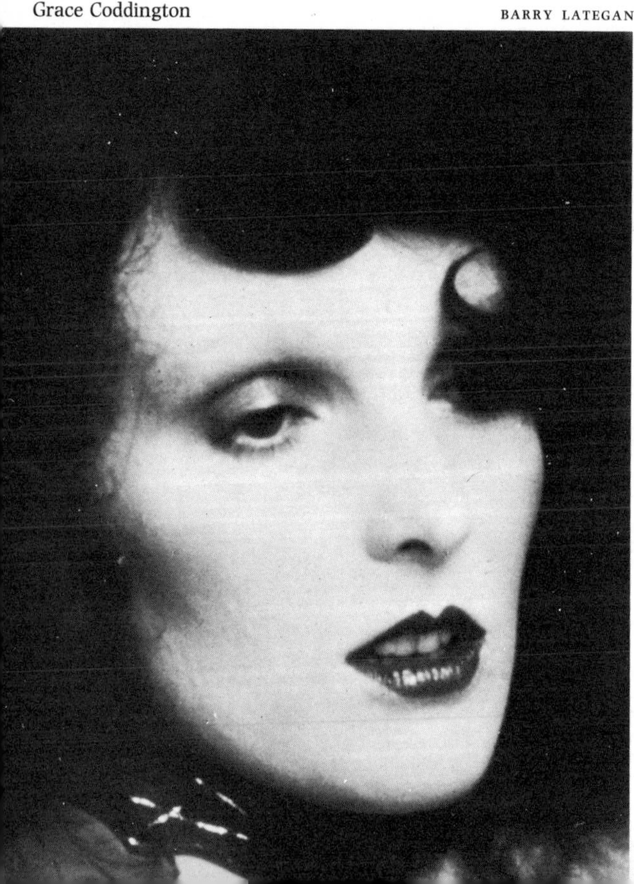

Lauren Hutton EVA SERENY

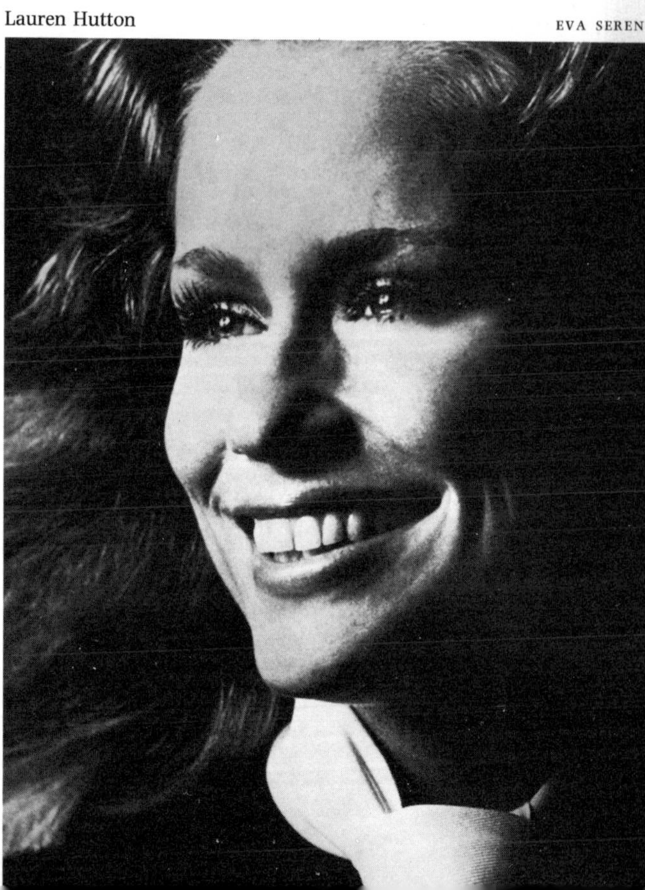

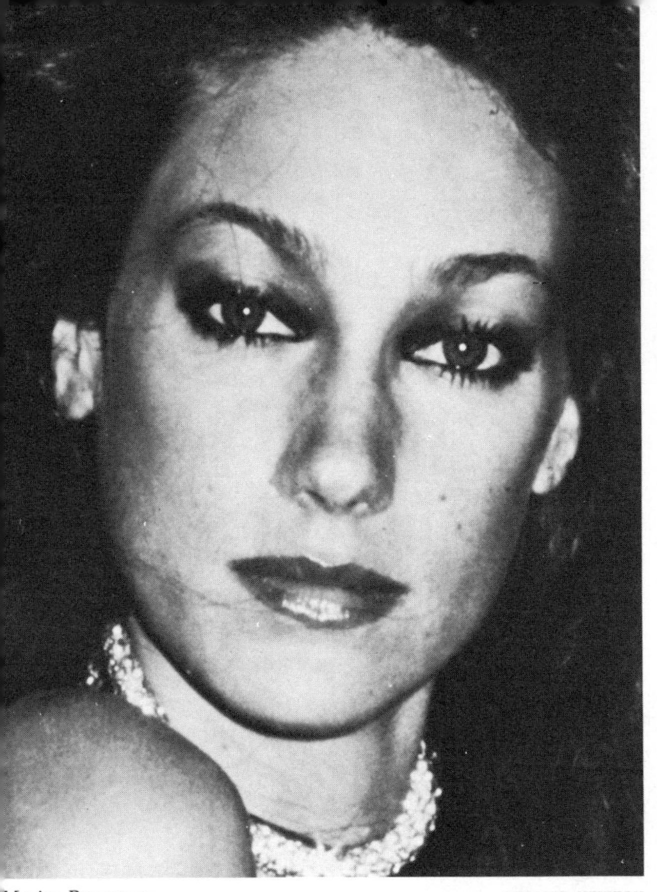

Marisa Berenson HELMUT NEWTON

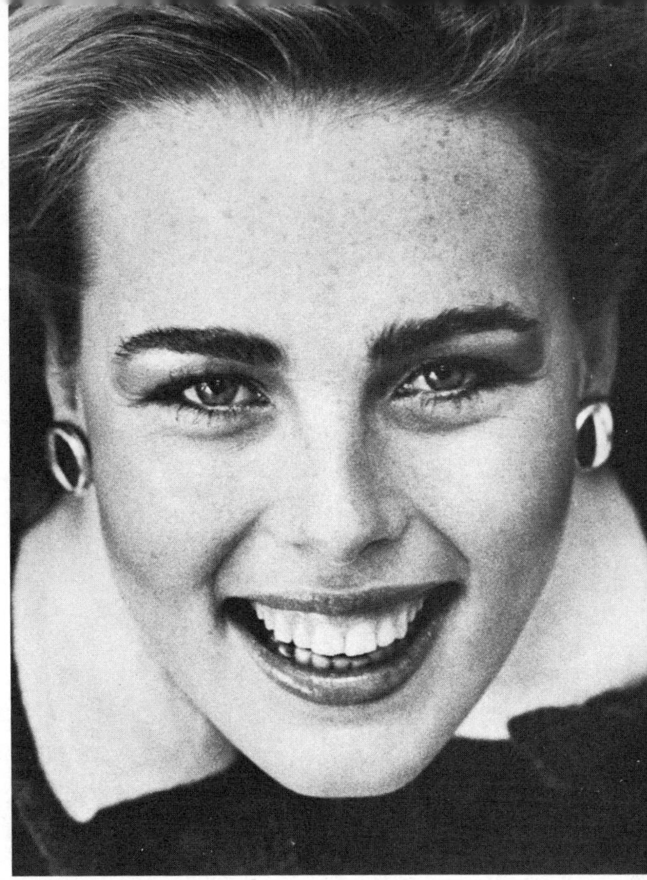

Margaux Hemingway TOSCANI

Bianca Jagger DAVID BAILEY

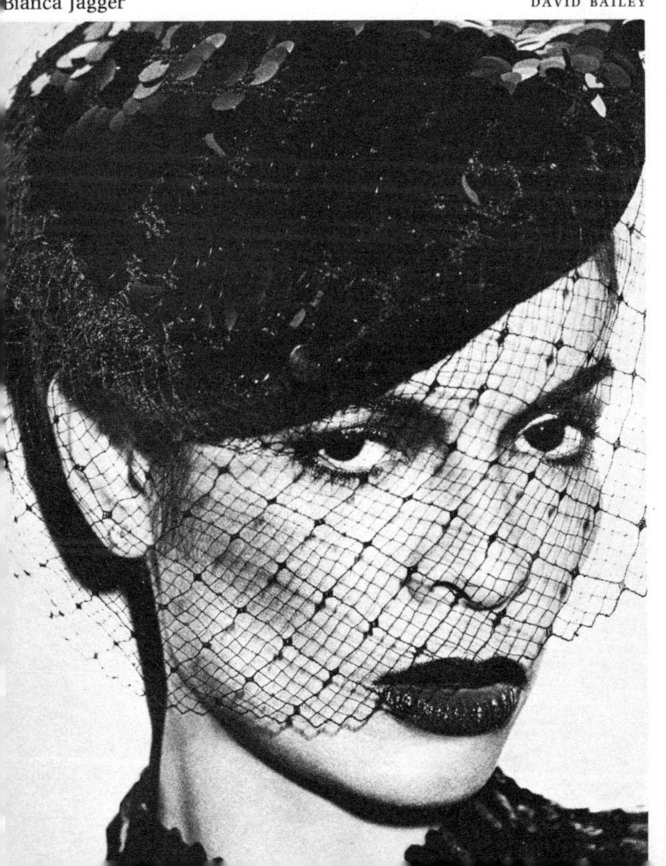

Marie Helvin DAVID BAILEY

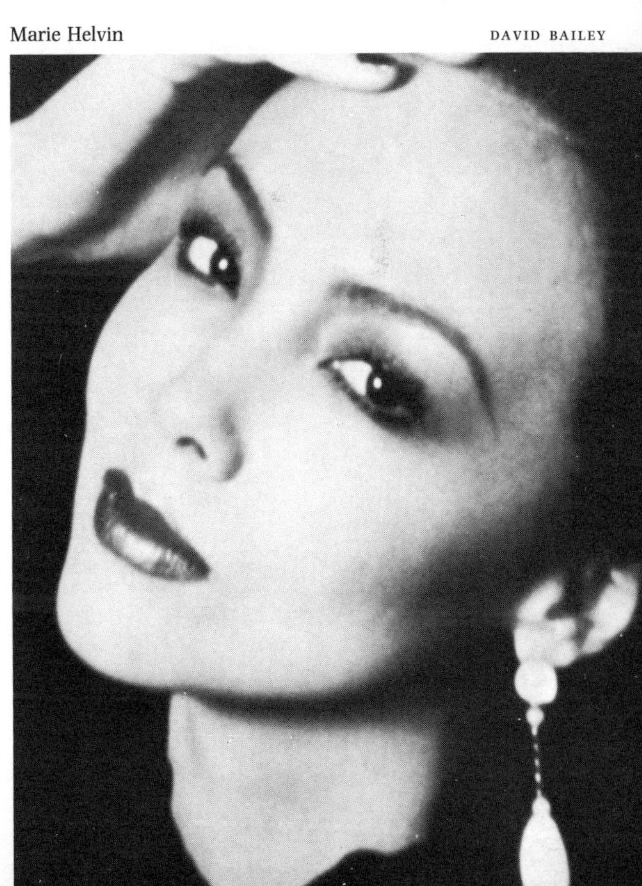

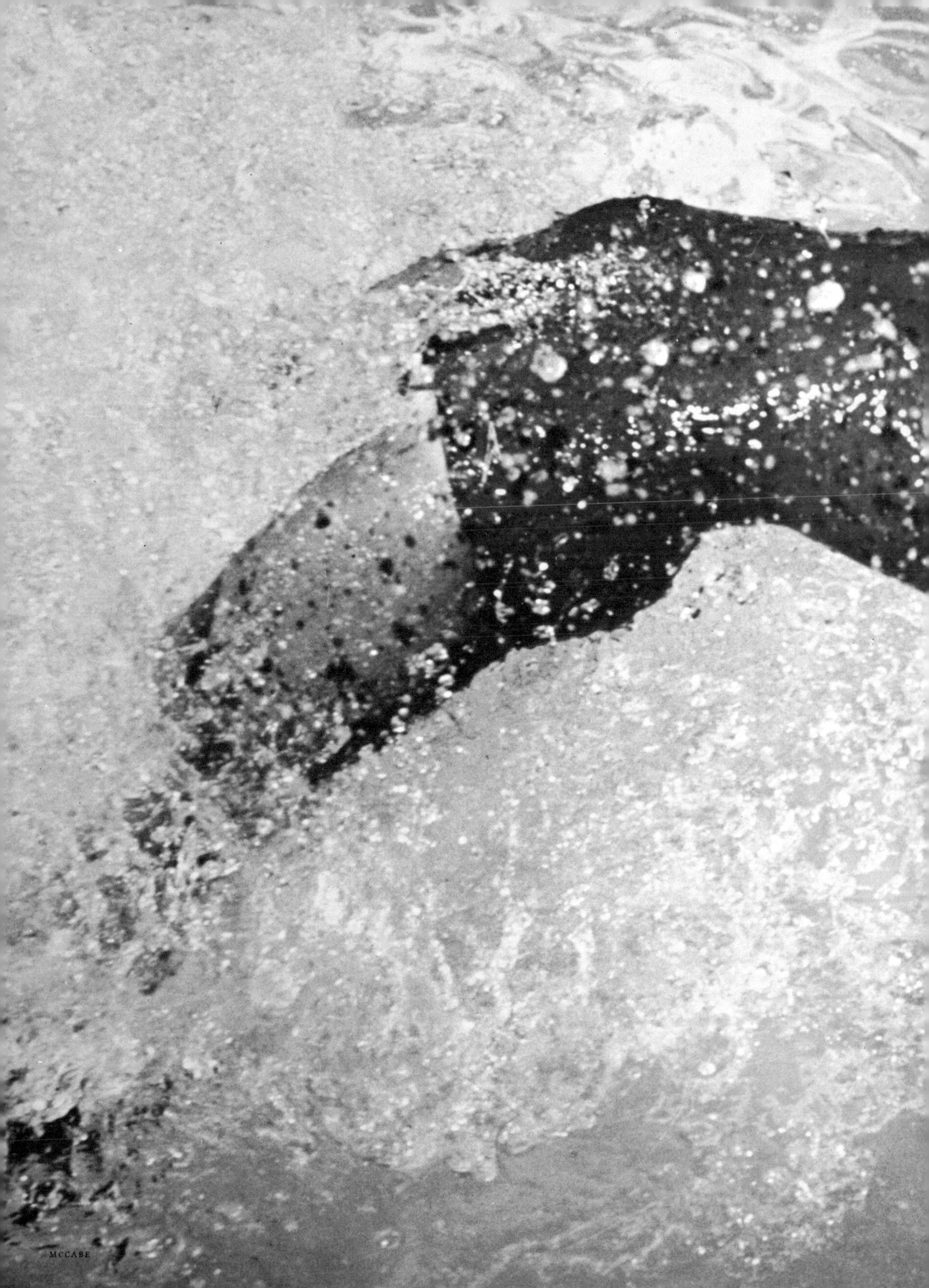

MCCABE

PART II THE AESTHETICS

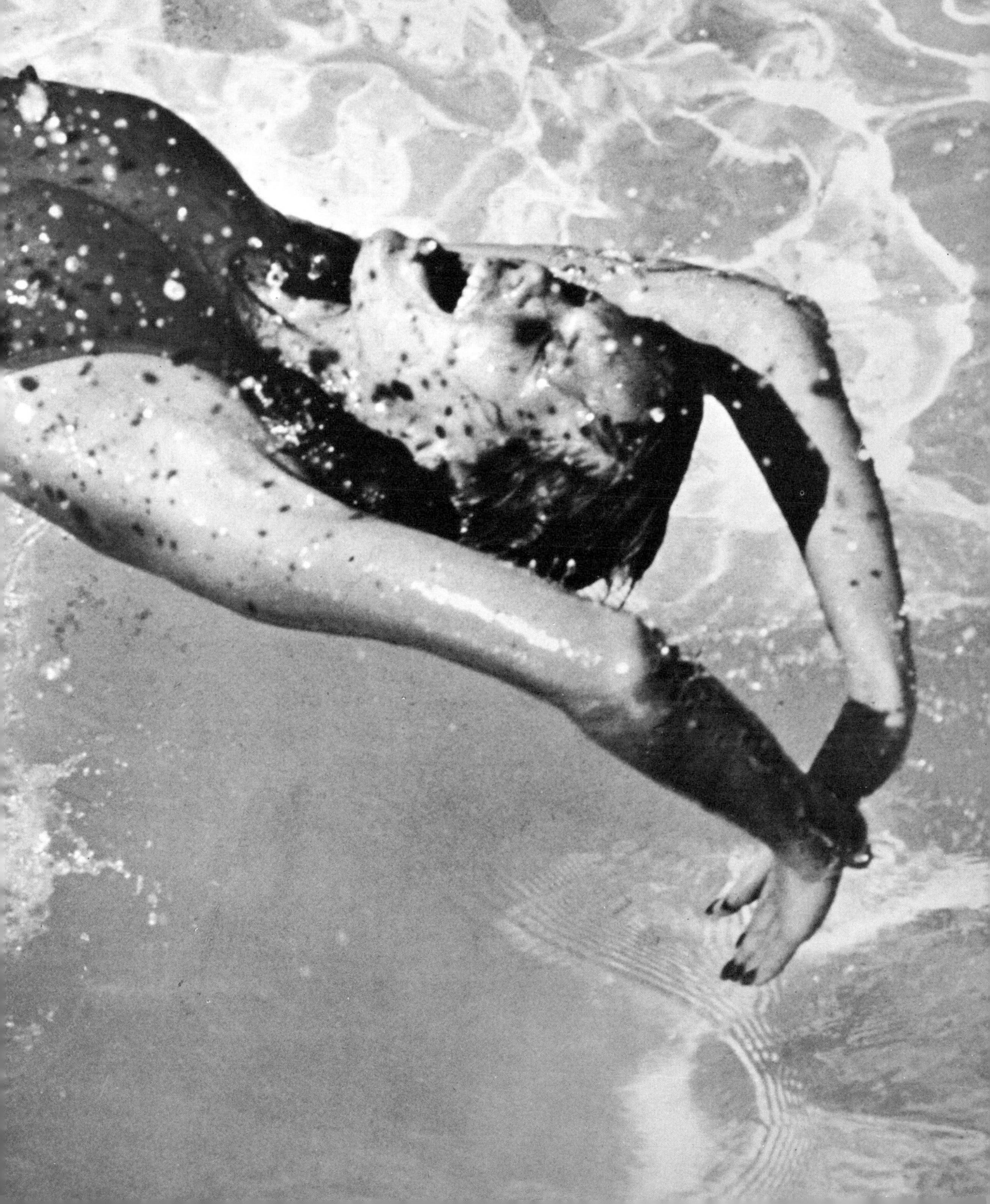

1

NATURAL PREPARATIONS

Some of the most satisfactory beauty products – facials, cleansers, conditioners, tonics – are those you can make yourself with familiar ingredients from formulas handed down, added to and improved upon over the years. It will take time to determine which are the best formulas for your particular skin. Not every recipe will be right or bring exceptional results. You need to learn to adjust the ingredients, to meet your own specific requirements; climate conditions often alter textures.

Home made skin preparations lack the usual preservatives of chemical additives, so will not last long. Make small quantities, and keep chilled any recipe containing perishable food, such as milk, eggs, wheatgerm.

The following recipes are classified according to their function. They are limited to the more simple preparations requiring the minimum effort in the making and in the search for ingredients.

CLEANSERS

Almond Cleansing Cream

4 oz. (120 g.) oil of sweet almonds
1 oz. (30 g.) hydrous lanolin
1 oz. (30 g.) petroleum jelly

Melt the fats slowly in a double boiler; remove from heat; beat until cool.

Lotion for Dry Skin

1 oz. (30 g.) mineral oil
2½ oz. (75 g.) glycerine
4 oz. (120 g.) milk of magnesia
4 oz. (120 g.) witch hazel

Stir slowly together all the ingredients; keep in a tightly covered glass bottle and shake before use.

Lotion for Oily Skin

1 oz. (30 g.) spirits of camphor
2½ oz. (75 g.) glycerine
4 oz. (120 g.) eau-de-Cologne
2 oz. (60 g.) distilled water

Mix together, adding the water last. Shake before using.

Apricot Cleansing Cream

4 tablespoons apricot oil
2 tablespoons sesame seed oil
2 tablespoons butter
1 tablespoon distilled water

Beat the ingredients, by hand or in a blender, until completely smooth and creamy. Keep in refrigerator.

Olive Cleansing Cream

4 tablespoons green olive oil
2 tablespoons sesame seed oil
2 tablespoons lard (vegetable fat)
2 drops of any essence

Beat the ingredients together until creamy. Keep in refrigerator.

Almond Meal Cleanser

½ cup oil of sweet almonds
½ cup corn or powdered oatmeal
½ cup grated Castile soap

Mix ingredients together without any liquid. Keep in jar and on use add just enough water to the handful necessary for cleansing.

CONDITIONERS

Night Cream

3 tablespoons almond oil
2 tablespoons hydrous lanolin
2 tablespoons cocoa butter
2 teaspoons rose water
½ teaspoon honey

In a glass bowl placed in a pan of boiling water, melt and smooth the almond oil, lanolin and cocoa butter. Remove from heat and add the rose water and honey; cool, then beat until blended.

Strawberry Conditioner

½ cup fresh or frozen strawberry juice
1 dessertspoon lanolin
1 dessertspoon powdered oatmeal

Melt lanolin in a bowl over water, add the oatmeal and when mixture is smooth stir in the strawberry juice, beating until creamy.

Lettuce Cream

1 cup chopped lettuce
½ cup lanolin
2 drops rose geranium oil

Heat lanolin over water in a small bowl. When it has liquidized add lettuce and beat until blended. Remove from heat and perfume with rose geranium oil. Strain.

Elder Flower Cream

(Freshly picked flowers give the best results)

1 tablespoon lanolin
6 oz. (180 g.) sweet almond oil
1 cup elder flowers

Melt lanolin in a bowl in boiling water, add almond oil, blend well. Put in the elder flowers and simmer for 30 minutes; cool and strain.

Lily Cream

1 cup distilled water
2 tablespoons powdered lily roots
1 tablespoon honey
1 oz. (30 g.) lanolin
½ teaspoon rose water

Simmer the lily root powder in the water for 30 minutes. Strain, add the honey. Meanwhile, melt lanolin in a glass bowl in boiling water, remove from heat; add the lily, then the rose water.

Cucumber Cream

½ oz. (15 g.) white wax
2 oz. (60 g.) oil of sweet almonds
1 cucumber

Melt the wax in a glass jar standing in boiling water; add the almond oil. Peel and chop the cucumber very finely, and add just enough to the jar so that it is covered by the wax. Cover with foil and leave simmering for one hour. Remove from heat and stir thoroughly. Strain.

Enriched Avocado Cream

2 eggs
1 teaspoon glycerine
½ teaspoon lemon juice
2 teaspoons avocado oil
½ teaspoon cider vinegar
2 egg yolks, beaten
2 tablespoons distilled water

Blend the eggs, glycerine and lemon juice; slowly add enough avocado oil to thicken the mixture to a heavy cream, then stir in the vinegar. Add the beaten egg yolks and water – slowly, blending all the time. Keep refrigerated.

Honey and Almond Cream

4 oz. (120 g.) natural honey
8 oz. (240 g.) hydrous lanolin
½ cup oil of sweet almonds

In a double boiler warm the honey, blend in the lanolin, and as it melts add the almond oil. Stir well; remove from heat and beat until thoroughly creamed. Refrigerate.

RESTORERS

Mayonnaise Facial Masque

1 egg
½ teaspoon sea salt
2 tablespoons lemon juice
1 cup olive oil

Blend half a cup of the oil with the remaining ingredients; whip until thick, pour in the remaining oil very slowly. Keep refrigerated. After applying to face, allow 15 to 30 minutes before rinsing off.

Oatmeal Masque

½ cup milk
2 tablespoons unprocessed oatmeal
2 teaspoons elder flower water

Cook the oatmeal and milk as though it were porridge, until soft. Take off the heat, add elder flower water. Beat together and when just warm, spread over the face. Leave for 20 minutes.

Cucumber Masque

1 cucumber
¼ teaspoon lemon juice
1 teaspoon witch hazel
1 teaspoon alcohol
1 egg white, whipped

Peel the cucumber and extract the juice, add lemon juice, witch hazel and alcohol. Stir well; then blend in the whipped egg. Allow to dry on face for a minimum of 15 minutes. Rinse.

Wheat Germ Facial

1 egg yolk
½ teaspoon wheatgerm
¾ cup oil of sweet almonds
1 teaspoon distilled water

Beat the first three ingredients together, add the water, beat again. Brush on the face, leave 20 minutes.

Honey Masque

1 tablespoon honey
1 egg yolk
1 teaspoon olive oil

Beat the egg yolk into the oil, then blend in the honey. Apply to the face and leave for 15 minutes before rinsing away.

Parsley Facial

2 handfuls parsley
1 cup distilled water
1 tablespoon honey
1 egg yolk

Boil the parsley in the water for 15 minutes; strain. Stir in the honey and beaten egg yolk when liquid has cooled. Brush on face, leave for 15 minutes.

Honey and Oatmeal Paste

1 oz. (30 g.) honey
1 teaspoon lemon juice
2 unbeaten egg whites
½ teaspoon oil of sweet almonds
2 tablespoons powdered oatmeal

Mix everything together except the oatmeal. When smooth slowly add sufficient oatmeal to make a paste moist, but not sloppy. Apply to face and neck for 20 minutes before rinsing off.

Apricot Wrinkle Cream

2 tablespoons lanolin
1 tablespoon apricot oil
1 teaspoon lemon juice
3 drops tincture of benzoin

Melt lanolin in a glass bowl in a pan of simmering water; stir in the apricot oil and lemon juice; blend very well and finally add the benzoin; beat again.

Almond Refining Paste

4 oz. (120 g.) blanched almonds
1 egg white
1–2 tablespoons rose water

Pound the almonds into a smooth paste; add the egg white, unbeaten, and enough rose water to make a malleable paste. Leave on the skin for about 10 minutes.

Pimple Clearing Cream

2 pints (1 l.) rose water
2 sliced apples
2 tablespoons chopped fennel
2 tablespoons chopped celery
¼ oz. (7½ g.) barley meal
3 egg whites
1 teaspoon lanolin

In a double boiler simmer in the rose water, the apples, fennel, celery, and barley meal; when mushy, add beaten egg whites and lanolin. Strain; beat until smooth. Keep in refrigerator.

Basic Pimple Cream

1 tablespoon castor oil
1 tablespoon glycerine
1 tablespoon lanolin

Melt all ingredients together in a glass bowl placed in simmering water. Cool and keep in glass jar.

French Freckle Cream

1 oz. (30 g.) grated Castile soap
3 tablespoons distilled water
3 teaspoons lemon juice
¼ oz. (7½ g.) oil of bitter almonds
¼ teaspoon cream of tartar
4 drops olive oil

Put the grated soap and water in a double boiler, melt over low heat; when all water has evaporated, blend in thoroughly the rest of the ingredients. Rub over freckles, leave for 30 minutes.

Paste for Blackheads

8 oz. (240 g.) powdered oatmeal
4 oz. (120 g.) ground almonds
2 oz. (60 g.) powdered orris root
½ oz. (15 g.) grated Castile soap
2 tablespoons water

Mix dry ingredients well together, then add 2 tablespoons boiled water to make a paste. Rub into blackheads and leave 1 hour.

Lotion for Blackheads

1 tablespoon Epsom salts
3 drops white iodine
1 cup boiling water

Dissolve Epsom salts and iodine in the boiling water. Apply hot.

Freckle Removing Cream

¼ cup of sour milk
½ teaspoon of grated horseradish
1 tablespoon of cornmeal or powdered oatmeal

Mix all ingredients together into a paste; put between two layers of gauze, then apply to freckled areas. Don't let it get too near the eyes. Leave for 30 minutes.

STIMULATORS

Raspberry Vinegar

2 cups raspberries
1 cup rose petals
1 teaspoon honey
2 pints (1 l.) cider vinegar

Steep the first three ingredients in the vinegar for one month – in a covered earthenware pot. Strain, dilute with an equal part of distilled water. Use as a toner.

Oily Skin Astringent

¼ teaspoon boric acid powder
1 dessertspoon witch hazel
2 oz. (60 g.) glycerine
2 oz. (60 g.) alcohol
1½ oz. (45 g.) rose water
¼ teaspoon friar's balsam (benzoin)

Dissolve the boric acid powder in the witch hazel, add other ingredients. Mix thoroughly.

Lavender Water

2 cups lavender flowers
1 oz. (30 g.) powdered orris root
1 pint (6 dl.) vinegar

Steep the dry ingredients in the vinegar for three to four weeks; strain, dilute with the same amount of distilled water. Use as a toner.

Rose Vinegar

4 cups dried red roses
½ cup essence of rose
1 pint (6 dl.) vinegar

Put all ingredients in a lidded glass jar; allow to stand for three weeks, often shaking it. Strain, dilute with equal parts of distilled water. Use as a toner.

Cucumber Toner

1 peeled cucumber
1 teaspoon witch hazel
1 teaspoon rose water
egg white

Mash the cucumber, add witch hazel and rose water; beat the egg white to a froth; mix very well. Refrigerate. Strain before use.

Elder Flower Rinse

1 cup elder flowers (fresh or dried)
1 pint (6 dl.) boiling water

Pour boiling water over the flowers and allow to steep for a minimum of eight hours. Strain. Use as a toner.

Peppermint Vinegar

1 pint (6 dl.) cider vinegar
1 pint (6 dl.) distilled water
1 cup mint leaves

Bring all ingredients to the boil, remove and place in a glass container. Allow to steep for five days; strain. Use as an astringent.

Sage Astringent

½ cup dried sage
½ cup alcohol
1 teaspoon glycerine
3 tablespoons witch hazel
¼ teaspoon friar's balsam (benzoin)
¼ teaspoon boric acid powder

Steep the sage in the alcohol for a week; strain. Dissolve boric acid powder in the witch hazel, add this and all other ingredients to the sage extract.

PROTECTORS

Sesame Tanning Lotion

¼ cup lanolin
¼ cup sesame oil
¾ cup distilled water

In a double boiler, melt the lanolin; take off the heat and blend with sesame oil and water. Keep in refrigerator.

Sun Protection Lotion

1 peeled cucumber
½ teaspoon glycerine
½ teaspoon rose water

Extract the juice from the cucumber and mix the liquid with glycerine and rose water. Refrigerate.

Anti-Sunburn Cream

1 egg white, beaten
1 teaspoon honey
½ teaspoon witch hazel

Blend all ingredients together until even. Smooth over bad sunburn. Always refrigerate.

Iodine Bronzing Lotion

1 cup olive oil
10 drops iodine
juice of a lemon

Blend all ingredients together very well and always shake before using.

FRAGRANCES

Lavender Toilet Water

½ oz. (15 g.) oil of lavender
2 pints (1 l.) ethyl alcohol

Mix the lavender essence with just a little of the alcohol until thoroughly blended; then slowly add the rest of the alcohol. Keep in sealed jars – mature for a minimum of 6 weeks before using.

Cologne Water

1 pint (6 dl.) ethyl alcohol
1 teaspoon orange water
1 teaspoon lemon essence
1½ teaspoons oil of lavender
1 teaspoon bergamot

Blend all the oils and essences, then gradually mix in the alcohol. Allow to mature for 6–8 weeks; keep in firmly lidded bottles.

Rose Essence

3 handfuls of dried rose petals
sweet almond oil as needed

In a glass bowl or jar, put dried rose petals and cover with the oil. Put the pot in a pan of simmering water, heat until the oil has removed all the colour of the petals. Strain; keep tightly lidded.

Herb and Flower Cologne

¼ oz. (7½ g.) bergamot
¼ oz. (7½ g.) orange oil
¼ oz. (7½ g.) balsam of Peru
¼ oz. (7½ g.) essence of cloves
¼ oz. (7½ g.) thyme
¼ pint (1·5 dl.) orange flower water
2 pints (1 l.) ethyl alcohol

Put all herbs and essences into a glass jar, pour over the alcohol very slowly and stirring all the time. Allow mixture to mature for two weeks before using – jar must be tightly lidded.

After-bath Splash

1 cup fresh rose petals
½ cup alcohol
1½ tablespoons lemon peel
1½ tablespoons orange peel
½ tablespoon dried basil
1 tablespoon dried peppermint
1 cup boiling water

Steep rose petals in alcohol for 1 week; strain. Steep lemon peel, orange peel, basil and peppermint in the boiling water – make as tea – for 12 hours; strain. Combine two liquids, cover tightly, always shake before use.

Fresh Floral Cologne

1 oz. (30 g.) rose water
3½ teaspoons oil of lavender
½ oz. (15 g.) oil of cloves
6 oz. (180 g.) ethyl alcohol

Blend the two oils with a little alcohol until thoroughly united; beat in the remaining alcohol. Add the rose water. Bottle tightly and mature for 6–8 weeks.

Spicy Toilet Water

2 cups rose water
2 cups wine or cider vinegar
2 bay leaves
½ tablespoon crushed cloves

Boil all ingredients together, but add a little extra water all the time to keep the liquid at the original volume. Allow to mature for a month.

FOR THE HANDS

Protective Cream

(to be worn under gloves)

1 dessertspoon fuller's earth
1 dessertspoon almond oil
2 egg yolks

Mix all three ingredients together into an even blend; keep chilled until use. Keep on during work, then rinse off.

Cuticle Softener

2 tablespoons fresh or frozen pineapple juice
2 tablespoons egg yolk
½ teaspoon cider vinegar

Mix together – a very sloppy texture in which nails should be soaked for 30 minutes. It can be preserved for a while in the refrigerator.

Chapped Skin Cream

½ oz. (15 g.) white wax
6 tablespoons sweet almond oil
2 oz. (60 g.) rose water
1 teaspoon cod liver oil

In a double boiler melt wax and oils; add the rose water drop by drop, slowly beating all the time.

Honey Hand Cream

¼ oz. (7½ g.) white wax
¼ oz. (7½ g.) spermaceti
½ oz. (15 g.) sweet almond oil
4 oz. (120 g.) honey
few drops perfumed oil

In a glass bowl over hot water dissolve the wax and spermaceti; stir in almond oil and honey. Blend well, cool and then beat in perfumed oil.

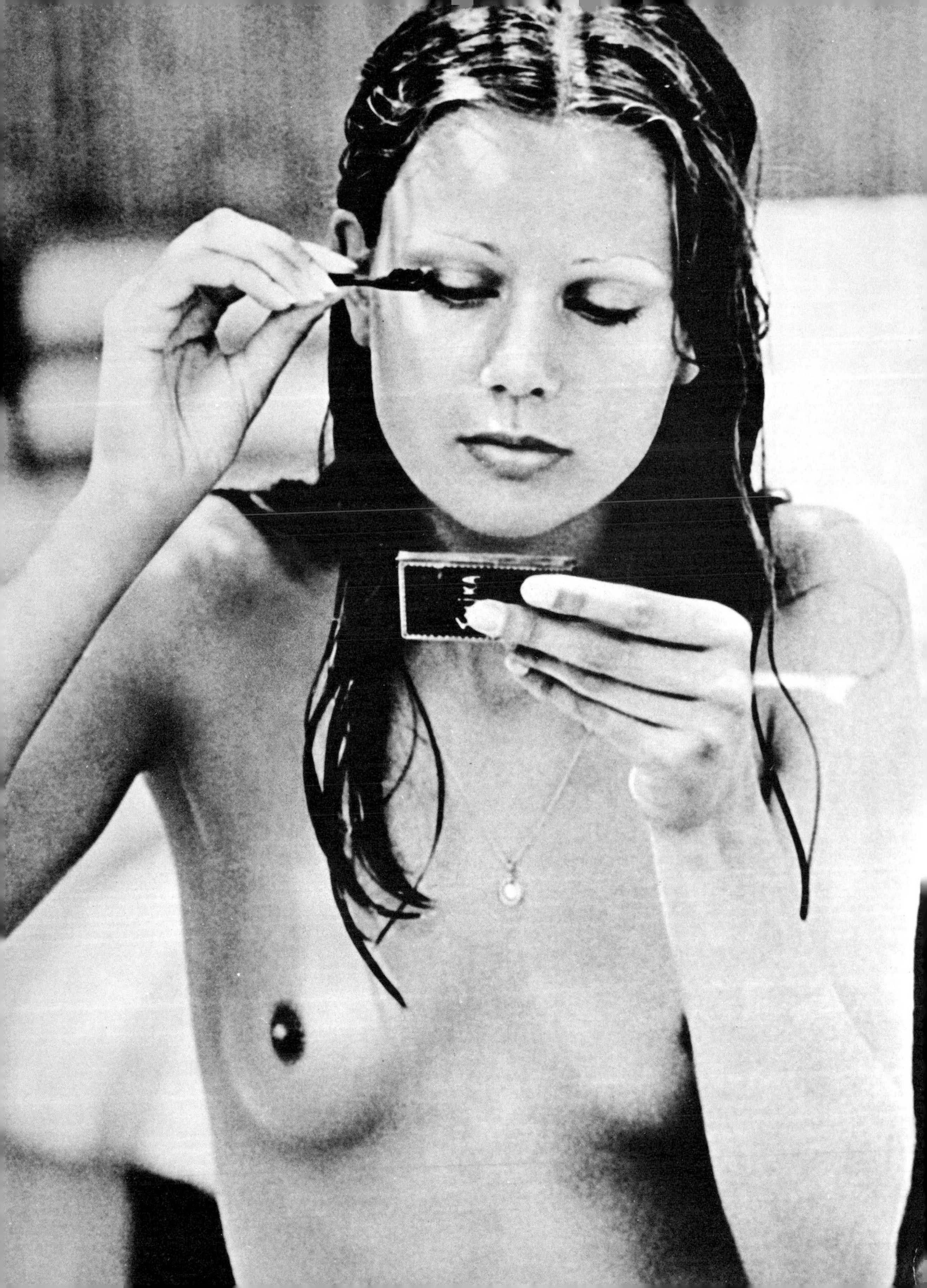

2

MAKE-UP

Make-up is any formulated preparation used for cleansing, treating, embellishing or altering the appearance. All contain a variety of ingredients, both natural and synthetic. The selection is vast, yet within the categories, compounds are basically the same. Differences are in the finer points – texture, colour, perfume, or in the addition of a special nutrient. Is there much difference between expensive and inexpensive brands? Performance does not vary a lot; it is usually how you use a product not what you use that determines the effect. It is true that more research goes into the more expensive items. Also the higher the price, the more attractive the containers, the better the depth and choice of colour, and sometimes ingredients are finer and perfumes rarer. But the real difference is psychological. If you think a certain product is more effective, it invariably is. The look, the feel, the smell, the image of a cosmetic – all contribute equally.

The make-up you use depends on what suits you. Some products are in agreement with your skin, others are not. There are also several ranges of hypo-allergenic cosmetics and manufacturers are increasingly concerned with purity. Cosmetics containing no chemicals whatsoever are likely to be more expensive because not only are natural ingredients often rarer, but the life of the preparation is usually limited.

SKIN PREPARATIONS

CLEANSERS: These contain oil to dissolve the grease of make-up and an emulsifying agent to make removal easier.

Creams – very good at removing make-up and dirt, but apt to cling to the skin. Generally better for dry and normal skins. Remove with tissue.

Cold Creams – more fluffy and can be used on oily skins too. Remove with tissue.

JUNE NEWTON

Liquids – contain more water than creams and come as lotions of varying creaminess. For all types of skin. Remove with tissue.

Rinsable Cleaners – light creams or liquids that can be rinsed off with water. Fine for all skins.

Pad Cleaners – thick wads of absorbent material saturated with a liquid cleanser. Good for special areas like eyes and for touch-up cleansing.

FRESHENERS: Remove last traces of cleanser, refresh and refine skin texture, sometimes acting as thinners of dead cells. They come in three strengths according to alcohol content. Apply with cottonwool wads.

Fresheners – the simplest, consisting of an aromatic substance dissolved in water, sometimes with a little alcohol. Soothe and cool the skin.

Toners – slightly more bracing because of higher alcohol content. Good for dry and normal skins.

Astringents – the strongest with highest percentage of alcohol. Tingle on skin and have a temporary pore-tightening effect. Good for oily skin.

MOISTURIZERS: A misnomer, as these products do not give moisture themselves, but promote moisturization by sealing in the available water. They do so by filming the skin with the thinnest invisible layer of oil or grease. The most essential of all skin preparations, they come in different formulas for different skins, so read the labels. Apply with finger tips.

Creams – the heaviest, also act as lubricants and protectors in extreme climates. Good for dry skin, ageing skin and for use overnight.

Lotions – lighter but still mild lubricants. Go well under make-up as they fill in surface irregularities, thus allowing foundation to adhere more smoothly and evenly.

CONDITIONERS – Also called: emollients, lubricants, nourishing, treatment, enriched or night creams. Eye creams and throat creams also come into this category, as do body and hand lotions. All are heavy duty preparations aimed to help skin that needs oil or moisture or both. They do three jobs – lubricate, moisturize and protect.

Creams – all contain oils or greases or both; the main difference between the many types is the concentration and proportion of the two. All oils and greases, whether of animal, vegetable or mineral origin, will act in much the same way.

They are tenacious, forming a protective barrier while the skin absorbs the fatty molecules; they smooth the surface and provide an anchor for moisture. They are applied with fingertips and massaged gently into the skin. They should not disappear, but be visible on the surface. The effectiveness of these heavier creams is increased by pre-wetting the skin. Leave on for a minimum of an hour. Tissue off, then cleanse the face.

Many creams contain extra ingredients claiming special properties. Most are intended to encourage the skin into increased cell renewal. Skin is capable of absorbing certain outside elements, but which and to what degree is controversial. Some of the more common additions are:

Hormones – satisfy the skin's need for oestrogen during and after the menopause. The hormone content of creams is too small to affect the whole system, and there is a legal limit as to how much is permitted in an ounce (30 g.). They do improve skin condition to an extent as they change metabolism of cells, causing them to expand, thus plumping and smoothing the surface.

Tissue extracts – include tissues from the embryo, placenta and ovaries of young animals. Their action is to increase capillary circulation and stimulate metabolism. Their content in cream is limited, but they can help to hydrate and nourish ageing skin, also remedy excessive dryness and oily problems.

Collagen – in its natural state is an important part of connective tissue and responsible for smoothness and resilience of the skin. It is used in creams to improve elasticity and help skin retain natural fluids.

Eye Creams – particularly concentrated conditioners with a high percentage of a finer oil. To be patted around the eye area.

Throat Creams – not very different from regular conditioners, but sometimes a little richer in oils. Apply with fingertips, massaging with upward strokes.

Body Lotions – water-based emulsions that are really diluted creams, but often containing additional aromatics and sometimes a freshener to give a cool feeling. They perform the same service as any other conditioner – smooth, lubricate, moisturize and protect. Apply by hand.

Hand Lotions – water-based emulsions of varying degrees of thickness. The same basic formula as a body lotion but often of a heavier consistency. Some hand creams are glycerine based, formed into a jelly substance by gum tragacanth. Protection properties are important; they also lubricate and moisturize. Apply by hand.

SUNSCREENS: These consist of a chemical screen plus a base which may be a water-alcohol mixture, a lotion, a cream, an oil or a grease. The type of base makes little difference, though the oily and greasy ones are more water resistant, and many women prefer creams because they also soften the skin. However the criterion for a sunscreen should be its efficiency at protecting the skin against sun and light. They work by selectively blocking out the ultra violet rays that are responsible for skin damage.

They fall into three groups; the names of the chemicals are impossibly difficult but to be selective you must read labels and recognize them.

The best – para-aminobenzoic acid, but with the disadvantage of being poorly soluble, so alcohol is needed to keep it in solution. This means that sunscreens containing it may be drying to some skins. It also tends to stain fabrics.

Pretty good – para-aminobenzoic derivatives such as iso-amyl and glyceryl, also benzophenone derivatives. These are available in all bases, but beware of a heavy application of benzophenone as it will almost eliminate tanning completely.

Fine – menthyl anthranilate, homomenthyl salicylate, triethanolamine salicylate, cinoxate, digalloyl trioleate. Found in all bases, don't stain and approved for limited amounts of sun. Apply liberally everywhere including lips.

Fake Tanning Creams – emulsions containing a chemical agent that darkens the skin. On the whole they work well, but some skins are inclined to go orangey instead of brown. Colour is temporary.

MAKE-UP PREPARATIONS

FOUNDATIONS: Their purpose is to provide the look of better skin colour and texture. They leave a film on the skin covering minor imperfections and unify colour. Generally made from a water-in-oil formula, the basic idea is that each drop of water is surrounded with drops of oil. The proportion of each varies to produce different textures and effects, but all give an even tint. They range in colour from flat white to the deepest mahogany. Some can be used without powder.

Liquids – provide a light protective film, can be of the creamy moisturized kind ideal for dry and normal skins, or oil-free formulas for greasy skins. They do not cover well, therefore are not good for camouflaging blemished skin. Sometimes difficult to control, and more efficient when applied with a sponge.

Creams – thicker and heavier with consistency varying from milky to whipped cream. Give the glossiest look, and easy to apply with fingertips or sponge. Usually waterproof.

Opposite: Guy Bourdin, 1974
Overleaf right: Norman Parkinson, 1972

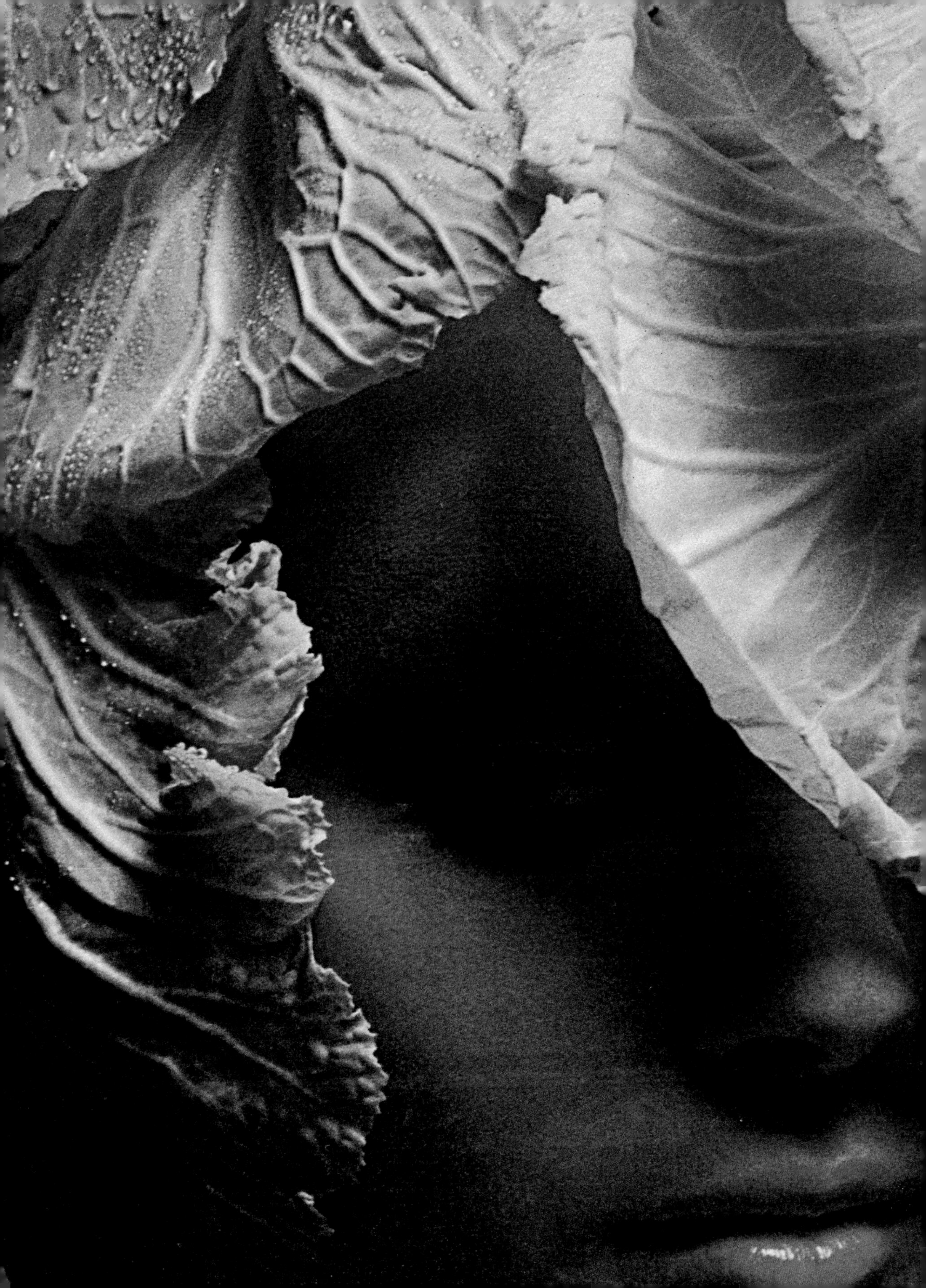

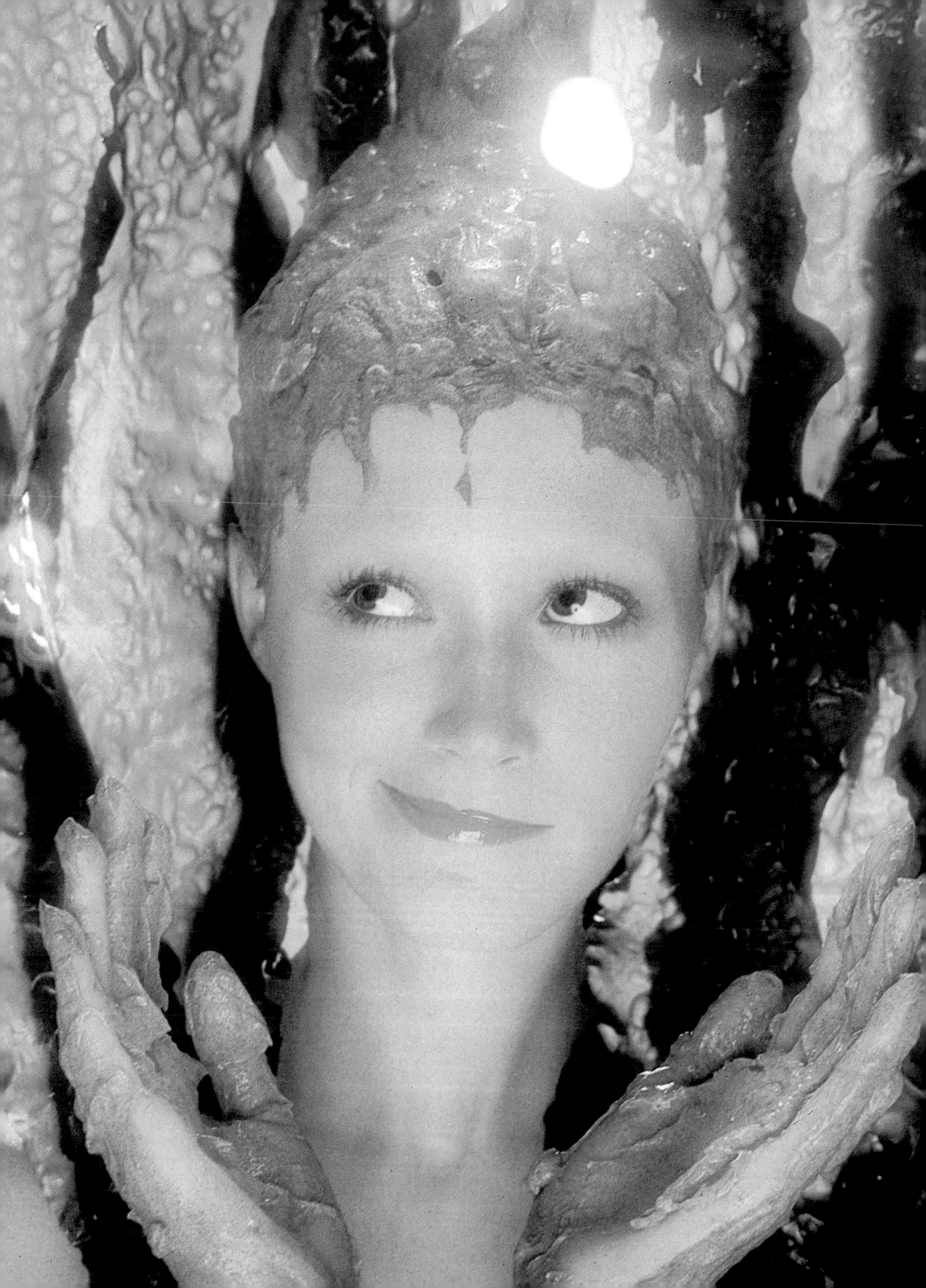

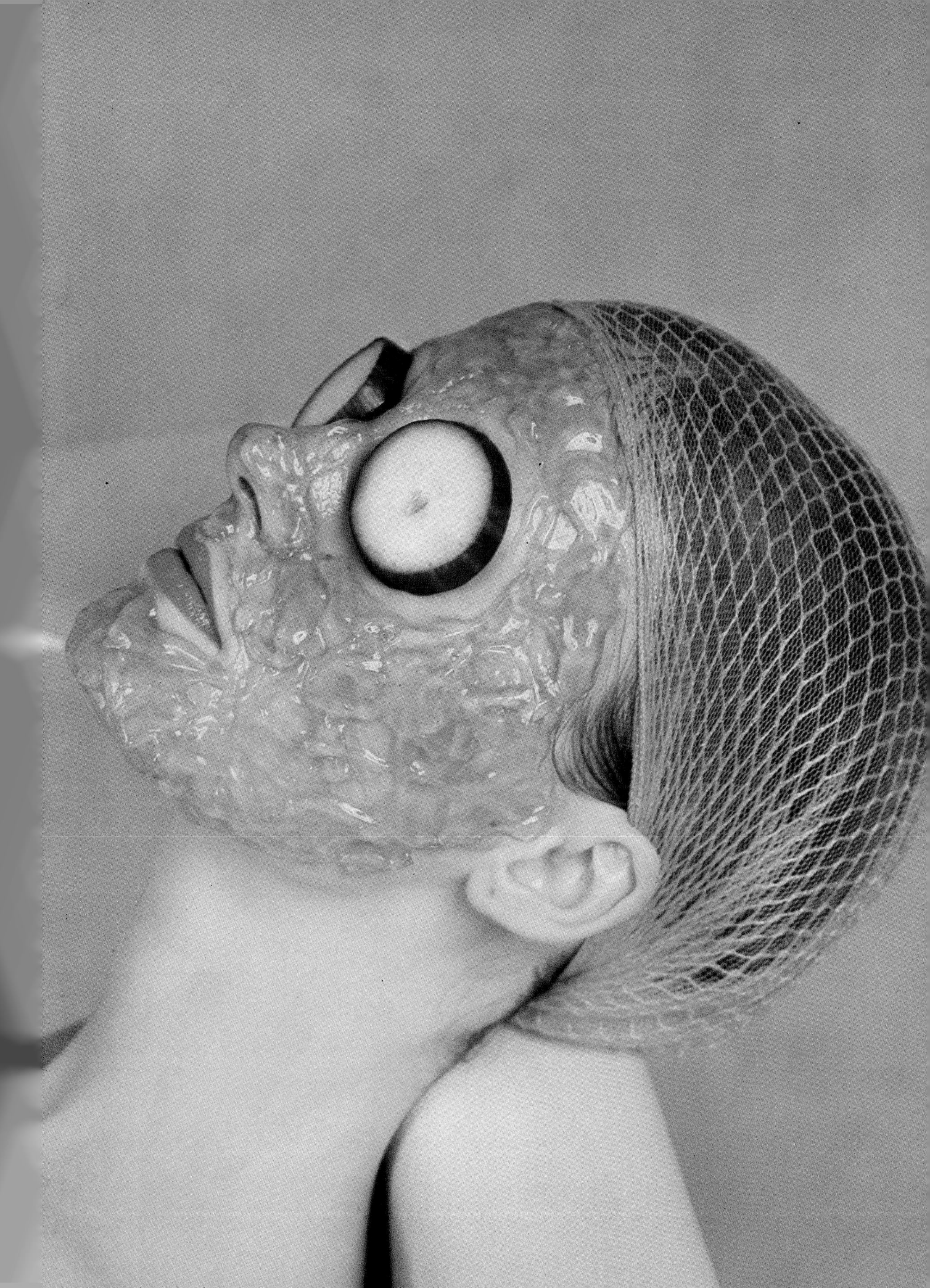

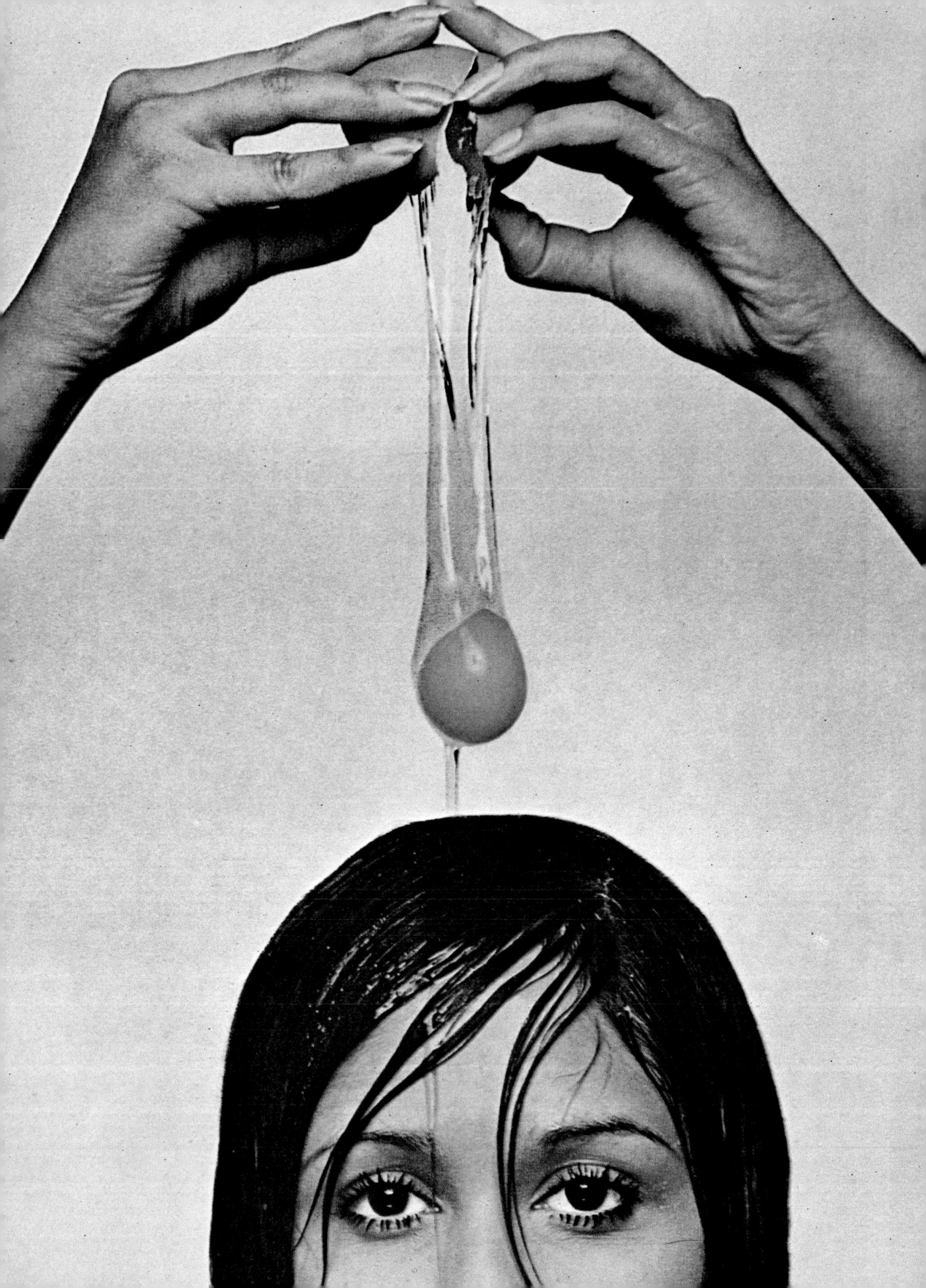

All-in-One Bases – a mixture of cream and powder, often more difficult to apply as they tend to drag the skin; a damp sponge eases application. Not suggested for dry skins. Do not require fixing with powder, but finish is drier.

Cover-Ups – very dense creams that feel like putty and often in stick form. Used to cover skin blemishes and alleviate dark circles under the eyes. Pat on with fingertips. All cover-ups require extensive blending afterwards.

Solid Cream Sticks – very thick formula, add the most colour, hide blemishes, dark circles, freckles. Stroke on directly, then blend with fingers.

Gels and Glossies – like a more fluid petroleum jelly, but coloured and scented; easy to smooth on with fingertips, provide a transparent shine, good for adding colour and a healthy looking gloss.

Cakes and Blocks – dense dehydrated formulas, add a lot of colour, good for covering blemishes. They can be drying so are not advisable for dry skins – but a great help to oily ones. Apply with a damp sponge.

POWDERS: Set make-up with a sheen or matt look. Translucent powders are usually preferred as they do not affect other make-up colours. Otherwise the colour spectrum is in four groups: the neutrals, the pinks, the goldens, the browns. If you use a colour, the general rule is to choose one shade lighter than the foundation.

Loose Powders – best for the final finish to make-up; apply with a puff or cottonwool wad.

Pressed Powders – usually in compacts and convenient for touch-ups, but do not apply layer upon layer, it will cake.

BLUSHERS: Used to be known as rouge. Now also known as shaders, contourers or, when light, as highlighters. Function is to add colour, warmth, shading or luminosity. Rosy, peach and tawny colours tone the cheeks; the deep tawny and brown shades are used to give the illusion of fading out undesirable features and hollowing cheeks. Apply powders with a brush, others with fingertips.

Creams – add moisture as well as colour. Blend in with fingertips; use over foundation but under powder.

Powders – brushed on face after powder; translucent varieties reflect more light and appear to glow.

Gels – transparent colours for a glossy look; apply over foundation, but don't cover with powder.

Opposite: Barry Lategan, 1969

EYE-SHADOWS: Add colour and dimension to the eyes, the look of which can be dramatically improved by intelligent shading. Often known as highlighters in the white and creamy tones. Full spectrum of colour.

Creams – oil based, soft spreading and easy to blend on skin. Should be set with powder – translucent or talcum – to prevent crease lines. Apply with fingertips or brush.

Sticks – more solid creams with oils dispersed in a waxy base. Like lipsticks, apt to go soggy in hot weather and hard to spread in cold. Apply stick directly to lids, then blend in with fingertips. Set with powder.

Liquids – usually provided with a built-in brush or wand applicator. Contain more water than creams and sticks, long-lasting when dry but difficult to apply as they're inclined to run.

Gels – easy to apply but often more gloss than depth of colour, so a couple of coats are required. Apply with fingertips.

Powders – based on compressed powder with a moisturizer added to give cling. Staying power is good, sometimes feel taut on dry skins. Apply with brush or sponge applicator.

Water-Colours – cake-like shadows applied with a wet brush. Long-lasting and painting-on property facilitates artistic effects. Some powders can be used in this way, but once water has been added there's no returning to using it as a simple powder.

Crayons and Pencils – waxier and softer than for brows, so easy to apply without pulling or dragging over the skin. Colour is drawn on with strokes or curves, blended with fingertips.

EYEBROW COLOURINGS:

Pencils – waxy narrow leads that have to be sharp to be effective. Draw on colour with tiny diagonal strokes.

Powders – like compressed powder, moisturized a little. Apply with slant-edged brush.

EYE LINERS: Define outline of eye by colouring all or part of the rim.

Liquids – oil-based in water; difficult to control unless applied with a fine sable brush.

Cakes – block of water-colour powder; one of the best ways to draw eye lines. Use fine brush, dampen powder.

Wands – contain a creamy fluid and built-in brush. Can be a bit gooey; allow time to dry otherwise they smudge.

MASCARAS: Generally oil-in-water formulas, giving colour and thickness to lashes.

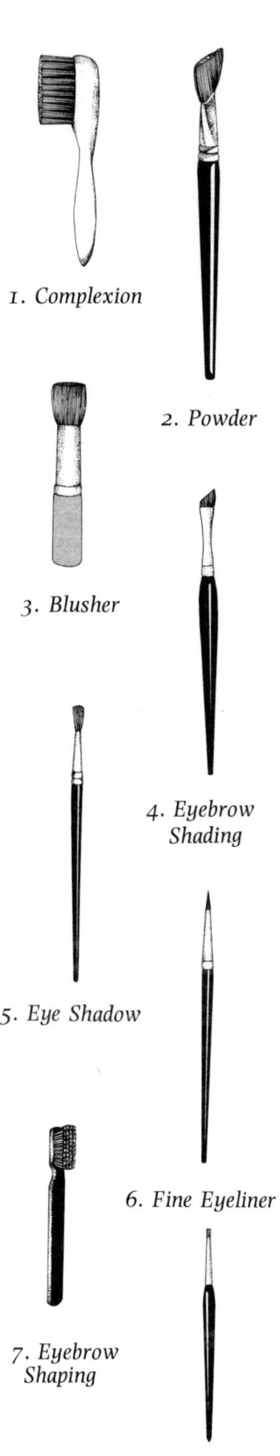

Cakes and Blocks – one of the oldest kinds and still one of the most efficient. Apply with a wet brush. Build it up slowly and gradually allowing to dry between coats. Long lasting, and lashes usually separate well.

Creams – thick, oil-based, waterproof. Messy to apply so use a brush.

Wands – contain creams that are rolled on either with a spiral brush or screw-like rod; some have teeth applicators and creams are combed on. Several have additions of fibres or filaments to build up lash length and thickness.

LIP COLOURINGS:

Sticks – basically colours and oils dispersed in a wax base, many colours combined to make one shade; lanolin is added for softness and pliancy. The creamy, lustrous looking lipstick doesn't stay on very long, but is good for the lips and prevents drying. Some shades slightly stain the lips. Application can be direct, but better with a brush.

Gels and Gloss – with glycerine or petroleum-jelly bases, they give lots of gleam but usually not much colour. Clear colourless gels are often used over lipsticks. Apply with brush or fingertips.

Pencils – soft, wax-base crayons used to outline lips.

APPLICATION

Think of features: look in the mirror, forget overall shape. What is your best feature, the most attractive, the most unusual?

Think of emphasis: eyes, mouth or cheeks; decide which. Avoid the pitfall of trying to play up everything.

Think of skin tone: is it right for you? Would you look better a little paler, beiger, darker, browner, blacker? Think of the best blushing tone to go with it – pink, peach, amber, tawny, plum.

Think of change: a common fault is to go on believing in one particular look too long. Slight alterations can give the face a new contemporary look without losing its basic image.

The art of contemporary make-up lies in putting together all the separate parts to give an overall impression. It is not difficult but it takes know-how. Decide what to emphasize, then work on the background. The art is in the blending – textures, tones, shadings, colours, lines, features. A lot of make-up blended well looks more natural than a little make-up slapped on. Blend mostly with your fingertips, but also with brushes. It is easier, more accurate and more effective to apply make-up with brushes, and there are special ones for each application.

THE BASIS: COLOUR TONES

Skin tones can be altered only within a shade or two. Lighter skins have the advantage over dark, as the range of going deeper through make-up is far greater than that of going lighter. Skin tone controls other colour areas too: the cheeks and lips always, the eyes sometimes.

The choice and blending of colour tones is the most important part of make-up and various tints can be mixed together before application. Use the palm of the hand as a palette and work with fingers or brush. If the consistency is a little too thick, thin it by adding a drop of moisturizer or non-alcoholic freshener.

Generally the foundation shade closest to your natural skin tone is best and the darker the skin the more transparent looking it should be.

Pale – needs a delicate touch, a film of creamy ivory for the foundation; a blush of pink or amber; pastel lip tone.

Creamy – often an oriental skin, needs a bisque or golden beige make-up base; peach or rose tints for cheeks and lips.

Beige – a medium-tone skin that can take many shades – beige, golden and suntan tones; coral, rose-reds, bright pinks and tawny shades to balance.

Olive – golden colours with a touch of rose in the foundation; cheeks and lips need warm corals, deep rose tints or tawny shades.

Brown – the darker the skin, the less make-up base it usually needs, often the shine of a gel is the best. Dusky tones can be covered with cool brown or earthy shades of foundation; amber, cinnamon and grape tints for blushing, for lips.

Black – gels give glow and bronzing sticks are good for the darkest skins. Cheeks can be buffed with amber or plum shades, the same for lips which can often take a vivid rose too.

FOUNDATION

Use sparingly, two thin coats are preferable to one heavy layer. Creams, liquids and gels can be broken down on the palm of the hand first to give a smoother and finer application. Then dot on nose, each cheek, chin, forehead. If you are using a cream stick, put a stroke in each place. Blend very well with fingertips – upward and outward across the chin, outward over the cheeks, across the forehead, down the nose, under the tip and very lightly around the eyes and on the lids. Continue foundation just under the chin. There is no need to cover the neck area, but make sure there are no demarcation lines. Cake foundation is applied with a damp sponge. Sponging over all make-up bases evens out the film.

CORRECTING

Blemishes and dark shadows can be concealed; facial planes and dimensions can be corrected by light and dark shading.

Blemishes – use an opaque cover-up product. If flaw does not contrast too much with the skin – broken veins for example – use a shade that matches foundation. To cover a reddish scar or dark birthmark, use one shade lighter. To cover a lightened area, such as a white scar or pigment loss, use one shade darker. Apply concealer to the exact spot, gently stroke and blend the edges in with the foundation. If necessary cover with a thin film of foundation.

Shadows – usually under-eye circles which can be camouflaged by lightening. It is better to do this with a very light foundation or with a thick white crayon stroked on, then blended with the fingers. Blend until the whitened area merges with the make-up base.

Contouring – emphasize the best and diminish the least using light and dark shadings interspersed with a red tone: moving down from the eyes, the rule is – white first, red in the centre (see make-up for cheeks) and the beige-browns underneath. It is easy to make a mistake, as the inclination is to do too much. Concentrate on the highlights: automatically the rest of the face will recede. Use a white base (on the palm first) or a soft greasy crayon. Lighten the ridge of the nose, the upper edge of the cheekbones (out from under the eye up to the hairline), put a stroke in the crease by each nostril, a dot centred under the bottom lip. Blend. Be cautious with shading. Use one shade deeper than foundation: narrow a broad nose by shading the sides from eyebrows to nostrils; subtract from prominent jaw or chin by shading the outer edges. And blend.

CHEEKS

This is quite a large area and it is more practical to consider it two levels – upper and lower. The upper is a small oval area high on the cheekbone and slanting outwards from under the eye; the lower is a larger oval starting in the hollow of the cheek at nostril level and going up and out towards the hairline. The upper cheek is for highlighting, to give radiance during the day and luminosity on an evening face. The lower area is for contouring the face, using a muted tint to give dimension. The one smoothly flows into the other, remembering that the upper cheek colour has to be blended into the previously lightened area under the eye.

Creams and gels – are preferable for the upper cheek as they reflect more light. Put a little on the palm, mix with an equal part of foundation and blend. Apply to the cheek, blending up and out towards the temple. Don't let colour stray, but let it merge. The same substance can be applied to the larger lower area, but make the colour a little deeper. Don't go below the nostril level, blend off the face into the hairline. For evening use, luminous and frosted tones can be applied.

Powders – effective for lower cheek shading, but not always for the upper area. They are brushed on after face powder. Suck in cheeks to indicate natural hollow, brush up and out from there. If cream colour is used for the lower cheek, it is often advisable to brush on extra shading at the end of complete make-up to adjust depth and dimension.

FACE POWDER

This sets make-up, giving it a finished look and staying power. Translucent powders (with talcum and baby powder as alternatives) are more reliable as tinted powder can change colour according to skin chemistry.

The puff is a matter of preference – swansdown, velour, cottonwool, sponge or brush. Take a generous amount of powder and starting at the chin apply upward with gentle press-and-turn motions. Cover the entire face, eyelids too. Now with the other side of the puff or a fresh one, dust across forehead, down cheeks and nose, across the chin. Brush or whisk away any excess. Powder should be an all but invisible film.

EYES

Eyes give your face much of its personality and most women emphasize their eyes above other features. The general idea is to shade down the minuses and shine up the pluses. It is done with shadow, lightener, liner, mascara and additional lashes. It is up to you to decide which and to what degree.

First Degree – the casual eye: smudge shadow on the lid, blend up and out towards the brow until it fades away; carry a touch of shadow round the corner to tuck just under the bottom lashes. A suggestion of eyeliner, mascara.

Second Degree – the contoured eye: achieve extra dimension by intensifying shadow colour and adding a deeper tone in the crease of the eye, following the natural curve of the socket. Lighten under the brow line; give a smudgy outline to the eye; mascara and scattered extra lashes.

Third Degree – the evening eye: planned to shine under artificial light. More vivid, stronger colour for shadow, a very definite line in the crease of the eye; luminous highlight under the brow; eyeliner and much fuller lashes with a false section added if necessary.

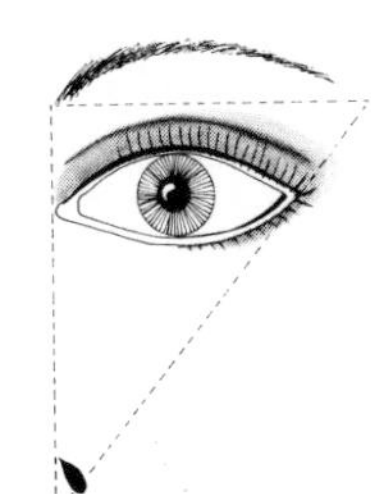

Eyebrow Proportions

EYEBROWS: Eyebrows give expression and balance to a face. They require grooming and definition but try not to alter their basic form. Some eyebrow hairs are temperamental and once plucked don't grow back again. The brow should start at a point above the inside corner of the eye; the highest part of the curve above the outer rim of the iris. The arch should be gentle with the end of the brow never lower than the beginning. It should terminate at the extension of the diagonal from nostril to outer eye.

Brush eyebrows into shape, up first, then across; pluck out hairs between and underneath the brow lines, never above. Tweeze with a quick, firm tug, always from underneath. Apply cream first, then astringent.

Define brows with a pencil or brush-on powder. The pencil must be sharp; apply in short diagonal strokes. The brush for powder application has a special slanted edge; make short feathery strokes. Colour looks darker on the brow, so select a shade lighter than your own colour. Dark brown is better than black; light brown for fair hair.

EYE SHADOW: This gives the eye its shape and shine. Bear in mind the colour-contour rules: deeper tones de-emphasize and brighter, pale ones emphasize eye features. All contouring is more effective with neutral and pink tones. If you can not resist blues and greens, keep them pale, so they are almost grey or tinged white. Any texture of shadow can be used, but blend and blend; strips of colour are most unattractive. Cover the eyelid, blend colour up and out. Define the crease, the curve of the eye socket with a thick crayon, smudge and blend. Lift the eyebrow and reflect light to the whole eye area by blending a highlighter under the brow, either at the outer or inner edge depending on the shape of the eye. White, creamy or pinky tones are best, or a transparent gel. For evening, dark colours can go deeper, light ones more luminous or pearly, and the crease definition stronger. Here are the best ways to make-up eyes.

Deep Set

Eyes can be brought forward by applying pale shadow over the lid, carrying it to just above the hollow. On the bone between lid and brow put a little brown, taupe or grey shading; highlighter under the brow and a

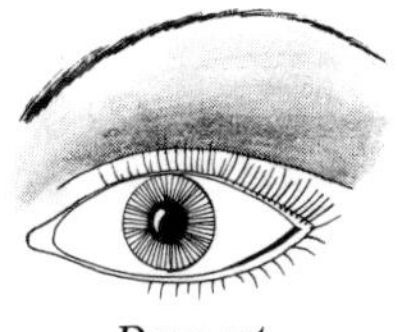

Deep-set

dot on the centre of lid. A smudged socket line above the natural crease. A light eyeliner in a fine line under upper lashes.

Prominent

The lid must be pushed back by covering with a deep tone of matt eye shadow, blending into lower brow area and curving around just under the bottom corner of the eye. Use a fleshy or pink tone on the underbrow section. Define a dark crease line, smudge it. Eyeliner helps minimize lid; emphasize top lashes, first by curling, then adding many coats of mascara.

Small

To give more importance to the eye you have to lighten part of the lid and recede the area around it. Begin by applying dark shadow around eye leaving inside top corner free; build shadow out at the sides, but only a small rim underneath. A pale tone should go in the corner, taken up and across the lid. Lots of lashes – false ones help; highlight under brow.

Round

Shading gives the eye width, but should be kept light. Cover the entire upper lid with a pale shade then, in a deeper tone in the same colour range, fill in the socket area, extending at corners parallel to the brow line. Outline the eye extending both top and bottom lines; add lashes from centre of lid outwards. Lengthen and darken the crease definition.

Heavy lids

Here you need to reduce the emphasis on the lid and increase focus on the eye. Use a matt colour in medium tone; make a triangle starting at inside corner, going up near inside of brow and angling back down to outside of eye. Put a small highlight at centre of lid. Define socket crease, make darker and smudge towards end of lid. Mascara the top lashes only.

Close-set

The accent has to be shifted to the outer part of the eyes. Pluck a bit more between the brows; blend cover-up between inner corners and bridge of

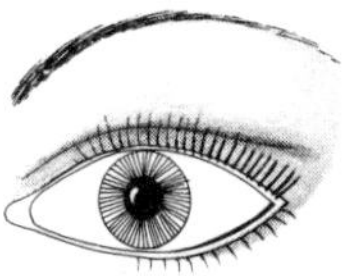

Prominent

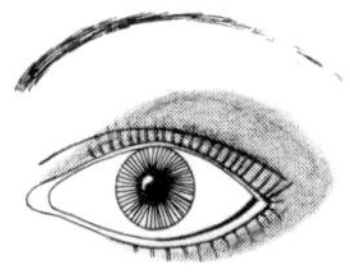

Small

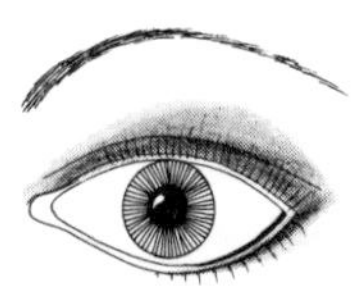

Round

nose. Start shadow towards the centre of the eye and blend outwards. Begin lid crease line at the same place and extend. Begin eyeliner half an inch in from the inner corner and extend. Add lashes to outer corners.

Wide-set

To bring eyes closer, use dark shading between eyes and the bridge of the nose, filling upwards to brow line; arch down, tapering to outer corner. Highlight a deep area under outside edge of the eybrow. Emphasize socket crease near nose, thicken eyeliner there but smudge to avoid harshness. Add extra lashes or heavy mascara towards centre of eye.

Droopy

Uplift is needed at the outer corners; it is more effective and less obvious to do it with shadow and a suggestion of eyeliner. Wing shadow out and upwards, almost touching brow line. Draw in a false socket line, raised at the outer edge, smudge. Feather an upswept eyeliner from centre of upper lashes; blend pale shadow at outer corner; curl up lashes, mascara.

EYELINER: Liner helps define shape and opens the eye, but it should be done with a delicate line. Black eyeliner is only for those with dark hair and dark skin, otherwise dark brown is deep enough. For fair skins, soft brown, taupe and grey tones. For evening, a coloured eyeliner can be effective when it tones with eyeshadow.

Apply with a very fine-tipped brush. Look down, and with one finger holding the eye taut, draw a fine line along the upper lid and as close to the lashes as possible; end at the outer corner, do not extend. Most women should use liner on the upper lid only; just dot or feather strokes on the bottom if you have no definition at all. Sometimes a line under the upper lashes is better, but keep it thin and even. Eyeliners often look better when smudged a little to blend in with lashes and shadow. Liquid and cake liners give a sharper line, pencil is more subtle.

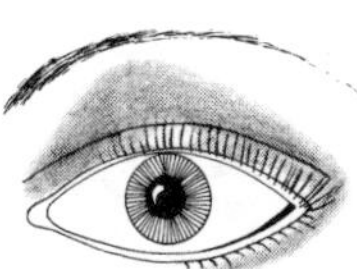

Heavy lids

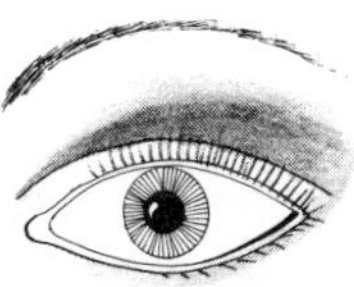

Close-set

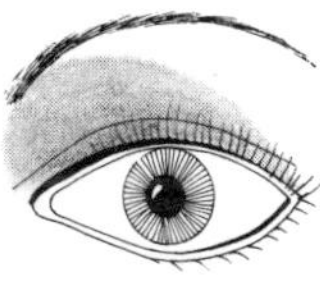

Wide-set

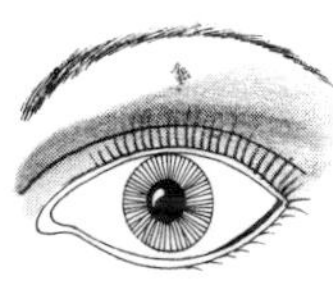

Droopy

MASCARA: Lashes need to be obvious, not spiky or thick, but long and feathery. Natural lashes are rarely long enough or dark enough to frame the eyes well. Mascara can be dark, and you can often take black even when your hair is brown; always use a shade much darker than your hair colour, in the brown, taupe or grey range.

Brush and lightly powder lashes providing a built-up surface for the mascara. It is often better to curl them first for a more fluttery look. Build up mascara in layers; many thin coats are better than a heavy one. Start by applying to the tips of the lashes, and working down to the base. Brush upper lashes downwards from the top, then brush up from below. This ensures both sides of the hairs are coated, and sweeps the lashes upwards. For the lower rim, brush up first, then down. Allow each layer to dry before applying another; you may need several coats depending on the fullness you want. It is important to keep lashes separated; should they cake and stick together, separate them with a fine, clean comb.

FALSE EYELASHES: Extremely effective and often more natural looking than layers of mascara. They can change a face considerably and make it more youthful. Use the same rule for colour as for mascara. The object is to supplement your own lashes, so they look thicker and longer, not stuck-on; put them on upper lids only.

There are three ways to supplement eyelashes:

A full strip: Check the length; lashes should begin a little in from the inside corner and not extend beyond the outside one. Cut with a razor if necessary.

If new, soak lashes 3 to 4 minutes in warm water to remove sizing that makes them stiff.

Flex base lightly to shape it to the contour of your eye.

Taking a wooden toothpick, dip in surgical glue and trail a streak of it along the lash strip. Let it get a little gummy. Pick up lash, hold as close as possible to natural lash line; using toothpick or emery board, press lashes downward in gentle vertical strokes until both lash lines meet.

Draw a thin eyeliner to fill-in any gap and cover up any excess glue. A very little mascara over the real and extra lashes blends them together.

Remove by peeling off gently beginning at outside corner. Pick off the adhesive. Lashes can be washed in clear warm water or a special liquid. To dry, roll in a tissue around a pencil.

Strip section: Cut off desired length from long strip with a razor.

Flex lashes around a finger so that they will follow the curve of the eye when applied.

Apply and remove as for full strip.

Lash by lash: Patience is required for this method. They are not attached to the skin but to your own lashes. The idea is to double the thickness of natural lashes not their number. Takes a minimum of half an hour for both eyes.

From a strip, select lashes – smaller ones for the inside of the eye.

Start from the inside and build outwards: with tweezers pick up lash, dip in surgical glue and using the hair base like a brush, stroke adhesive all the way down your own lash. Then press false lash base against natural lash base; hold a second.

Lashes should last a week, but do not use oily eye make-up. Mascara is not necessary nor advisable as it cannot be cleaned off without taking the lashes with it. To remove, apply an oily make-up remover.

LIPS

Lips need shine, colour, and careful shaping. Learn to outline lips, using a pencil or brush and a darker or lighter tone than that of the overall colour. It gives a cleaner, neater, fresher look than a stick alone. For greater control, rest elbow on the table using the hand like a lever. Outline bottom lip first, from centre to right corner, from centre to left corner. Extend slightly at the corners to give the mouth an upward lift. Outline the upper lip, again from the centre to the corners. Fill in with colour either with a brush or the lipstick. Don't run over the outline. For extra shine use gloss over the lipstick.

Making lip corrections is not always successful as alterations can be very obvious, particularly when lipstick starts to wear off. Never attempt to reshape the whole mouth; keep the colour subdued: These are subtle corrections:

Too big: outline just inside the natural line, using a light shade, fill in with a deeper but still lightish tone.

Too full: avoid bright, shiny or heavy colours, keep lipstick just inside natural lip line; outline in almost-matching shade.

Too thin: outline in a light shade just outside the natural lip line, stopping a little short at the corners; fill in with a deeper tone.

Uneven: when lips don't match in thickness, use two different shades – a darker one for the thickest lip, a lighter one for the other.

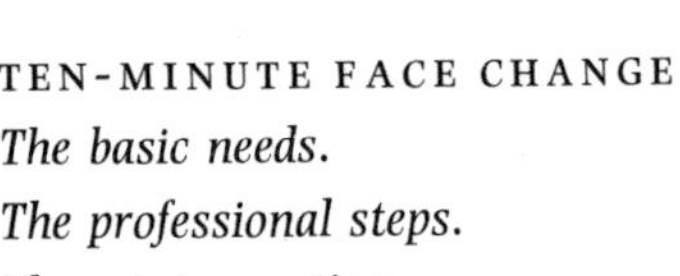

TEN-MINUTE FACE CHANGE

The basic needs.
The professional steps.
The minimum time.

Success depends on technique and that is only acquired through practice. The correct sequence of making up is of the utmost importance. Emphasize one area only – eyes, mouth or cheeks – keep the rest in subdued tones. The professional plan: a clean, well moisturized face, a simple range of cosmetics.

Equipment: tweezers, tinted foundation, pale cover-up or crayon, darker shading, cream blusher, translucent or baby powder, eye shadow, eye crayon, eyeliner, eyelash curler, mascara, eyebrow pencil, powder blusher, lip pencil, lipstick, gloss or petroleum jelly.

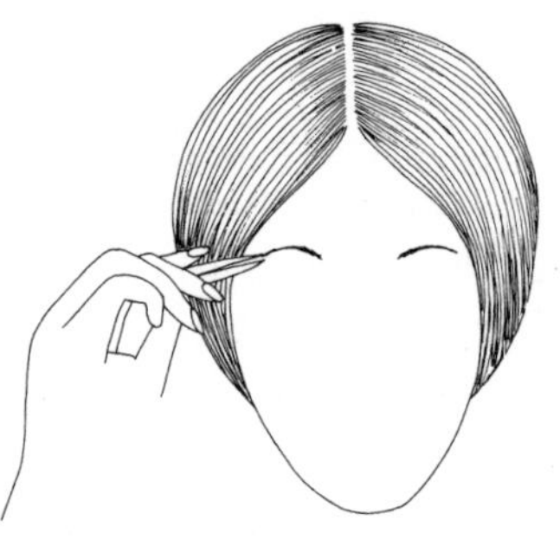

1. *Check brows* first to see if they are properly shaped, no stray hairs. Open up the arch, pluck only from underneath. The curve of the brow is important for the balance of the entire face; can be extended and colour defined later.

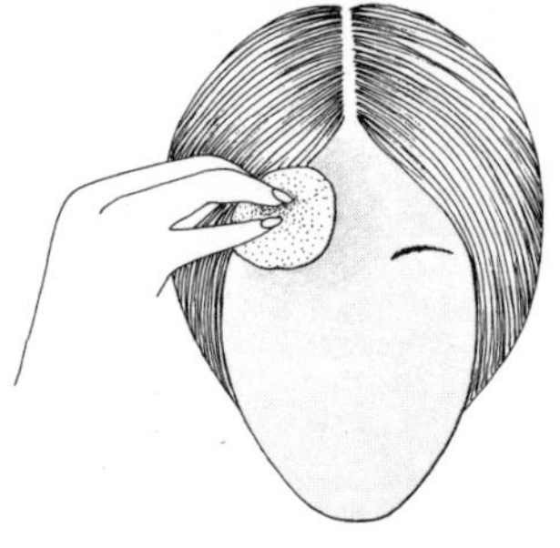

2. *Cover skin* with foundation smoothed evenly over face and under chin, blend well, no tide marks. Two thin applications better than one thick; use palm as palette to make consistency more malleable. Sponge for evenness.

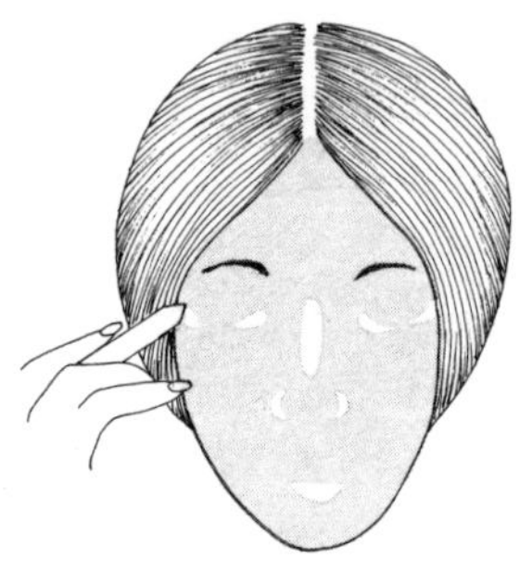

3. *Lighten up* dark areas under eyes, around nostrils, under lips, with light cover-up or white crayon. Also apply to high plateaux: ridge of nose, upper edges of cheekbones. Blend well until only a light shine remains.

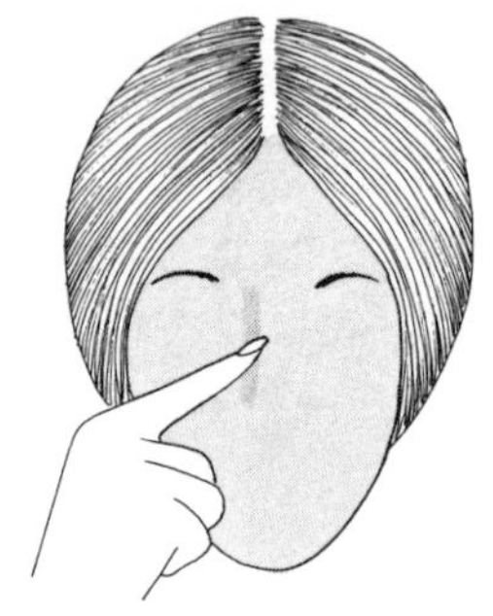

4. *Fade out* faults with darker tint, but very slightly as worse errors can result from doing this incorrectly. Sides of nose and heavy jaw lines can be eased away. Blend to almost nothing, mere shadows.

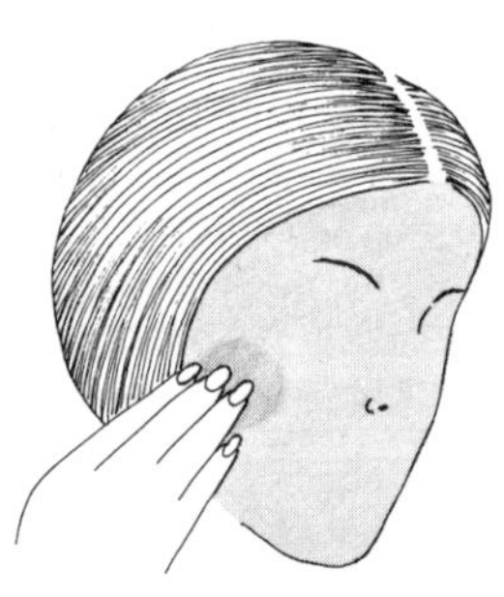

5. *Colour cheeks* with a cream blusher, applying in a diagonal sweep upward and outward towards the top of the ears along the top of the hollow. Blend so you can only see a radiance and no lines suggesting colour stops or starts.

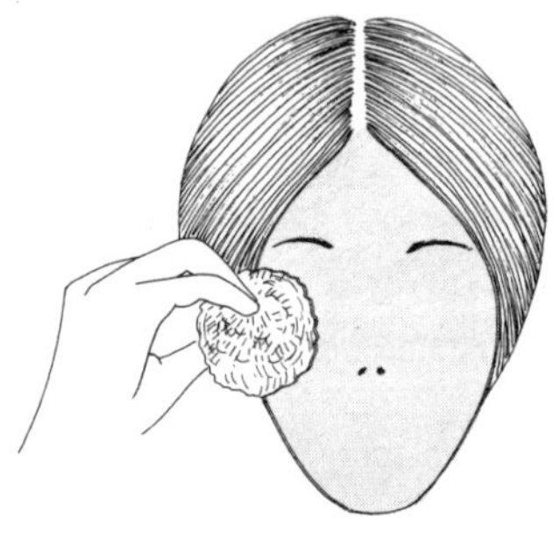

6. *Powder lightly* with a translucent or baby powder. Use cottonwool, puff, brush or dry sponge. Gently pat powder on with lots of tiny, circular press-in motions to ensure setting. Flick down to remove excess. Brush for lightest look.

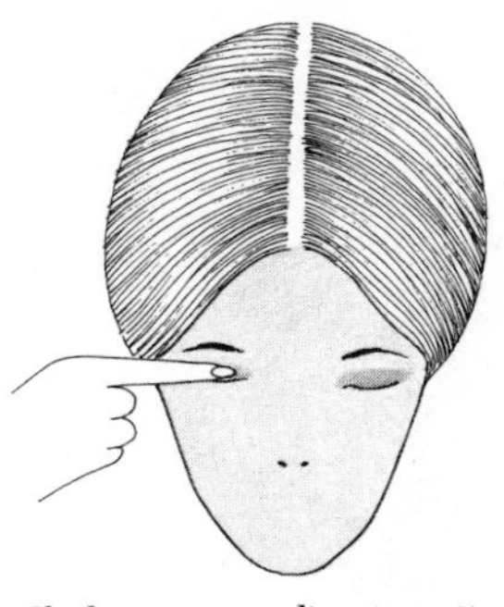

7. *Shade eyes* according to pattern decided. First apply colour to entire lid, then blend in swiftly with fingertips, adding and subtracting as you go. Look downward to prevent smudging. If cream, set with powder.

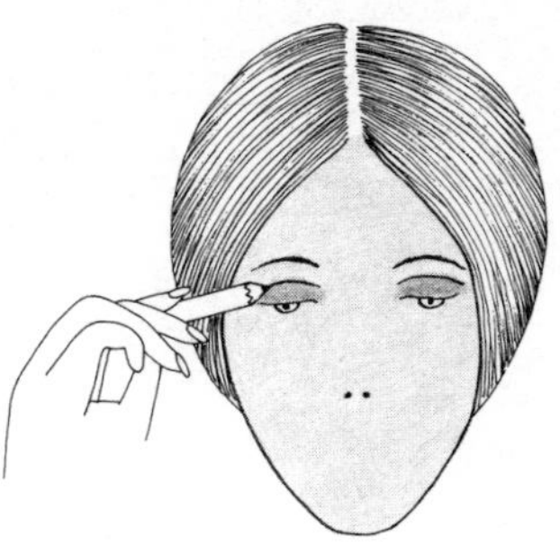

8. *Contour crease* of eye socket area to give dimension. Draw arc with thick eye crayon, using deeper shade than eye colour. Blend with fingertips or cottonwool swab. To emphasize eyes for evening, make line darker and definite.

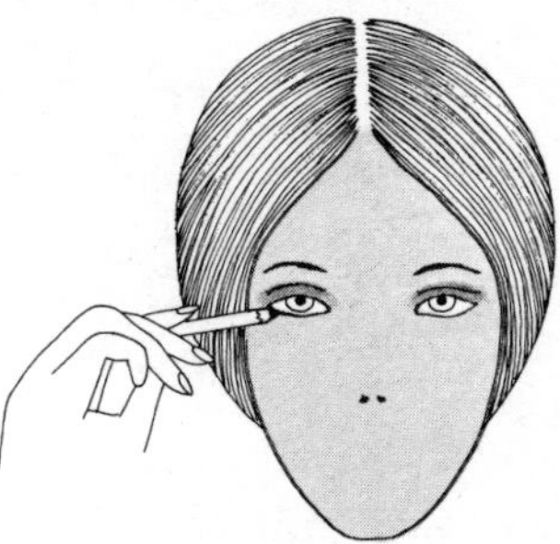

9. *Outline eyes* to define shape and make lashes look even thicker. Avoid hardness; softer lines are more effective. Consider it like shadow; dot and blend into smudgy line becoming darker and thicker towards outer corner of eyes.

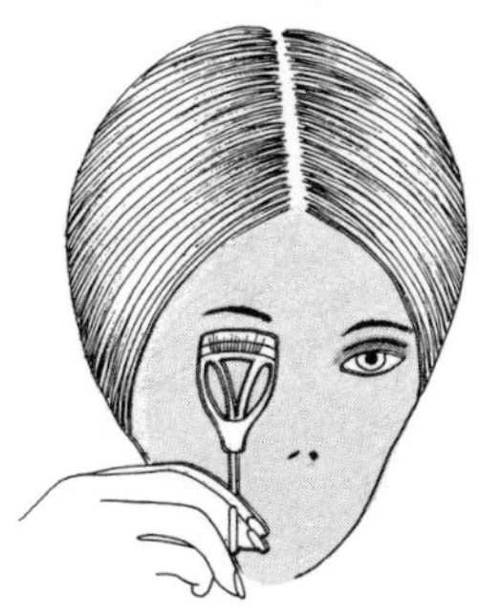

10. *Curl lashes* with special curling instrument. Eyes can be opened up, giving the illusion of more lash too; makes mascara application easier. Lightly powder.

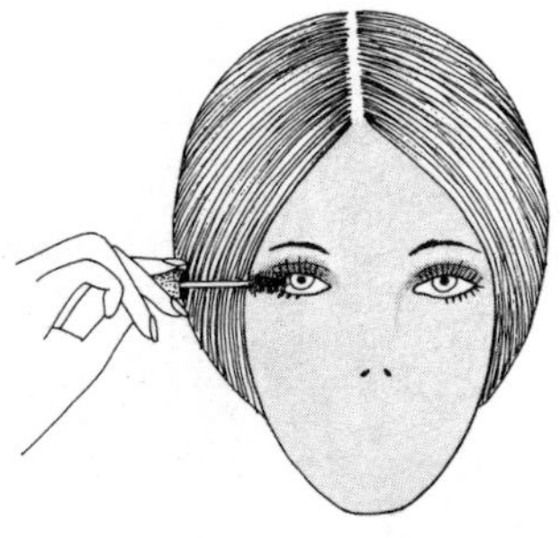

11. *Apply mascara* starting with tips of lashes and working to base for a feathery line. Brush upper lashes downwards from the top first, dry, then brush up from below. Lower lashes up first, then down. Use plenty but in thin layers.

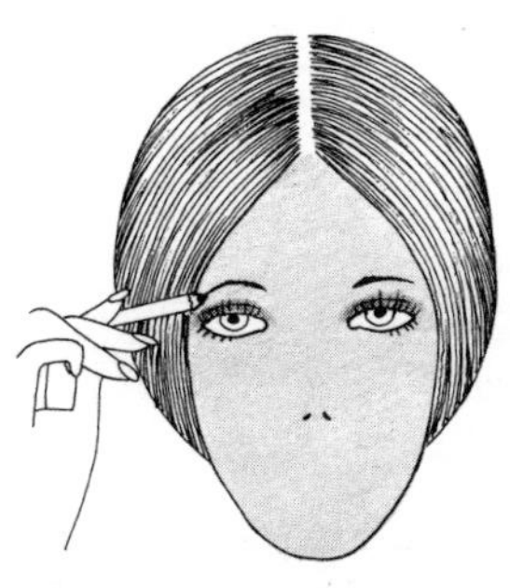

12. *Define eyebrows* after brushing to remove any trace of powder, up then across to smooth hairs in place. Apply eye pencil in light tiny diagonal strokes simulating a hair. Extend slightly at the end; brush to blend and soften line.

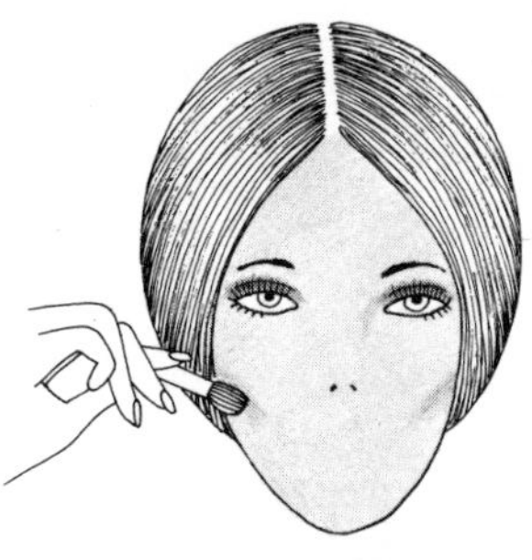

13. *Brush blusher* powder lightly over cheeks to stabilize colour and add a luminous touch. Suck in cheeks and flick the brush across the top of the indent, in upward strokes. Shade choice here can determine whether day or evening face.

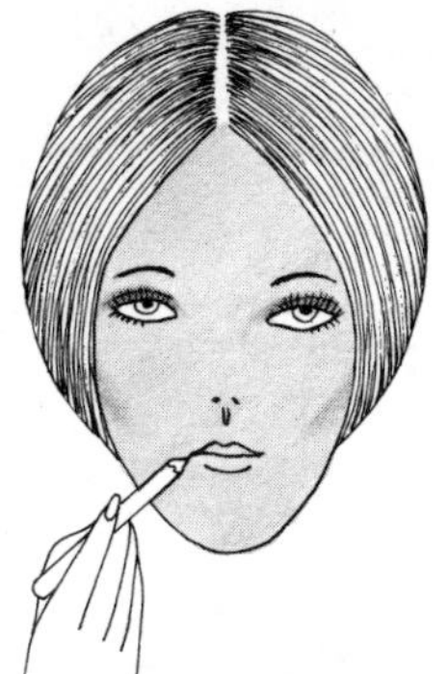

14. *Outline lips* with a pencil to establish shape, whether natural or not; the colour a little darker than lipstick. Draw in bottom line first, extending slightly at corners. Or do this with a brush using a deeper lipstick like paint.

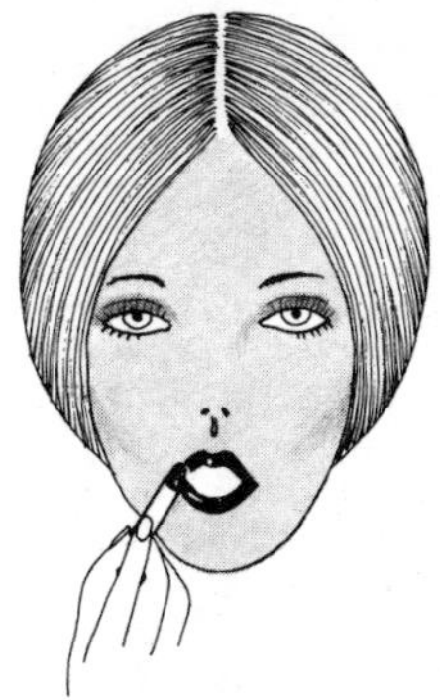

15. *Colour and gloss* lips, first filling in with the lipstick applied directly or with brush, blend into the outline but don't completely cover it. Blot. Apply another light coat. For extra shine, smear on a lip gloss or petroleum jelly.

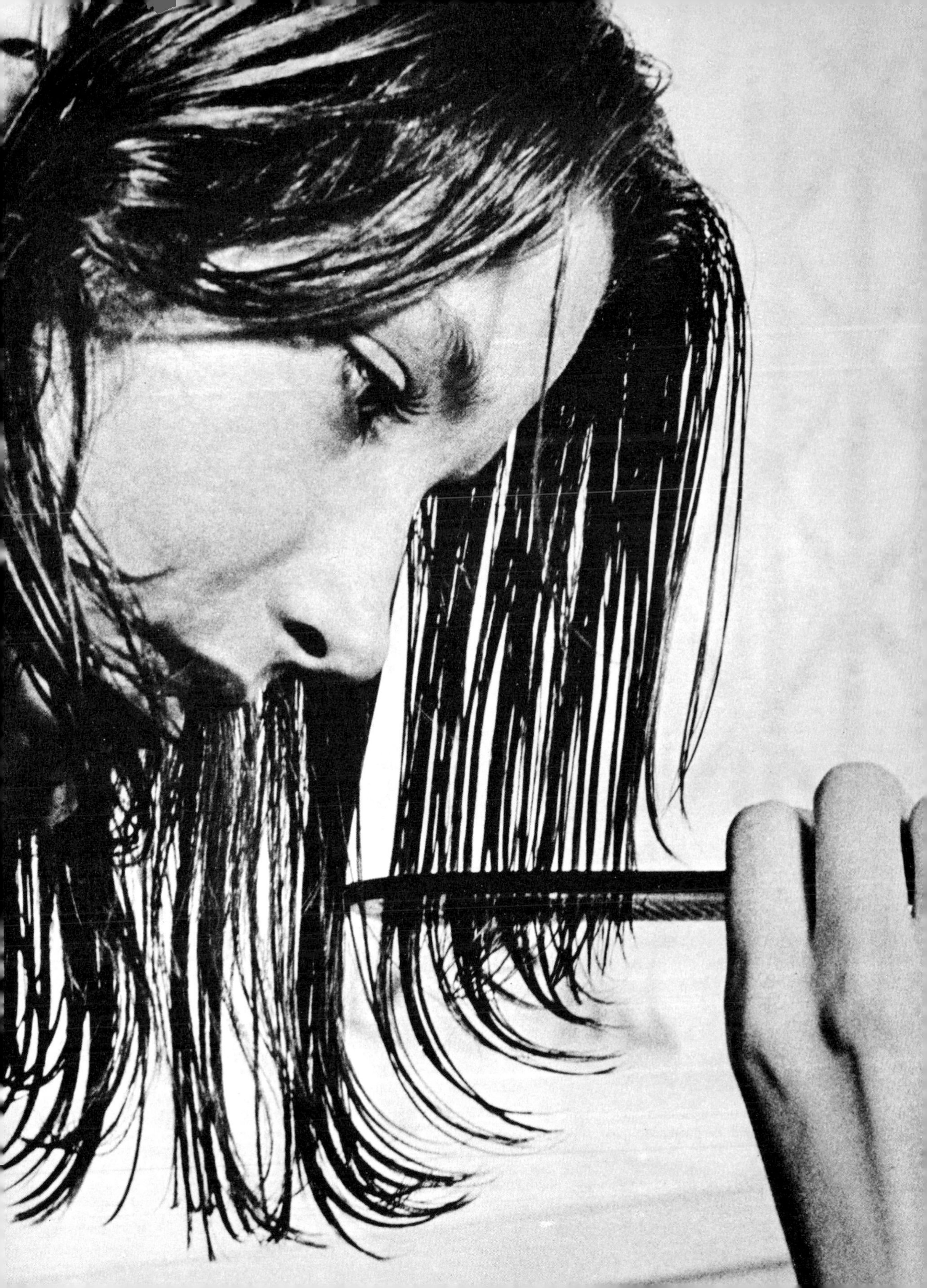

3

HAIRSTYLE

Before any decision can be made on style or colour, the first thing to establish is what type of hair you have. Three aspects have to be considered: texture, body and pattern.

TEXTURE — FINE OR COARSE

Fine hair is narrow in diameter, inclined to be weak, limp and lacking in body. It is usually thin and looks fullest and best when it is blunt cut and not much longer than chin length. Styling depends on how curly it is. Anglo-Saxons and Nordic people often have this sort of hair.

Coarse hair is fat, generally strong and sometimes wiry. It can be hard to manage and style depends on thickness and curliness. Women in hot climates – Mediterranean, African and Eastern areas – often have strong coarse hair. It can respond well to a longish cut, unless wiry and very curly. When straight or wavy, too short a cut will make hair stand out.

Medium hair is somewhere between the two extremes and combined with medium body has the fewest limitations of style.

BODY – THICK OR THIN

Thick hair means there's a lot of it. If it is coarse, it is easy to tell, but fine hair can be deceptive. Warm climates and thick hair usually go together. Straight thick hair can look marvellous cut to one length, but generally thick hair is better cut in different lengths to reduce bulk and give shape. If it is curly and thick, beware of cutting it too short – unless it is cropped Afro hair – because it is difficult to control.

Thin hair is usually best kept to short to medium length and cut evenly to give the illusion of bulk. Curls can also give the impression of body.

PATTERN – CURLY, WAVY, STRAIGHT

The more you take advantage of the natural tendencies of hair, the easier it is to take care of it.

EDWARD OLEKSAK

Curly hair, cut in layers, can work at most lengths, but don't let it grow beyond the shoulders, particularly if it is thick.

Wavy hair usually reverts to its natural state very quickly after being persuaded into a contrary style. It can be cut straight or tapered; looks best medium length. Hair with only a suggestion of wave has a certain fall and it is important to follow that in styling. When hair is wet, after being combed back from the forehead, push forward with hands – it usually falls into its natural parting, and it is advisable to keep to it.

Straight hair can be coaxed into turning up or under and if necessary will take to permanent waves and curls. When straight and fine, blunt cutting gives it body and fullness; short to medium lengths are best. Straight coarse hair can look very attractive long, it swings at medium length, but can be a problem when short.

PATTERN CHANGE

The body and texture of hair cannot be altered, but the pattern can. It is done through a combination of chemicals and heat. The more drastic the change, the more severe the procedure and the more care is needed to compensate the altered hair.

BODY WAVE

This gives a loose wave 1 to 2 inches (25–50 mm.) in depth; it doesn't give a curl and doesn't change the overall shape of the hair. It is done on large rollers.

PERMANENT WAVE

This gives a tighter wave; it is done on small bone-shaped rods and the curl pattern is every $\frac{1}{2}$ to $1\frac{1}{2}$ inches (12–35 mm.). The idea is not to provide rigid rows of waves, but to offer texture and a base for certain styles, particularly the short ones. It often helps fine, straight hair.

AT-HOME PERMING

A simple procedure if you follow the directions: most disasters stem from failure to do this. Read labels and instructions very carefully; don't take short cuts and don't omit any steps. Each product has its own specific directions, but follow these general rules:

Do a test curl; this is important to help judge timing for the strength of curl. Try one section on a narrow rod, another on a roller, to decide if you want a curly perm or just body.

Home permanents usually come in three strengths: for fine, medium or coarse hair – check. Some are done in two steps: a waving solution first, then a neutralizer to stop the action and stabilize the degree of wave. Others are one-step procedures, where a timing element is built in; the snag is, there's no individual control.

If hair structure has been previously altered in any way – tinted, bleached, waved – it is porous and more susceptible to the wave solution.

The coarser your hair the more it will take the curl; the finer, the less.

The bigger the rollers, the looser the curl. If hair is short you are forced into using the small rods. Long hair is easier to handle on large rollers. Avoid putting too much hair on the rods. The pattern for rollers is the same as for setting (see page 232).

Hair must be washed before perming, dirt and grease can affect action.

Try not to perm more than three times a year, and twice is better.

STRAIGHTENING

This is a permanent wave in reverse. The chemical method is by far the most successful, though waxes and gums are sometimes used temporarily to smooth out hair. Coarse hair is the easiest to straighten. It is not obligatory to do the whole head, the more problematic areas around the hairline and temples can be straightened separately. Straightening makes hair less heavy. It shouldn't be done more than once a year; it is preferable to do it at the start of summer, as curly hair is particularly affected by hot weather humidity. Afterwards hair should be protected from sun and sea water, and it can react to the chlorine of swimming pools.

Because it is a more complex and difficult procedure than waving, few women are capable of doing it at home. This is how it is done professionally.

Hair is shampooed, blotted dry and combed; the straightening lotion (mixed 15 minutes beforehand) is put on by brush or with fingers, soaking all surfaces; it is then combed through the hair. Head is wrapped in plastic for 20 minutes. Hair strands are now soft, and the next step – the most important and most arduous – is to continuously comb from 10 to 20 minutes, relaxing or altering the curl pattern. Afterwards hair is rinsed, towelled to remove excess water, combed; then a neutralizer is applied, combed through and takes about 5 minutes to stabilize straightness before being rinsed out. The process takes about 2 hours. Bleached, tinted or toned hair may not react as well as natural hair.

COLOUR CHANGE

No cosmetic can achieve a greater illusion of naturalness than hair colouring – if it is done well and suits your skin. The rule is not to change the colour too much; best is one or two shades lighter and it is rarely recommended to go darker. Very few women can take really drastic changes. Professional colourists prefer to mix at least three tints together which give three or four tones to the hair. This looks much more real than a solid mass – natural hair is always a combination of several shades. When deciding on colour you must consider the tone of your skin and the colour of your eyes. Experiment by trying on a few wigs and hairpieces. There are cool shades, ashen tones, warm shades with bright and reddish hues. If your skin is pale, choose a warm shade, but if your skin is colourful or if you want to lessen a too red or brassy look, try a cool colour. Even if you go to a professional colourist, have an idea of what you want and don't judge a new hair shade immediately. It takes a few days for natural oils to return and they can make quite a difference to the final colour impression.

Most women can handle toning that involves a temporary or semi-permanent colouring. Lightening within a moderate colour range is not difficult either, but a more drastic change should be done at a salon. During lengthy bleaching, hidden tones often come up – brown hair can prove to have a lot of red in it, for instance – and special toners are needed to eliminate brassy tones. If colouring is done correctly it does not harm hair, though it is important to condition it after washing. It often helps fine hair by giving it more body.

There are three basic kinds of hair colouring – temporary, semi-permanent and permanent:

TEMPORARY RINSES

These are the most short-lived of all forms of colouring and last only until the next shampoo. They contain no bleaching agent so do not lighten hair. They contain no penetrating agent so they simply coat the outside of the hair shaft. They make only subtle changes in colour, adding high-lights within the same colour family as your own. On light to medium brown, rinses can highlight, darken, tone down reddishness or add it. They are good for dulling brassiness in over-bleached hair. On darker hair, rinses have less effect but will brighten, darken or add highlights. Rinses won't cover grey, but will blend in adding a little colour. Rinses often have built-in conditioners, some also act as a setting lotion. They are generally hypo-allergenic and unlike other types of hair colouring require no skin patch test.

SEMI-PERMANENT TINTS

These work in the same way as temporary rinses, only more intensely; they also last longer, through four to five shampoos. They have no bleaching agents, so they cannot lighten. They contain a very mild penetrating agent so the hair shaft is diffused with a little colour as well as being coated with it. They substantially alter tones within the same shade range – fading gradually, leaving no appreciable demarcation line between the tinted portion and the new growth of hair. With each shampoo, a little colour is washed away. Finally it goes and you simply repeat the process. Semi-permanent tints can turn a muddy blonde into a golden one, add a sable glow or reddish tint to brown hair; and they can darken. Like temporary rinses, they usually contain a conditioner. There is some build-up colour which gives the hair a heavy unnatural look, but only a professional can spot this or know how to counteract it.

PERMANENT COLOURINGS

These last as long as the hair does, though exposure to sun and certain air pollutants can cause discoloration. They contain both bleaching and penetration agents. They can lighten hair and colour it by duplicating the process of natural pigment distribution. They alter the structure of hair, as the bleach not only strips colour but makes the shaft more porous and therefore more receptive to new additions. Any colour change is possible – lighter, darker and eliminating grey. Partial lightening can be very effective.

For a moderate change, from medium brown to medium blonde for instance, you can use either a shampoo or a cream formula. Shampoos are worked into the hair and they colour as they clean. Although more convenient than creams, they are much less effective. Cream formulas are brushed or swabbed on dry hair section by section. Both processes require mixing of two preparations: the colour, called an oxidation dye, and the bleach (usually 20 volume hydrogen peroxide), called a developer because this is what makes the colour develop in your hair; the chemical reaction takes place within the hair shaft.

To lighten your hair more than a few shades – from darker brown to very blonde – a two-step process is necessary which separates the bleaching and colouring actions. It should be done professionally. Hair is first stripped of all colour – called pre-lightening – and it can take up to an hour. After comes the colour – golden, fawn, red or whatever. If you want a really pale blonde look, a toner is rinsed through the hair after stripping to drab or ashen it, eliminating brassiness. The greater the degree of colour change, the longer it takes. From black to blonde – the extremes and not recommended – might have to be done in two operations with a day's rest in between. Hair suffers from bleaching and must be conditioned constantly to combat brittleness and breakage. There are also special shampoos for lightened and tinted hair.

Darkening hair is much simpler than lightening, and less hard on the hair because pre-bleaching is not necessary.

Any permanent hair colouring needs retouching every 3 to 4 weeks to cover regrowth. Just the roots are treated, then before washing the formula is quickly combed through the entire head of hair to ensure even colour.

PARTIAL COLOURINGS

These are alternative colour possibilities, all permanent, but growing out gradually and without the necessity of frequent touch-ups. They usually involve lightening strands here and there to produce a blend of light and darker shades that look like the natural effects of the sun.

Highlighting – also known as frosting. Hair is lightened in very fine strands beginning approximately one inch away from the parting. It can be done all over the head or just around the face. A perforated rubber cap is put on the head and selected strands pulled through the holes with a crochet hook; the number depends on how much highlighting you want. These strands are bleached then toned – the whole shaft or just the tip.

Streaking – several slender streaks are lightened along the movement edges of the hair, following the line of the cut. The bleach is usually painted on, then toned with an overall rinse.

Framing – just two rows of fine streaks are lightened and toned around the hairline, to frame the face. Of necessity this must be very delicate.

Tortoise-shelling – dark streaks are put in over lightened hair to bring it closer to a natural colour without the shock of a total darkening. It is done the same way as highlighting.

Collage – three shades are blended together in the front and at the sides. First, fine sections of hair are bleached. After shampooing, some of the natural hair is blended with the bleached hairs and treated with a toner. The result – if you start with brown hair – would be a blend of brown, honey blonde and caramel.

AT-HOME COLOURING

Temporary rinses and semi-permanent tints that are shampooed in are no problem; tints that require section application can be mastered with practice; bleaching and its complementary colouring or toning is better done by a professional. Before starting, check these points:

The examples of hair colouring found on many charts and packages show how that particular colour looks on colourless hair. The colour result changes according to the colour of hair it's applied to. Before buying be sure you have the right colour for the right type of hair.

Don't straighten or perm hair for two weeks before colouring.

Read directions carefully, be strict about timing, too many minutes or too few can greatly affect colour depth. After mixing chemicals, they must be used immediately.

Before treating the entire head, it is essential to make two tests:

Patch Test – for allergic reactions. In a salon this is done on the skin behind the ear. If you think this spot is difficult to observe, an alternative is just inside the crease of the underarm. Prepare a small amount of colouring; wash skin, swab on formula, leave for twenty-four hours being careful not to rub or wash it off. If there's no reaction, go ahead. If there's any sign of irritation, don't use that product.

Strand Test – to check colour reaction. Cut off two or three dozen strands near the scalp and using the remainder of the trial mixture prepared for the patch test, follow colouring procedure exactly as instructed. What happens to the strands will happen to your whole head. Look at the results in strong light.

NATURAL VEGETABLE COLOURINGS

Henna is totally vegetable with no chemicals at all; it is non-toxic and can also be used on pubic hair. It does not disturb the molecular structure of hair as it coats the hair shaft, and thus also increases body. It is slightly astringent, so it is a good idea to rub oil on the skin before using. The colour lasts several months.

Henna must be used with caution. It is difficult to stabilize the colour except with experience. Its intensity of colour varies according to individual hair conditions, and amateurs often have been left with strange shades. A strand test is an absolute necessity. It is a long tedious process but by experimenting you can achieve rich auburn, mahogany or red tones. Brown tones can be acquired when henna is mixed with other vegetable dyes. For example, one-quarter henna and three-quarters camomile will bring a warm chestnut to fading brown hair. A half-and-half combination of henna and camomile will give reddish tones.

Hair must be shampooed before using henna. Wear gloves because it can stain hands and fingernails. Mix 2 cups henna powder with 1 cup warm water into a thick paste; add 1 teaspoon of vinegar to help release the dye. Let it stand for an hour. Stir mixture in top of double boiler until well warmed, leave for about half an hour. Brush on hair divided into sections; comb through all strands. Wrap in towel. For a brown colour leave for about 3 hours, longer for reddish tones and keep checking until you get the colour you want. Wash hair and keep rinsing until water is clear, combing all the time.

Sage can give a brown tone to grey hair. Make a strong infusion, preferably combined with black tea; boil half an hour and let it steep for several hours. This liquid must be dabbed into the hair every day until it deepens to the correct shade.

Saffron or Marigold Flowers will give a reddish tint; use a steeped infusion as a rinse, putting it through the hair many times.

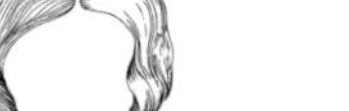

Round Face

STYLE

Contemporary hair styling stresses individuality rather than fashion. The aim is healthy naturalness. It is how hair swings and moves that matters.

The basis of all modern hairdressing is the cut: when that is done to perfection hair can be styled to swing and curl. The shape of your hair can change the shape of your face, emphasizing best features, minimizing others. This is why body is significant. Move your hair around to see what direction works best for your face. Where features are good, pull hair back to reveal them – eyes, forehead, ears, chin, throat. Where there's a fault of too much or too little, cover with hair – a low forehead, a high one, fat cheeks, strong jaw. Balance a prominent nose, a receding chin with hair so placed that the eye is drawn away from it.

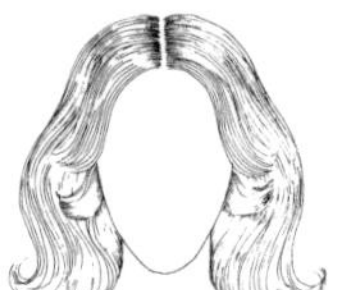

Long Face

Round Face – emphasize the top or cover the cheeks; usually short cuts work better.

Long Face – make width at the sides by fluffing out hair with waves or curls; best with medium-length hair, fullness starting around ear level.

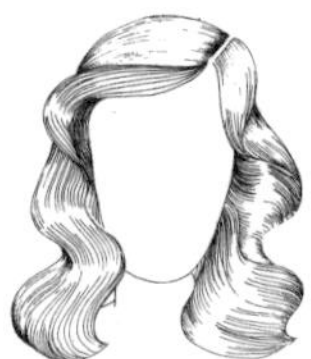

Square Jawed

Square-Jawed – cover the jaw line; straight hair can be cut to hang over the cheeks, wavy hair can break the line; leave forehead clear.

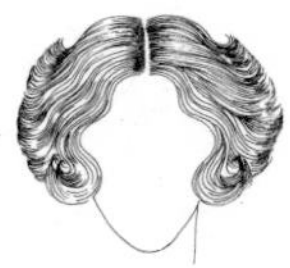
Heart-Shaped

Heart-Shaped – hair should be given volume over the fullest part of the cheeks; even straight hair can achieve this through good cutting.

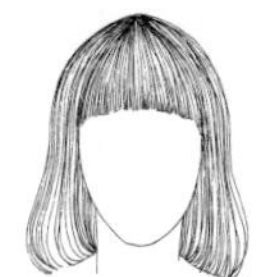
Low Forehead

Low Forehead – or one that narrows towards the hairline; simple to cover it with a deep fringe that only looks right when it almost reaches the eyes; it should start far back at the crown; the rest can be any length.

Small Face – providing features allow it, take all hair away from face, framing it with height and width.

Big Face – let hair fall over the face, covering part of the cheeks, possibly at an angle over the forehead.

Prominent Nose – balance it by drawing the eye to the other side of the head; emphasize the crown, giving bulk to short hair or arranging long hair into an up-swept style.

Receding Chin – hair must be long enough to arrange fullness along the jaw line.

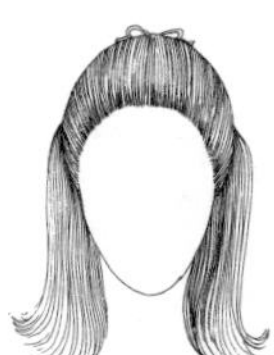
Small Face

THE CUT

Whatever the length of hair, it should be cut about every six weeks, more frequently for a very short look. It should never be allowed just to grow long. This produces split ends and a straggly appearance.

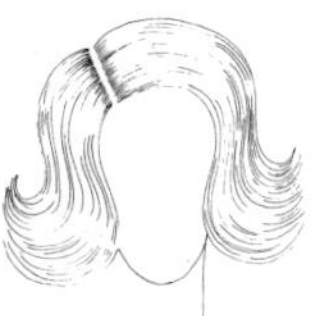
Big Face

Hair should be cut wet, after it has been shampooed. It has to be done with precision. Hair is parted into half-inch horizontal layers and each piece cut in turn following the shape of the partings. Cutting starts at the neckline, the rest of the hair being pinned up and brought down piece by piece. Modern styling calls for scissors and a blunt cut which means hair is clipped straight across even when cut into different layers. This helps discourage split ends and achieves a clean, swinging line.

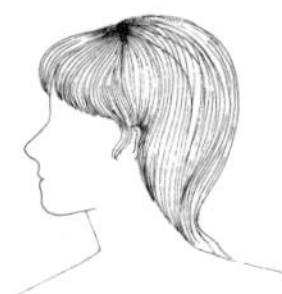
Prominent Nose

Hair can be cut all one length, which is good for thin fine hair in need of fullness, and for long straight hair. It can be shorter in certain sections, but in any segment hair is the same length. If hair is to be turned under it is usually cut shorter underneath; if hair is to be flipped up, the upper layer is cut shorter.

A layered cut is when hair is cut to different lengths all over the head. It is usually good for thick hair and encourages waves and curls. Hair is sectioned into layers – the shorter ones can be on top or underneath, depending on the style.

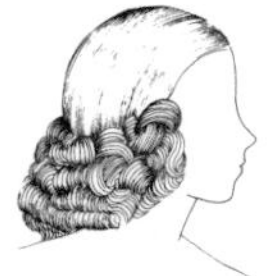
Receding Chin

These two basic ways of cutting can be used alone or in combination to create a variety of styles. Look at the sketches on the following pages.

SHORT

The most contemporary cuts are usually short; the best ones are those you can care for yourself. The expertise of the cut is vital; shape is everything and even short hair can look like lots of hair if done right. Curly hair is usually better short, thin hair too. To change the pattern of short hair is, of course, easier than at other lengths, and this is one of the main advantages of keeping hair at a minimum:

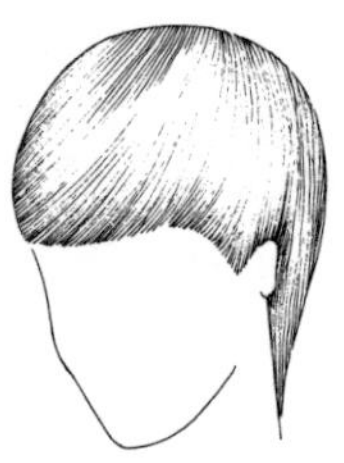

1. Cap cut brushed forward over forehead; good for straight hair whether fine or thick.

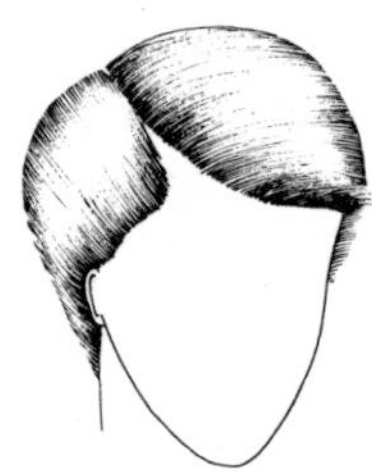

2. Hair brushed back like a boy's, flicked over forehead; hair must have some body.

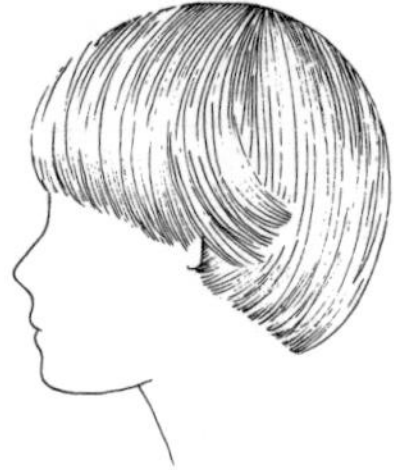

3. Classic fringed bob, hair almost touching eyes; straight hair only, thick or thin.

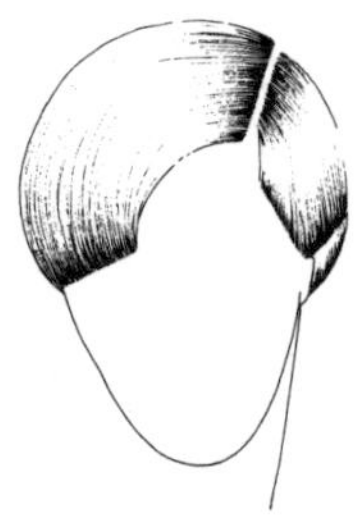

4. Angled cut, side-parted and geometrically shaped; best with straight thick hair.

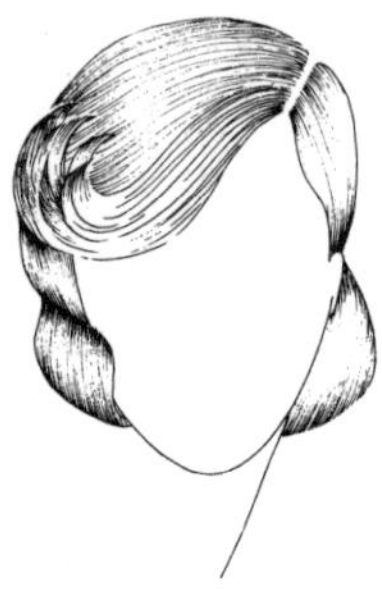

5. Hair is actually blunt cut, but waved with curling iron for layered effect; needs body.

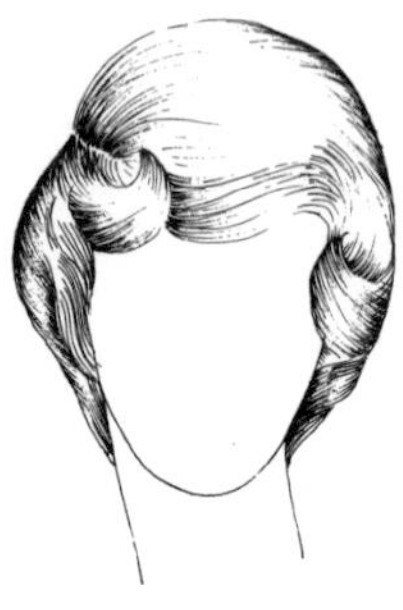

6. A layered cut for wavy hair, good for thin hair to give illusion of more bulk.

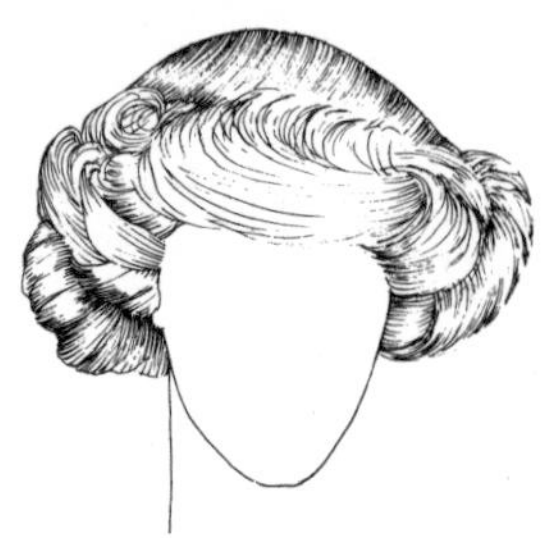

7. For wavy hair with lots of body, cut in sections to give maximum side width.

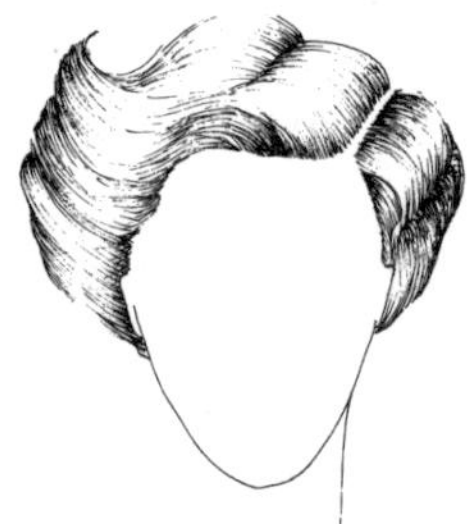

8. Hair blunt cut for a one-sided flick; hair must have body, some wave.

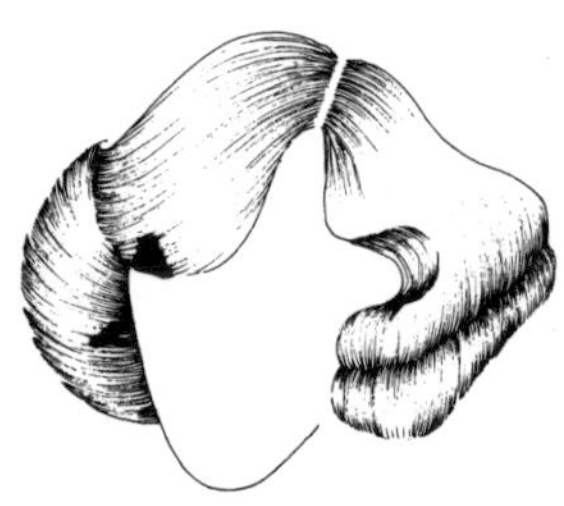

9. Only for thick hair; semi-wavy; blunt cut for side width.

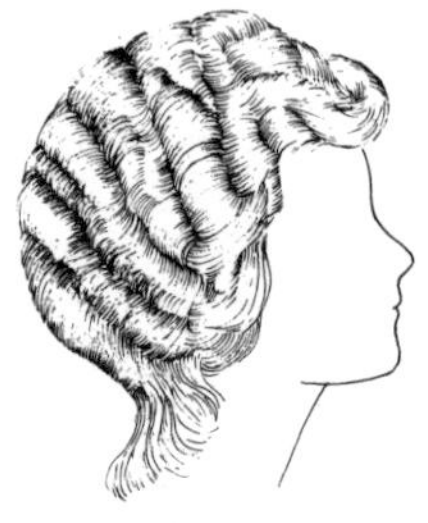

10. Curly or wavy hair cut in layers for wavy curls from forehead to nape.

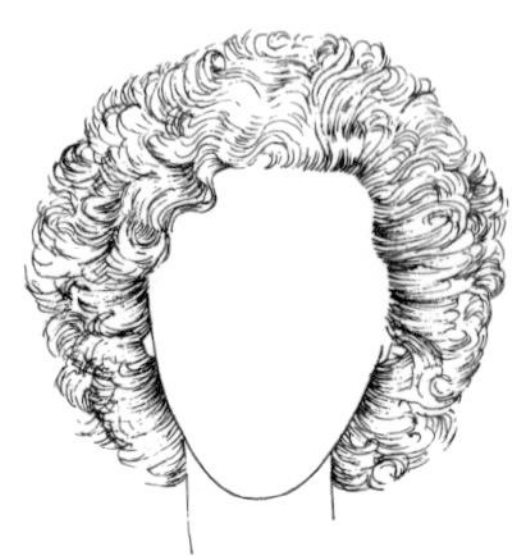

11. For curly or very wavy hair; the cut is the same even length all over, brushed up.

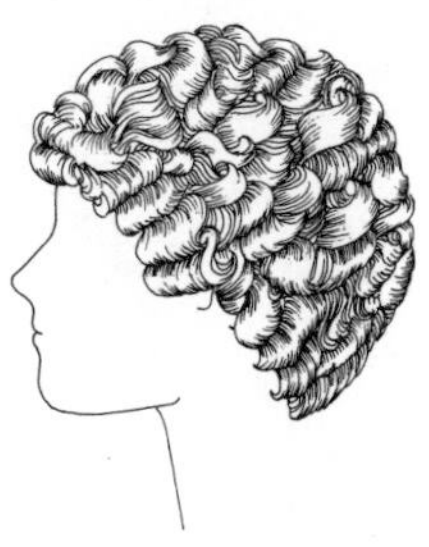

12. The only way to style very curly hair, the Afro cut with short tight curls massed over entire head.

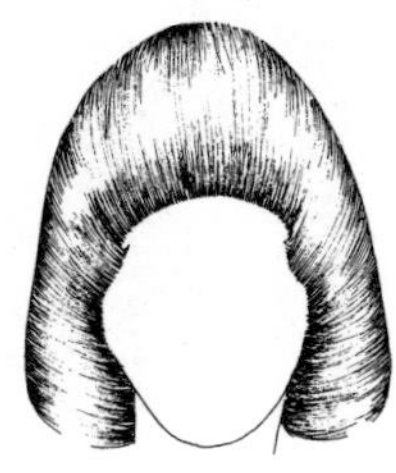

13. A cap page-boy ending just below ears; for thick straight hair with body.

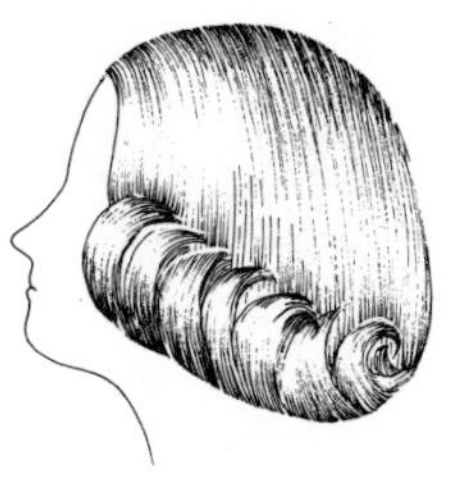

14. Classic flick-up bob looks best when moving over cheek; straight or wavy hair, all textures.

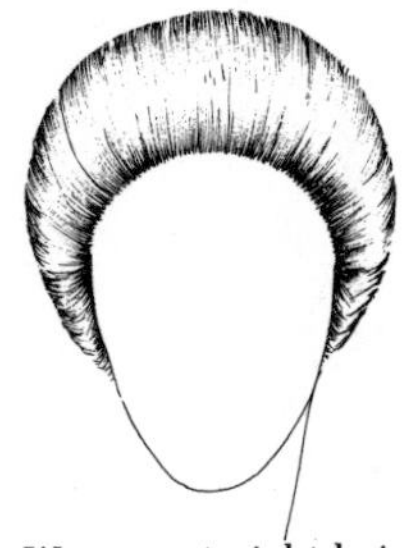

15. Wavy or straight hair can be done this way; hair cut to one short length; brushed up and back.

MEDIUM

In general, this is the most flattering length, but effect and staying power absolutely depend on the right cut for your type of hair. Note that at this length hair is more likely to fall into its natural ways faster, so follow its inclinations; a continual pattern change is not advisable. Cut and style according to texture and pattern; wavy hair is best at this length, so is thick hair. Medium length styles require the most upkeep.

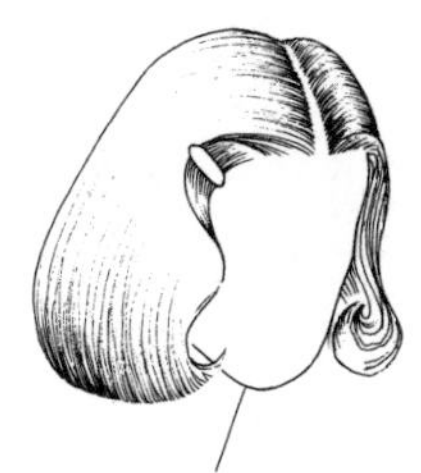

1. Hair blunt cut to same length; straight hair or a slight wave, all textures.

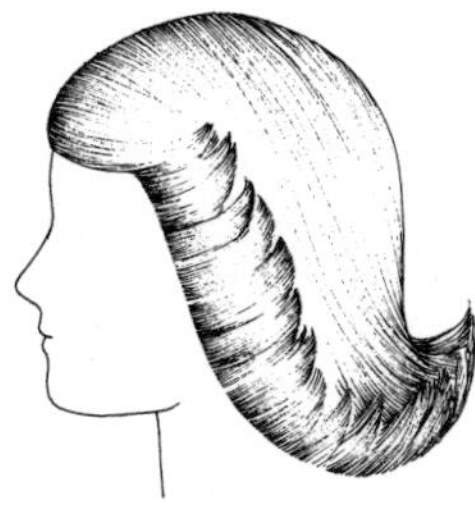

2. Body needed for this style, minimum wave; blunt cut in a graduating curve.

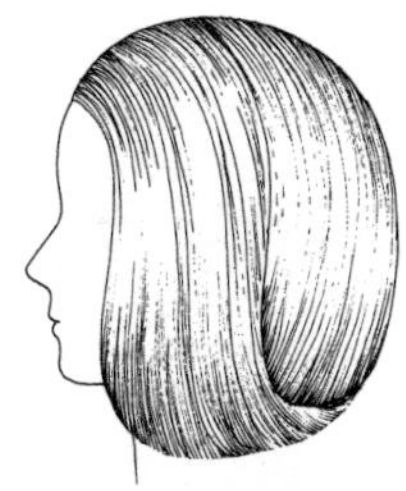

3. Good for straight hair, any texture; even length blunt cut coaxed to turn under and back.

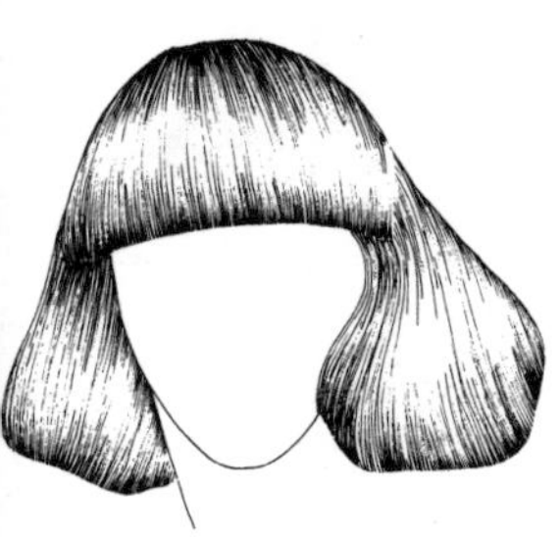

4. Hair must be thick and straight; it's the under layers that provide fullness.

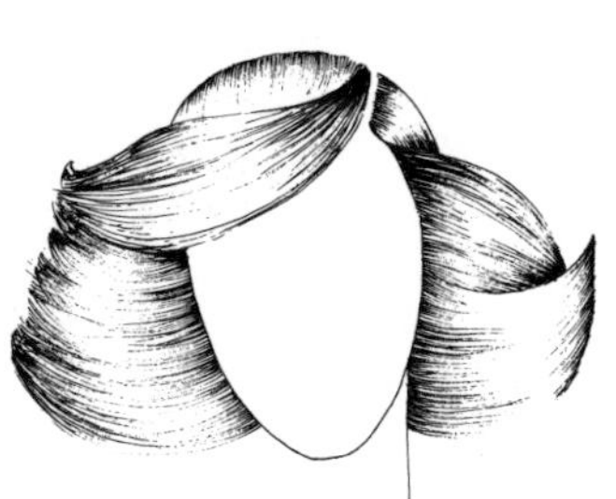

5. Works well on semi-wavy or straight hair, but body is necessary to maintain width.

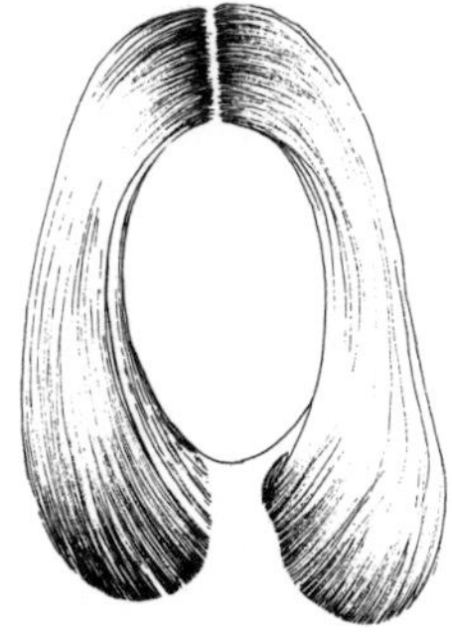

6. For straight hair only, thick or thin as hair is turned under to provide fullness at base.

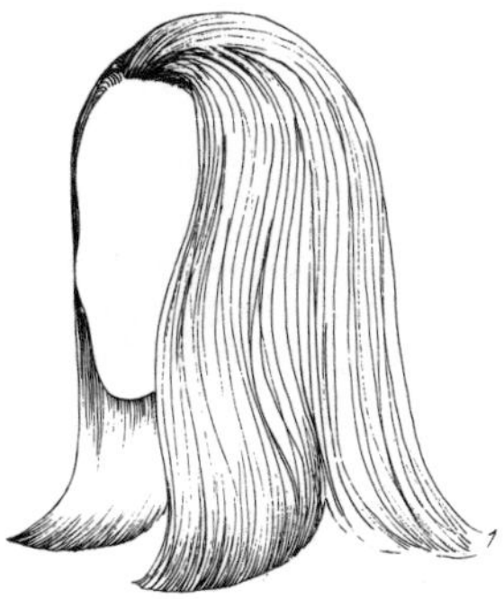

7. Straight or wavy hair of all textures can adapt to this classical fall of hair.

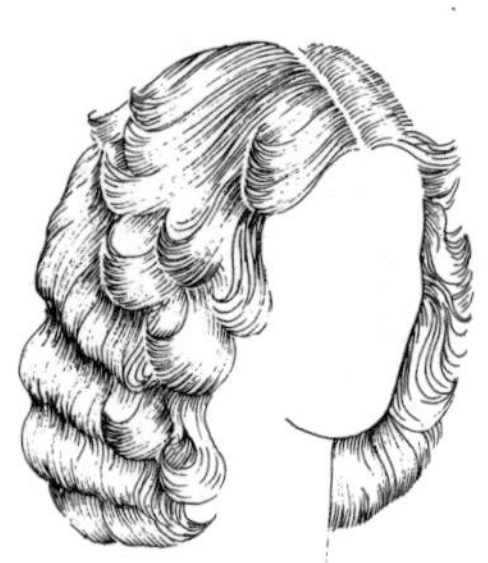

8. A layered cut for curly or wavy hair; centre parting here, but easily adaptable to side combing.

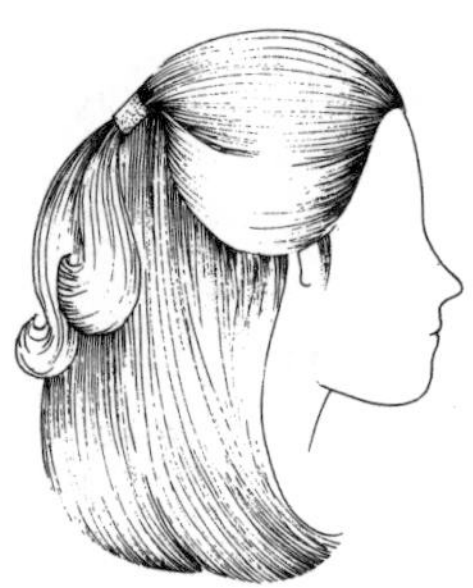

9. Blunt cut to one length, upper section drawn back; for all textures, straight or semi-wavy.

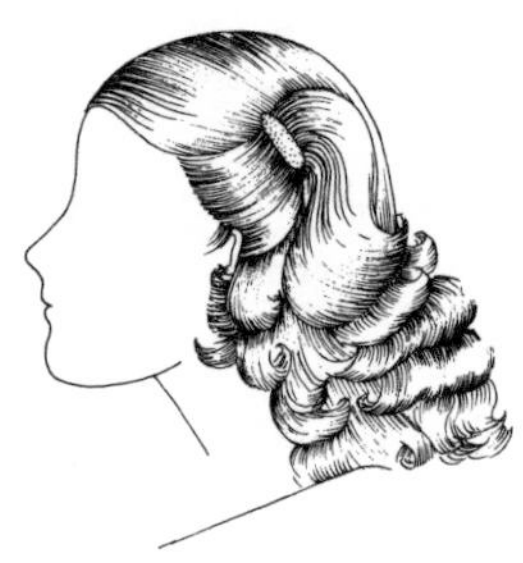

10. Semi-wavy hair cut in layers from the ears down, the crown left smooth; body not necessary.

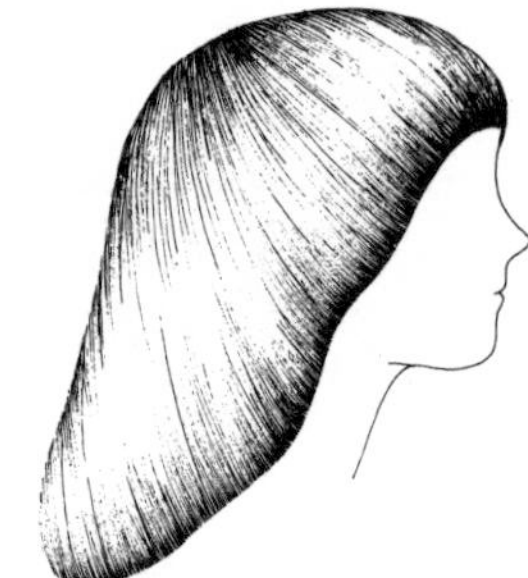

11. Page-boy cap only for straight hair and better if some body; blunt cut in graduation.

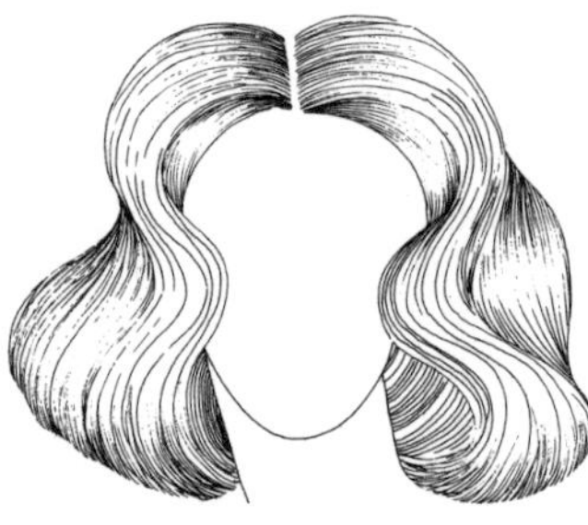

12. Only for thick wavy hair; the basic cut is blunt of even length; parting easily switched.

LONG

Often the easiest to control, long hair can provide the widest range of styles. The trick is knowing how to handle it: manipulate hair in sections, secure the main bulk with pins or covered elastics, use the free pieces to drape for interesting effects. All textures of hair can achieve sculptured effects; straight hair is easier to place, but even curly hair can be coaxed into sleek shapes. Most styles here can also be done with medium length hair plus hair pieces.

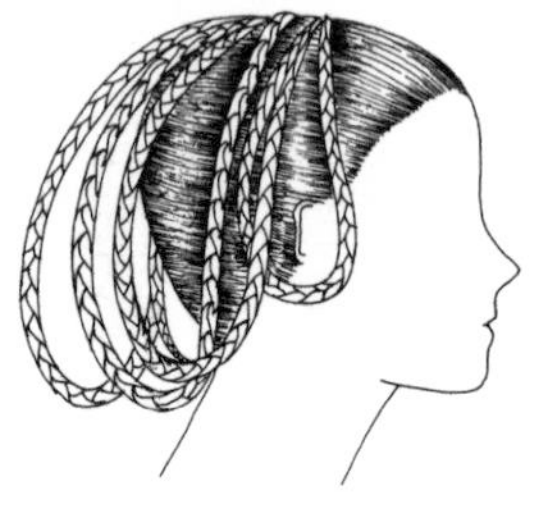

1. Coarse frizzy hair plaited in a series of narrow looped plaits; can remain until next washing.

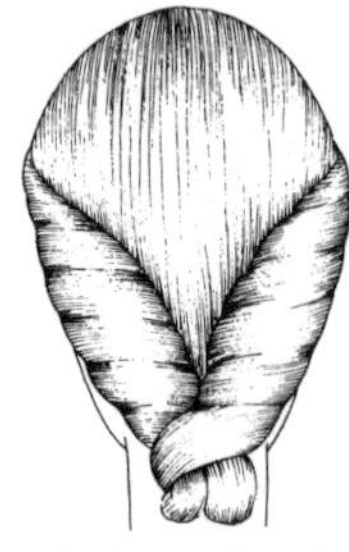

2. Straight hair only, plus addition of hairpieces; centre plait at crown.

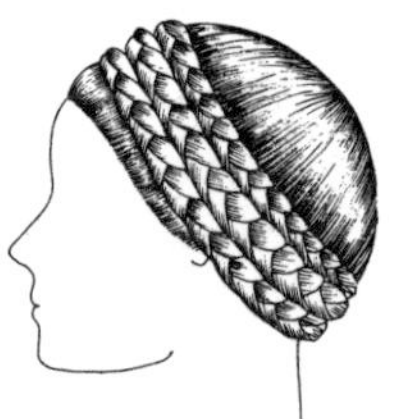

3. Renaissance feeling, plaits true or false are wound around head.

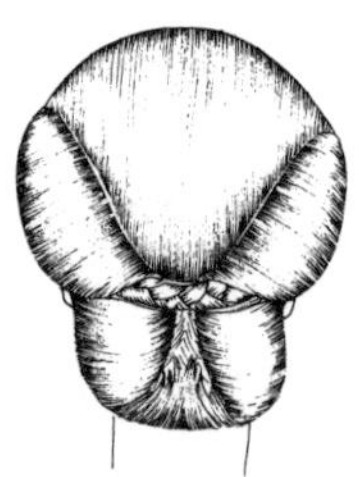

4. False plait pinned in semi-circle is the base for wrapping of hair in rolls.

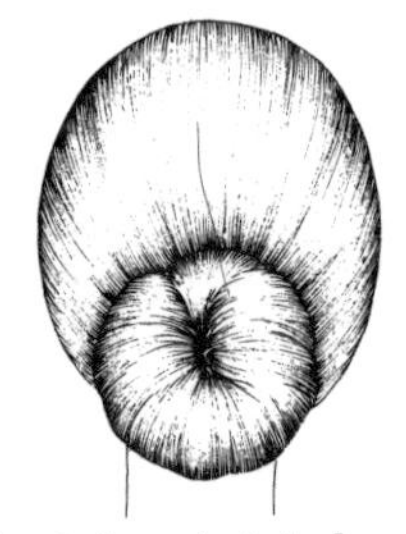

5. Classic bun; hair is drawn back in elastic, back combed and curved under.

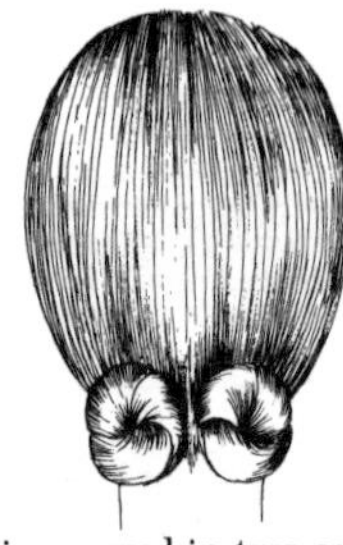

6. Hair secured in two sections at base of neck, back combed and pinned in two circles.

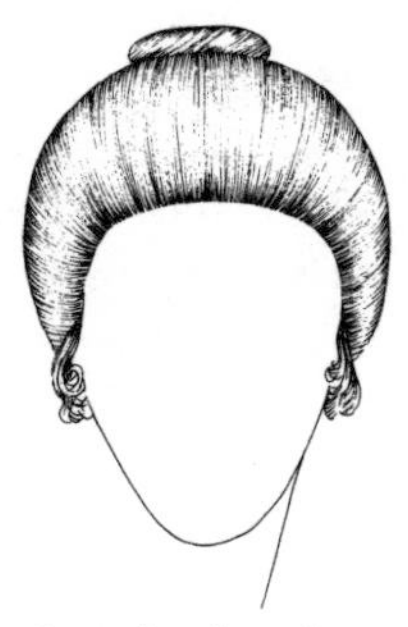

7. Edwardian idea, hair drawn high and evenly from face, a circular top knot on the crown; a few strands over cheeks.

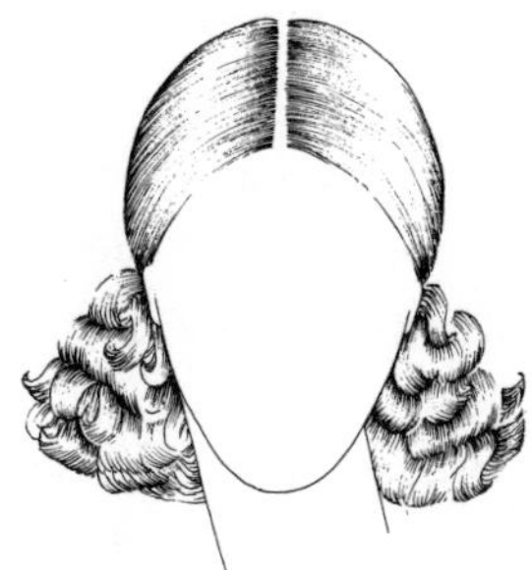

8. Wavy or curly hair can be tautly forced back into a band. then curls allowed to spray from there.

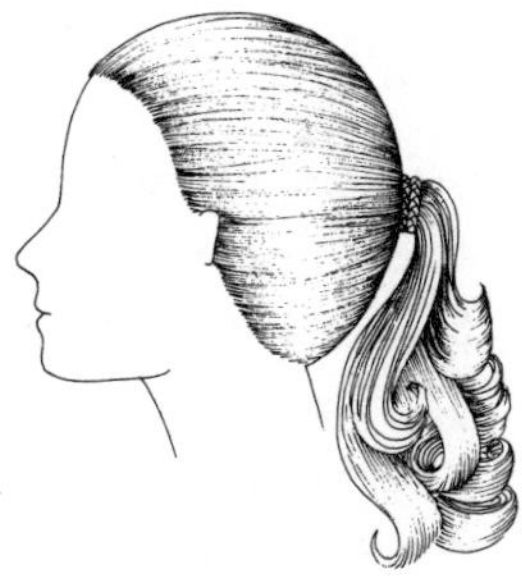

9. A simple pony tail, covered with a fine plait at the knot, the rest curled.

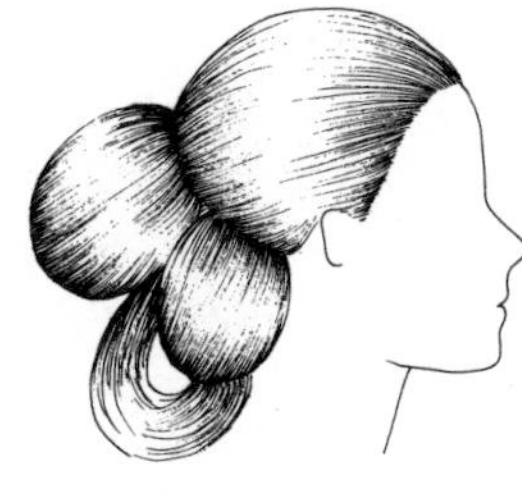

10. Hair is secured with a band at nape of neck; divided into three parts and formed into giant loops.

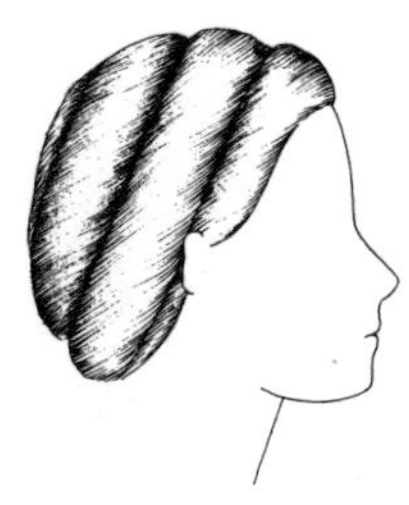

11. Straight or wavy hair can be divided into sections and pinned in parallel rows; strings on crown help control.

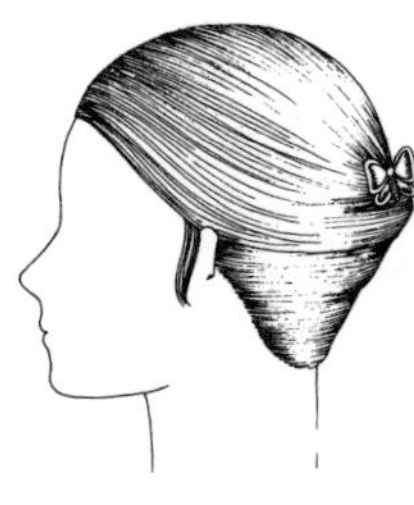

12. The classic French twist softened by cheek strands; for straight or slightly wavy hair.

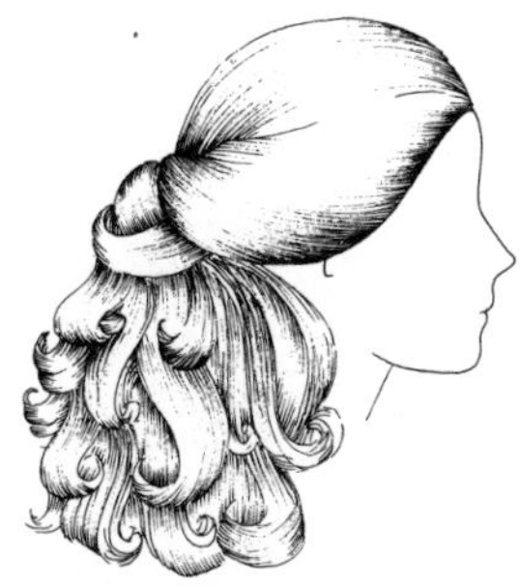

13. Wavy hair caught in a loose knot; side sections are draped over covered elastic band.

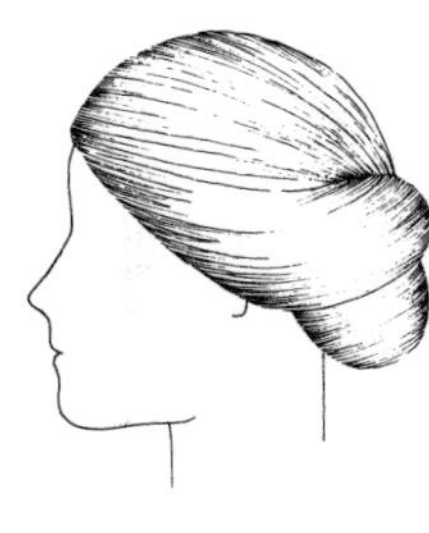

14. Very simple and only achieved with thick straight hair; two side sections and lower one form large rolls.

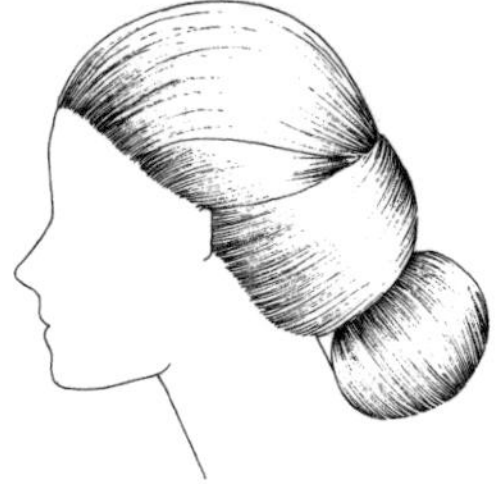

15. Centre section pulled into low pony tail; folded under, side sections swathed over band.

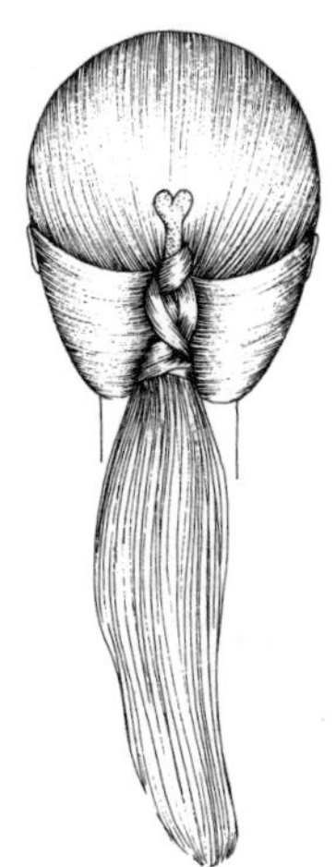

16. Only straight thick hair can be rolled like this; side sections are twisted across each other at nape.

17. False pony tail added to sectioned hair; natural hair draped over pin conceals attachment.

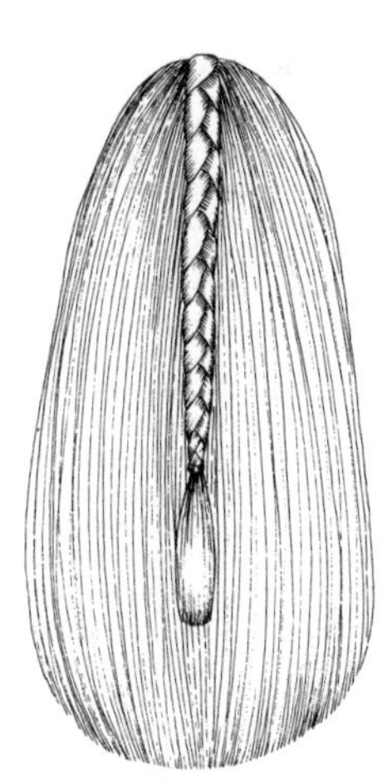

THE SET

There are two ways to transform your wet cut into a living manageable style – by setting in rollers or blowing dry into shape. Curly, wavy and thick hair is often better controlled through rollers.

1. For no parting or centre division, roll crown hair back from hairline. Six rollers are average to reach nape; four rollers, wound down, in double rows either side. Six flat clip curls at nape, two more at ear level – substitute rollers if hair is long. Fringes can be incorporated in crown rollers; when brushed forward they give a fuller effect.
2. For side division of hair; three diagonal rollers wind downward from side part across crown. Side hair rolls down, top back hair winds down. At nape and sides near ear, clip curls or rollers according to length.

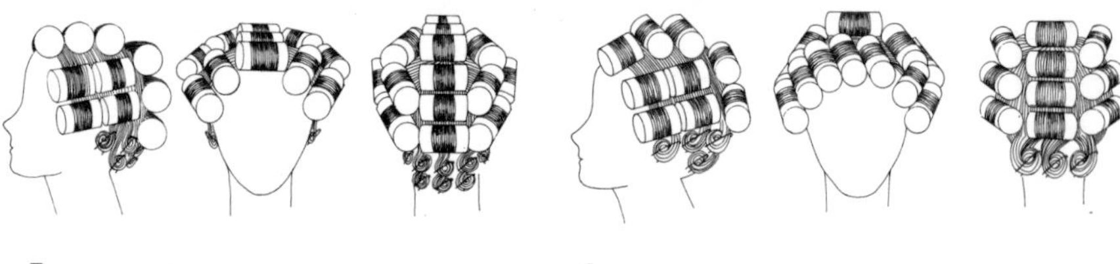

1 2

3. For a flat straight fringe, comb forward while wet, hold in place with tissue or cottonwool secured with clips or transparent sticky tape. Other rollers as for first pattern.
4. For getting long hair as straight as possible, use the head as though it is a huge roller; set two big rollers at crown, hair wound down and back; wrap hair firmly around the head securing it with clips. When almost dry, take down and wrap in the opposite direction; dry completely.

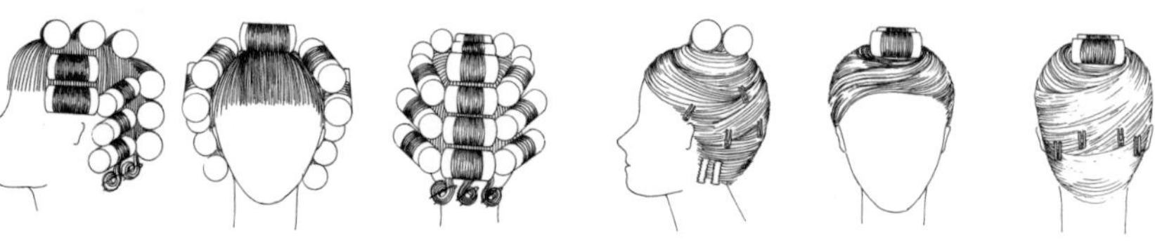

3 4

SOME GENERAL RULES

Setting lotion makes hair more manageable and easier to handle.

Rollers with brushes inside are rough on hair.

End papers help hold ends of hair smoothly and prevent crimping.

Be sure hair is smooth and taut, but not tight on rollers; stretch it a little first by pulling in the opposite direction from which it is to be rolled.

Divide the hair and work with thin sections of one-and-a-half to two inches (40–50 mm.) wide, well combed out.

The bigger the roller, the looser the set; the smaller the roller, the tighter. Most hairdressers use six sizes ranging from three-quarters to two inches (20–50 mm.) in diameter.

The coarser or curlier the hair, the larger the roller you need.

BRUSHING OUT

Before taking hair down, allow hair to cool off at room temperature after a hot dryer. Take the bottom curlers out first. In brushing out, always brush straight back to evenly distribute the curl. Put into final shape with minimum of back combing; use hand dryer and brush, or curling iron for special curling or straightening effects.

BLOW DRYING

A precision haircut is a necessity for a good blow dry result. If straight, time can be saved by towel-drying first; if curly and you want to get hair as straight as possible, you must start to blow dry while it is soaking wet. One very important point – do not pull wet hair too taut in an attempt to smooth and straighten it; this destroys hair and can cause hair fall-out. Don't have the drier near the scalp so hot that it almost scorches. Never concentrate too much heat on too small an area.

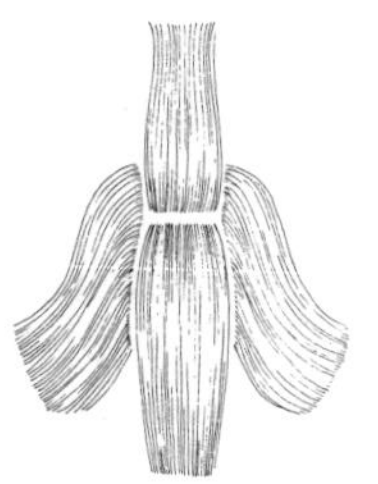

You can style with a circular brush and a hand dryer, though some dryers are equipped with built-in brushes. This is the procedure:

Divide hair into four sections – crown, back and two sides; keep separated with clips.

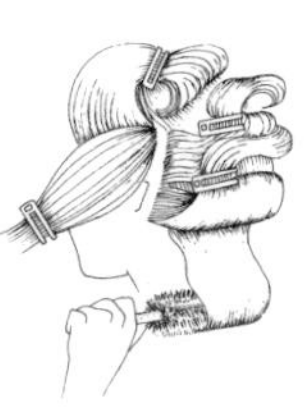

Start blow drying at the back at the nape; place brush under hair at the roots and blow over it. Dry roots first, then middle strands, then ends.

Dry upper back section layer by layer; move to sides and dry in the same way, beginning at neck; finally dry the crown.

For extra bounce, blow hair in opposite direction to the way you want it eventually to go, until almost dry; then switch direction for final minutes.

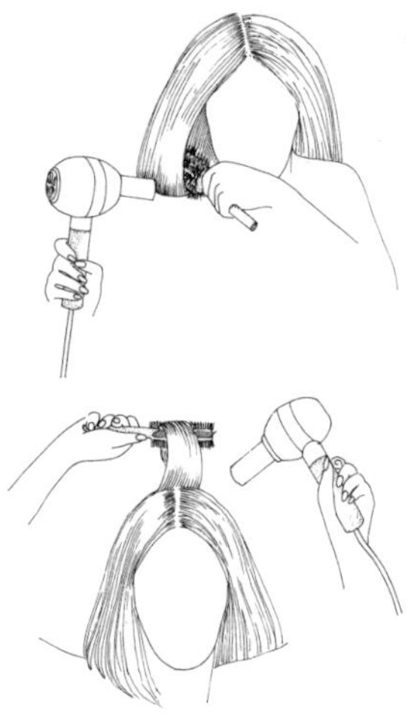

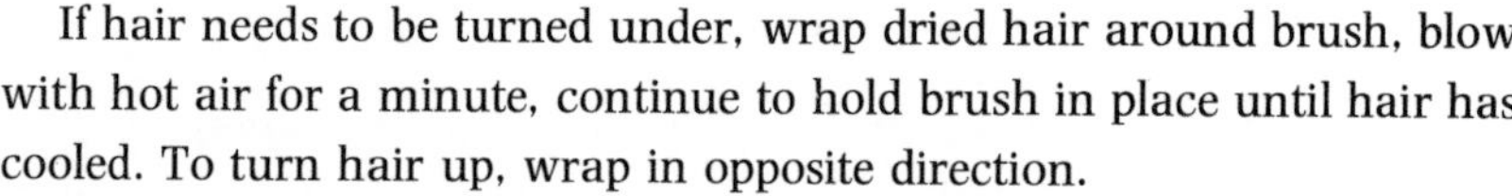

If hair needs to be turned under, wrap dried hair around brush, blow with hot air for a minute, continue to hold brush in place until hair has cooled. To turn hair up, wrap in opposite direction.

If hair is layered, brush all hair over head while drying to give a lift; when hair is not quite dry and you have the necessary height, brush and dry in direction of style.

Short curly hair should be brushed away from scalp.

For fringes – brush backwards first until almost dry, then bring forward twirling around brush, dry and let air cool hair completely before removing brush. For straight fringes, brush flat on forehead.

ELECTRIC ROLLERS

These are used on dry hair to restyle and shape hair between shampoos. They are fast and effective but should not be used every day as they are inclined to dry out the hair, even those with a 'mist'. They can be used for the whole head or certain sections to give curls, a wave or smooth according to the size of the rollers. This is how to get the best results:

In general electric rollers will make curls about twice as large as those with the same size ordinary rollers.

Large rollers make loose, casual waves, medium rollers bouncy waves, small rollers tight waves, curls or ringlets.

The more hair you wrap around each roller, the looser the curl will be.

The use of end papers ensures a smoother set.

Some electric roller units recommend a special conditioner to use while setting – check instructions.

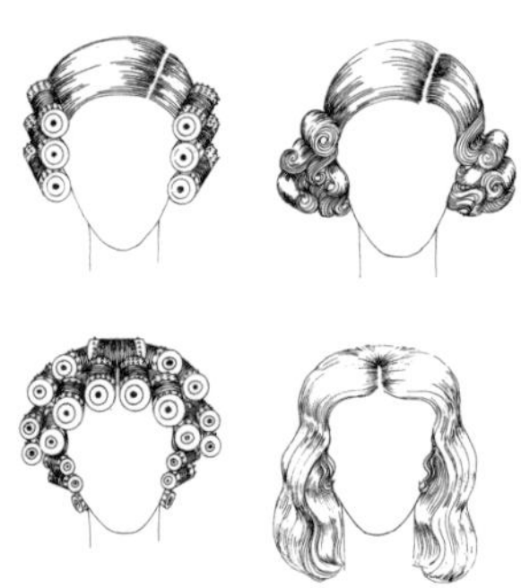

Rollers remain active for about 15 minutes after you have taken them off the heating rods.

When putting in rollers, start at the top of the head, working neckwards; when taking out vice versa.

Allow the hair to cool in curled rolls before brushing them out.

CURLING IRONS

A quick and successful way to pick up a dropping curl, shape fringes, organize ends and lift the hairline. Use with caution as they can easily scorch hair. Plastic or Teflon-coated irons minimize risk. Don't put a metal iron on bleached hair.

Time-test a strand, building up from 2 to 20 seconds to judge how much heat it can tolerate and how quickly it curls. A good idea is to briefly dip iron into diluted setting lotion as this provides protection for the hair. Curl hair in the same direction as you would if it were going in rollers. After curling, clip strands until cool.

WIGS

A wig can either improve the way your hair looks naturally or create a totally different style. The most important thing is that it should look natural, have swing and motion.

Your first wig should be close to your own style and colour. Choose one that is relatively simple to handle. All wigs can have a professional haircut and it is not essential to invest in a human hair wig; some of the synthetic fibres are very convincing, but check colour in daylight and check its springiness. Fibre has the advantage of being more stable than real hair, does not react to the environment and is easy to care for.

Take time selecting a wig; proper fit is crucial – too tight a wig will ride upwards, too big a wig will roam around on the head. A well-fitting wig should not need to be clipped or pinned to your own hair. If you prefer hair away from the face, a more natural look is achieved if an inch of hair at the hairline is combed into the wig; of course colours have to match perfectly. If the colour is different, a wig should have a fringe or be styled in such a way that hairline is invisible. Shape and untangle a wig with a wire brush, there is less fibre loss than with a comb and less static electricity than with a nylon brush. Before putting on a wig, your own hair must be securely pinned back and up; long hair can be wrapped around the head, a net or cap securing it if necessary.

Human hair wigs should be washed and set by a hairdresser, but fibre wigs can be done at home:

Shampoo every month, using a mild shampoo. Follow instructions of the manufacturer.

Dry on a wig block.

If you want more curl, set on conventional rollers, dry under a hair dryer. Follow the original curl and pattern, don't attempt a complete restyle.

HAIRPIECES

These help to add dimension or build up a style, and are particularly useful in creating imaginative up-swept effects. Colour matching must be exact and always checked in natural light. Fibre pieces are invariably as effective as real hair and less expensive. They are washed in the same way as a wig, dried and styled on a wig block.

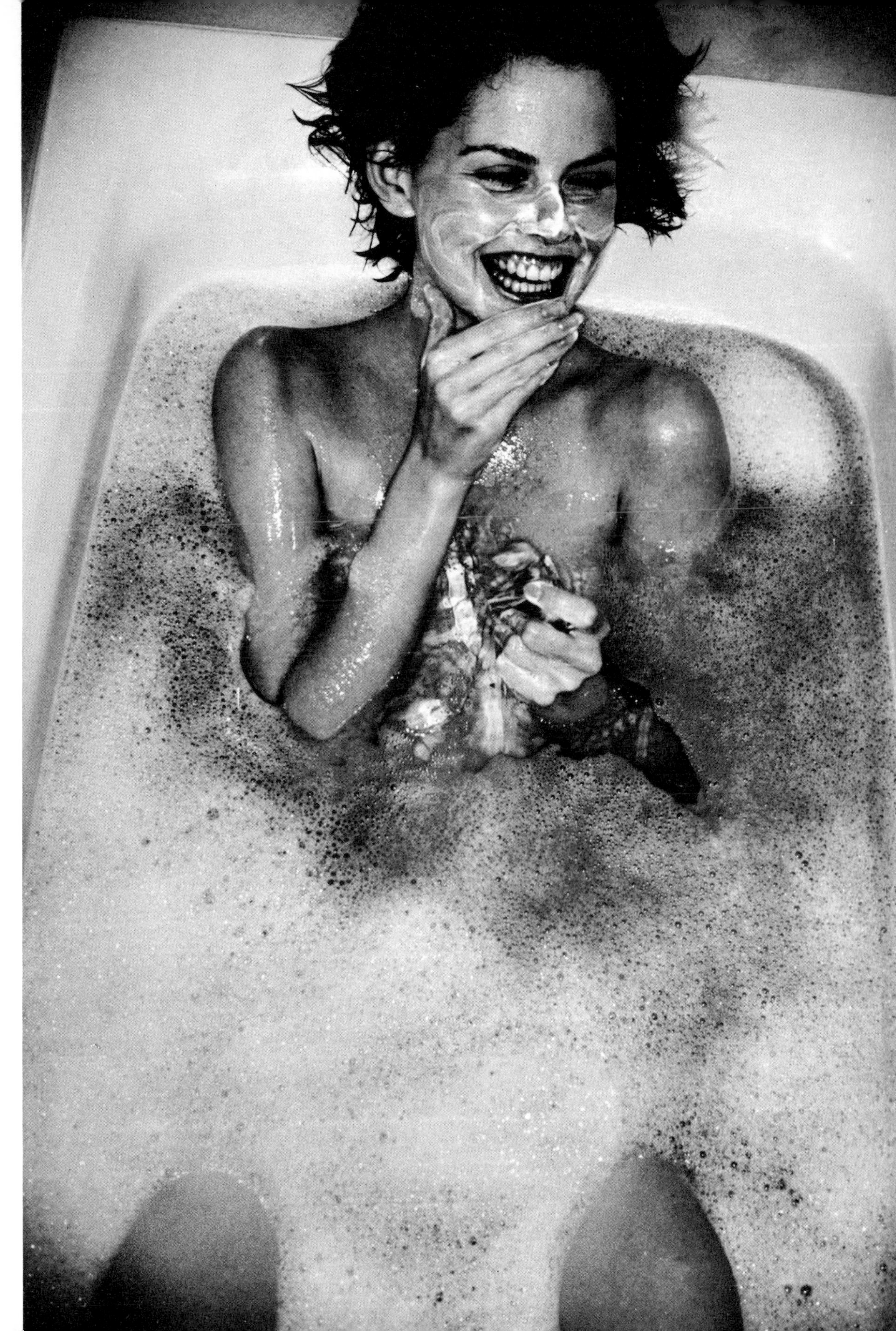

4

BATHING

Bathing is the only way to keep fresh and immaculate; it cleans the skin as nothing else can, it also refreshes and stimulates it. It is the first act of beauty and without it, all preparations and perfumes would be useless. If it is just cleanliness you want all you need is water, a bar of soap and a towel. But there's more to bathing than that.

A bath is therapeutic. It can be used to relax, soothe, stimulate, exercise and perfume your body – as well as clean it. Bathing is one simple daily event that can impart a feeling of luxury. To be a pleasure it must be sensually appealing to the touch, to the eye and to the sense of smell. It must be an exercise in relaxation and tranquillity.

There are times when speed is the criterion. Then it's a quick bath or, better still, a shower. A morning shower wakes you up in a brisk, invigorating manner and takes no time at all. Turn on the water full force to stimulate circulation and to give you a warm glow. It gets you going, it refreshes, it cleanses – but it's quite a different thing from a bath.

Many people think of a luxurious bath or a luxurious bathroom as extravagance – something to feel guilty about. Bathrooms reflect this feeling, and are usually the smallest and most miserable-looking rooms in the house. We are changing though and the message is getting across that a large, comfortable bathroom is an investment in well-being.

So first rethink your bathroom. What can be done to make it more appealing? In these days of washable carpets, protective papers, and treated metals, it is not necessary to make it strictly a tile and chrome set-up. Try cotton or nylon carpets, waterproof paper; instead of an ugly medicine cabinet use interesting cupboards and shelves, framed mirrors – many, not just a functional one above the washbasin; hang prints and paintings, attractive lamps; cover chairs, stools, and hampers; have potted plants, a table for books. Some of the best bathrooms are those that were once bedrooms, porches or terraces; they have space, light, large windows, a view. They are places of beautiful efficiency for cleansing, relaxing, thinking. The true benefits of the bath begin like this:

BATHTUB

Bathtubs should be deep and long enough to stretch the legs, but not so long (as some are) that you have trouble touching the end with your toes. A non-slip mat is a good idea, so is a comfortable foam pillow or folded towel on which to rest your head.

IMPLEMENTS

Body groomers for the bath all have to do with scrubbing and rubbing.

Loofah – a very dry rough-textured vegetable gourd that swells and softens when wet; it is perfect for rubbing off dead skin and leaves the body tingling. Natural loofahs are usually from twelve to fifteen inches long, and able to reach any part of the back.

Friction strap – usually made of hemp, blended with horse hair; long and flat, stringy-looking with strap handles at each end; it is gentler than a loofah but serves the same purpose.

Sponge – an elastic porous mass of interlacing fibres that was once the skeleton of a marine animal; comes in various shapes, sizes and porosity. If a sponge becomes too clogged with old soap, it can be cleansed by soaking overnight in vinegar, then rinsed. There are silk sponges for really delicate skins and nylon sponges in all colours.

Flannel or wash-cloth – a small square of cotton towelling used for rubbing on soap, rubbing away dead skin and rinsing; launder frequently.

Bathmitt – basically two kinds: one has soap in it, or a pocket in which you can slip soap or any cleansing product; the other kind has a rough surface and sometimes contains an abrasive or a stimulant; good for giving skin a rub down.

Body brushes – preferably made of stiff, natural bristles; long-handled ones for the back, smaller ones for arms, legs, fingers, toes, nails.

Pumice stone – a piece of ultra-porous volcanic lava; rubs away skin on elbows and particularly on heels and soles of feet, also sides of fingers that may get work stained; modern substitutes are synthetic friction blocks, as effective but not so sturdy.

ROUTINE

Drink a glass of water to encourage perspiration before you step into a steaming bathtub. Set your hair, cover it with a cap and it will be fresh and bouncy when you comb it out. Take off make-up, apply any treatment that is necessary (masque, lubricant – see page 121). If it's a morning bath, or pre-going-out bath, put on make-up beforehand; it will set in the bath, look more natural and oddly enough, fresher; it will also last longer. Lower yourself into the bath slowly; allow your body to drift in the water with spine immersed, head on pillow. Soak first, and exercise at the same time if you wish to take this good opportunity to work-out muscles (see Bath Exercises – page 250). Then wash, working up a fine lather with soap, stroke limbs with a loofah underwater, this helps firm flab as well as getting rid of dry flaky skin. Brush and pumice where needed. Rinse well, with a hand shower of fresh water if possible. The soaking time varies depending on the type of bath and the temperature.

VERSATILITY

A bath can be relaxing and intoxicating, or energizing and circulation building. With the addition of oils and softeners, it can help prevent the skin from getting rough, replacing moisture, oil, and acidity. With the addition of herbs, it can be soothing, healing, calming or reviving. Bathtime is a treatment for skin and muscles. The heat urges pores to open, making them more receptive to skin lubricants and cleansers; the warmth and humidity relax muscles, relieve tension and increase the stretch and contract capabilities of muscles. Warm water calms because it temporarily lowers blood pressure; cold water quickens circulation and gives you an extra spurt of energy.

TEMPERATURE

Depending on the temperature, water can be a great relaxer or a great revitalizer. Meticulous bathers use a thermometer; the rest rely on the elbow test or how it feels to the hands. Anyone with circulatory complaints should never expose themselves to extremes of temperature.

Hot (100° to 110°F, 38° to 43°C) – this is de-energizing and drying; it can bring out the little surface veins on legs and thighs, and if your bosom is covered, hot water can soften it and encourage sagging.

Warm (85° to 100°F, 29° to 38°C) – this is the best temperature for relaxing and perfect for treatment baths – herb, mineral, oil and aromatic additions. It's the bath to soak in, to read in for up to twenty minutes but not too much longer, otherwise the skin begins to crinkle. Keep water at an even temperature by replenishing it often. Choose which temperature you prefer; the exact body temperature, 98.6°F (37°C), is recommended. At its warmest, this range is fine for unstiffening muscles, or warming you when you are chilled to the bone.

Tepid (75° to 85°F, 24° to 29°C) – relaxes, revives, and refreshes in hot weather; prolonged for 10 to 15 minutes it gives the circulatory system the chance to expand and release internal heat through the skin. Such a bath can keep you cool, or at least cooler, for five to six hours; a colder one may cool you only temporarily.

Cool (65° to 75°F, 18° to 24°C) – a quick pick-up after a day's work, or if you feel sluggish in the morning and can't stand a cold bath or shower. Don't stay in for more than 10 minutes.

Cold (less than 65°F, 18°C) – really stimulating; should be an in-out plunge with quick soaping and rinsing. It's better as a bracing shower with the shower power turned on at its fullest – the high water pressure exercises muscles, gives circulation a real boost.

TIME

Convenience and your way of life dictate bathtime. Whether you are a night or morning bather is a matter of taste, but make it a daily routine.

Morning: If you like a morning bath – and it is a gentle easing into a heavy daily schedule – use an oil or milky powder, or if you prefer a brisker start, try a salt or seaweed bath. Soak, exercise if you like, wash, scrub and finish with a lukewarm splash followed by a quick colder one.

End of day: After a day's work, many women find it ideal to unwind in a soothing bath, to ease tension for a quiet evening at home, or to recuperate for an evening out. Have a mineral, herb or aromatic bath; exercise first, then relax for 10 minutes. A cooler rinse will give you extra energy.

Night-time: To encourage a good night's sleep, laze in a milky, foamy or protein-enriched bath (oatmeal, for instance); if it's perfumed, choose a drowsy, sweetish one. Rinse with water of the same temperature; dab dry, don't rub vigorously.

TYPE

There are four basic baths – nourishing, toning, lubricating or restoring. All are more rewarding when perfumed. Some general rules are: mint and rosemary for energy, sandalwood for tranquillity, cedar and pine for meditation, jasmine for soothing nerves, and rose for calming – carnation is said to be an aphrodisiac. Over the ages, there have been dozens of stories about famous beauties and their special use of herbs and aromatics in the bath to maintain their beauty. It is simple to work out your own formula from kitchen items and everyday herbs. Below are several recipes which may be made up as stated or with an addition of a favourite herb or fragrance.

Nourishing: Usually protein-based baths that soften and enrich the skin and combat dryness. These are soothing baths, good for morning and evening.

MILK:

A cup of powdered skimmed milk in a bath of warm water – the modern version of the ancient milk bath.

OATMEAL:

Stir 1 lb (½ k.) of oatmeal into a deep bath. It contains oils that smooth and nourish. Rinse well afterwards.

OATMEAL BATHMITT:

1 lb (½ k.) oatmeal
¼ lb (120 g.) bran flour
¼ lb (120 g.) powdered Castile soap (finely shredded will do)
¼ lb (120 g.) powdered orris root

Mix thoroughly and put into a muslin or cheesecloth bag, then into a towelling bag or mitt.

This can either be used as a bathmitt and directly rubbed on to the skin, or soaked in the bath itself.

OATMEAL, ALMOND, OR BRAN BAG:

Make a muslin bag, and fill it with oatmeal, almond meal or bran, and let soak in the bath the way tea bags soak in water. Put the bag on a long string hanging from the tap and use for two or three baths.

MILK AND HONEY:

This is probably the most expensive home-made bath, but has become a weekly ritual with several well-known beauties.

1¾ oz. (55 g.) bicarbonate of soda
3 pints (1·5 l.) dried milk
1 lb (½ k.) honey
4 oz. (120 g.) salt

Dissolve soda and salt in a pint (6 dl.) of lukewarm water. Make 3 pints (1·5 l.) of milk from dried milk, following proportions indicated on the package; warm it, and dissolve in it the honey. First put the salt-and-soda mixture in a warm bath, then stir in the milk and honey.

STARCH:

Hard water can be softened with the addition of a couple of teaspoons of ordinary laundry starch, which also gives a milky, softening texture to the water and in turn smooths skin.

Toning: Mineral salts help stimulate circulation, making the skin tingle; they are invigorating and recommended as a start to the day; they are especially reviving during bleak winter months when one cannot get to the sea. They aid in the removal of toxins, and often help get rid of liquid weight.

SEAWEED:

Fill a muslin bag with seaweed (preserved from summer or found at a health shop) and let soak for 10 minutes in a warm bath before getting in.

SEA SALT:

Rub handfuls of coarse salt over body – everywhere except face and genital area. Salt can be contained in a mitt, if preferred. Rinse salt off with warm water, then wash in bath with lubricating additions.

EPSOM SALTS:

Use ½ lb (240 g.) in a warm bath; this is additionally therapeutic if you add mint, pine or eucalyptus extract or oil.

TEA:

A colour toner this, for it tans the skin and keeps up the shine of summer; make a strong tea (just ordinary tea) with four dessertspoons to a quart of boiling water; let it steep for 10 minutes, then pour into warm bath – not too deep, otherwise tea becomes too diluted and less effective.

Lubricating: Oil in the daily bath is the easiest way to counteract skin dryness; it gives the body a silken feeling, and helps restore moisture. Oils that disperse in water are few (though there are now many commercial combinations) but it doesn't matter, as floating oil will cling to the skin and lubricate it equally well. Just a few drops of oil are effective.

AROMATIC OIL:

Mix ¾ cup castor oil or almond oil or avocado oil with ¼ cup any aromatic oil. Suitable fragrances are: rose, jasmine, lavender, mint, pine, lemon flowers, citron. Use only a few drops in each bath.

KITCHEN OIL:

1 cup corn, sesame or olive oil

1 tablespoon liquid detergent shampoo

½ teaspoon aromatic oil

Pour all into a bottle, shake well; use a couple of tablespoons for each bath, remembering to shake again before use.

SHAMPOO OIL:
Oil-base shampoos are as beneficial to the skin as to the hair; it's a quick and inexpensive way to lubricate the skin; a couple of dessertspoons are enough for a deep bath.

Restoring: Herbs and other natural botanical sources are the bases of the restorative bath. These are treatment baths in the tradition of the spa. They are always warm baths, which draw out the beneficial elements. Some are relaxing, some reviving; they are ideal for recuperation after a day's work or for soothing before going to bed.

HERBALS:
There are many herb baths, simple or compound ones, the recipes of which have been handed down over the generations. Don't throw herbs into the bath; they will stick to your body and play havoc with drainage. There are two ways to use herbs in the bath:

1. Pouchette – put herbs in a bag of porous fabric such as cheesecloth; to please the eye more, put this in a patterned silk or muslin sack and hang over the tap for several consecutive baths.

2. Infusion – crush or break-up herbs and make an infusion as you would tea; a pint (6 dl.) of boiling water to 2 tablespoons of leaves or flowers. Never boil the herbs themselves – pour the water over them and let them steep for a minimum of 15 minutes. The longer you allow a herb to steep the more effective it will be but 3 hours is the maximum. Keep pot covered; use ceramic or glass pots, never enamel-lined pans.

LAVENDER MIX:
Dried lavender flowers mixed with smaller amounts of mint leaves, rosemary, comfrey root. Put in a muslin bag and pour on boiling water. Steep for 15 minutes, pour liquid into bath and also hang pouchette from tap into bath.

ROSEMARY MIX:
Rosemary, fennel, sage and yarrow; make an infusion or pouchette.

CAMOMILE:
This mild yellow-white flower contains azulene which is very soothing and restoring to the skin. Use fresh or dried flowers. For an extra zing, add dash of rosemary and pine needles (infusion or extract). Camomile also protects you from insect bites.

ELDER:
Restores nerves and calms, as well as healing and stimulating the skin; either an infusion or pouchette.

COMFREY:
Good for healing scars – make an infusion from the leaves.

LADY'S MANTLE:
An infusion in the bath is said to help menstrual difficulties.

BLACKBERRY:
Spring tonic to restore a dull skin, use several nights in a row. Make a strong infusion, add to warm bath.

PINE:
Boil pine needles for 20 minutes and allow to steep for 12 hours.

Or – put needles in a vacuum flask, add boiling water and leave for 24 hours.

Strain and use a cupful per bath; add to basic lubricating bath.

LEMON:
Add slices of lemon to a lemon-scented bath oil (either commercial or your own concoction); use slices to rub over skin.

CIDER VINEGAR:
Restores the acid mantle to the skin and can be very important in keeping this balance. Add one cup to a bath; the water takes on a velvety quality, but the skin does not retain the smell of vinegar afterwards.

SOAP

Soap is the best way to cleanse the skin. Facial skin may need special care but rarely is a woman so sensitive to soap and water that she must use only cleansing oils or creams for her body. Soaps are made from fats and oils, combined with an alkali. This alkalinity is neutralized on contact with most skins. Talk about soap being too drying and the cause of flakiness is exaggerated, as this condition is usually brought about because of over-use or abuse and not because of the soap itself. Too much soaping is definitely bad and quite unnecessary. Every soaping must always be followed by a thorough water rinsing, and in the case of dry skins by an application of cream or a moisture-preserving lotion. Soap is neither old fashioned nor ineffective.

Conventional soaps are reasonably mild and there is a wide range of products to choose from. Choice is a matter of experiment; if one soap tends to make your skin taut, change to another. There are soaps based on olive oil as were the first soaps made in Castile, soaps using natural botanical sources, soaps rich in lanolin, soaps superfatted with cream. The fattier soaps are midway between regular soaps and a rinsable cleanser. They don't clean as well as regular soaps, but are milder. The rules to follow are: for an oily skin, use a drying soap; for a dry skin a superfatted one; for a normal skin, any good mild soap.

Cleansing detergents are not to be thought of as meagre substitutes for soap because they're synthetic. They come as bars, liquids, lotions and gels – and clean exactly the way soap does; they must be very well rinsed away. They are very effective in hard water, and also lather in sea water. For oily skin, use an alkaline detergent to strip away excess oils; for dry skin, a detergent with built-in moisturizer is best.

Home-made soaps are complicated to produce and frankly not worth the effort, but here is a recipe for liquid herbal soap that's simple to make, soothing and nourishing to sensitive skins:

HERBAL LIQUID SOAP:

2 tablespoons dried camomile flowers
12 tablespoons milk (fresh or made from powder)
1 egg
1 teaspoon honey
1 tablespoon almond oil
2 tablespoons herbal shampoo with oily base
2 tablespoons rubbing alcohol

Steep camomile flowers in the cold milk for three hours – covered with a cloth. Beat egg into almond oil, add shampoo, then honey and finally alcohol, beating all the time. Blend in the milked camomile. Put in a tightly sealed jar; shake always before use. If you want a more perfumed soap, substitute part of the almond oil with an aromatic oil.

PREPARATIONS

Bath products cleanse, soften and revive the skin and soothe the senses. Here are the general types, for bath and afterwards.

In the Bath:

Bubbles – soften and scent water; often not necessary to use soap.

Crystals – mineral salts, coloured and perfumed to soften water.

Gels – transparent cleansers that can be used as an alternative to soap, gentle and good for dry and tender skin; pour into bath to give a foam or squirt straight onto body before shower.

Milks – essentially water-conditioners, rich in fats and oils; soften water and smooth skin.

Oils – some float on the water, some mix with it; all lubricate well, leaving a film on the skin that acts as a conditioner and moisturizer.

Salts – those made from Epsom salts, perfume and colour water; some from sodium derivatives, soften water; some are carbonated and make water effervescent. Special herbal salts indicate therapeutic benefits.

After the Bath:

Bath oil spray – softens and scents skin, less drying than a perfume or cologne, therefore good for dry skins, or special dry areas.

Body lotion – a moisturizing creamy fragrance, important to help keep skin supple; smooth on all over when you are still a little damp as pores are clean, open and ready to soak up extra moisture.

Dusting powder – lighter version of talcum powder; to be shaken, sprayed or patted on; it cools and smooths, helps absorb moisture and enables you to slip more easily into clothes.

Splash and friction waters – tangy colognes and toilet waters that brace, cool, and stimulate the body.

Talcum powder – a smooth mineral powder, sometimes with antiseptic properties due to the addition of boric acid.

After-bath lotion to make at home:

3½ oz. (100 g.) of red rose petals steeped in 2 pints (1 l.) of white vinegar for fifteen days. Make in a ceramic jar, covered with gauze.

The same lotion can be made with lavender, orange blossom, mint.

DRY FRICTION BATH

This is said to be conducive to sleep and a cure for insomnia. Using a friction glove – made from hemp, horsehair, heavy cotton or plastic – massage the body gently in upward sweeping motions. Switch glove from right to left hand to reach all parts of the body. There is no need to massage roughly as the glove does most of the work with its heavy texture. Accumulated dead cells and surface dirt are brushed off; skin is given a chance to breathe, blood circulation is increased and consequently toxins lying on the surface are disposed of more quickly. Over a period of time, this can really cleanse and refine the pores. Done once a week, it's a real tonic for the skin.

SPIRIT SPONGE BATH

2 oz. (60 g.) spirit of ammonia
2 oz. (60 g.) of camphor
1 cup sea salt
2 cups ethyl alcohol
Put all ingredients into a quart bottle, fill to brim with boiling water. Allow to cool slightly.

Shake lotion before using, then with a cloth or sponge, rub the spirit all over the body, but do it gently as the liquid itself invigorates as it cleanses. Afterwards just dry with a towel, don't rinse or sponge over with water.

PERSPIRATION AND ODOUR

If you ask most people what causes body odour, they will answer perspiration or sweat. It's not true. Moisture excretion, which is the body's air conditioning system, is not to blame. Sweat is colourless and practically odourless when it appears on the surface of the skin. It consists for the most part of pure water and a few salts, which are responsible for giving a faintly salty smell that's rather attractive and considered aphrodisiac. What causes body odour is a group of bacteria that turns the innocuous moisture into stale smells through decomposition. This only happens if moisture cannot evaporate fast enough.

Areas exposed to air have no problem getting rid of surface moisture, but when perspiration is trapped next to the skin, body odour begins. The underarms, feet and outer vaginal areas are the usual problem spots. Synthetic materials hinder evaporation – tights, underwear, shirts, and sweaters shut off air circulation more when not of natural fibres.

Perspiration is caused by the activities of two different types of glands. They both secrete moisture through tubular ducts. They are:

Eccrine glands – these are evenly distributed all over the body, between 2 to 3 million of them. Their secretion is 99% clear water with a few salts. They act as the main temperature control and through thermal sweating endeavour to hold the body at an even normal temperature. Interfering with this process in any major way can be fatal.

Apocrine glands – these are less common and are concentrated in specific areas: underarms, groin, buttocks and the nipples. Their secretions are also mostly water, but they are cloudy and contain some protein and fatty substances which attract the bacteria. These glands are larger than the eccrine ones, and commonly associated with hair follicles; they usually develop during puberty. Apocrine glands take care of a certain amount of thermal regulation through sweat, but their activity is mainly due to nervous and emotional reactions: a slight argument, a tense conversation, a moment of agitation, is enough to get them going. Environment temperature doesn't make any difference to the apocrine glands. Whether it's 110°F (43°C) or below freezing, their secretion is the same.

All-over perspiration is adequately dealt with by regular bathing. Underarms need particular control for the problem here is not only odour but visible wetness. Extra precautions are usually necessary and this is one reason for shaving under arms though in many cultures it is considered a de-sexing procedure and therefore not done.

The problems of wetness and dryness have two basic solutions in the underarm area.

Deodorants and deodorant soaps which control odour by impeding bacterial action.

Anti-perspirants which limit both odour and wetness by reducing the volume of perspiration as well as fighting bacteria.

The safety of deodorant soaps has not been definitely established. They contain antiseptics which, when exposed to sunlight, sometimes cause an adverse reaction in the form of blisters and swelling.

Deodorants and anti-perspirants come in cream and liquid form and allergic reactions are extremely rare. They must be used regularly and are most effective when applied to a thoroughly clean area. It is helpful to remove hair, as this traps sweat and makes it harder for the controlling agents to reach the skin. Apply when the body is cool and at rest – not directly after a shower because the skin is hydrated and perspiration ducts are not sufficiently open; fifteen minutes later is better. One application a day is sufficient for most women, while an additional one gives complete 24-hour protection. For excessive sweating it is advisable to apply before going to bed with another application in the morning.

How well deodorants and anti-perspirants work depends on many factors – temperature, clothes, exertion, stress, tension, and whether you naturally perspire lightly or heavily. Odour is more easily brought under control than wetness, and no anti-perspirant is 100% effective. Nor should it be. 50% is a more realistic level, but it is quite enough for aesthetic reasons. Even if it were possible, it wouldn't be desirable to block completely the flow of perspiration. A deodorant or anti-perspirant does not last until washed off; its durability is limited.

Why use a deodorant instead of an anti-perspirant when the latter does two jobs instead of one? Some women are irritated by the additional chemicals that go into an anti-perspirant. A deodorant is simply a germicide (a very small amount, 1% or less), a fragrance and a mixer that makes it easy to apply. Anti-perspirants contain aluminium or zinc salts which penetrate the sweat duct openings, and it is this activity that prevents the delivery of a lot of the sweat to the surface. However these salts can sting sensitive skins. Allergic reaction to anti-perspirants is rare.

Irritations

Underarm irritation is not necessarily directly caused by a deodorant or anti-perspirant. It could be from a chemical finish or dye in fabric, from sensitivity to your own perspiration, from cutting or grazing your skin when shaving or because of a more serious disease. If irritation doesn't clear up or shows signs of spreading, it is important to check with a doctor right away. To help prevent irritation, the first thing is to make sure you shave correctly. A blade must be sharp, otherwise you drag off layers of skin. It is a sensible precaution to delay using a deodorant or anti-perspirant for 24 hours after shaving. If you have an acid skin condition, you are likely to get an irritation from deodorants – try many, as some are less acid than others. The cause of irritation may also be a particular perfume in a deodorant.

Natural deodorants

These help counteract odour, but cannot control wetness.

Chlorophyll has a marked effect on the bacteria that cause body odour, so eat foods rich in this substance, i.e. green leafy vegetables.

Rub underarms with leaves of parsley, watercress, outer dark lettuce leaves, tops of beets or radish.

Use an infusion of sage under arms or in bath.

Lovage in a hot bath acts as a deodorant and purifier; put shredded leaves in a muslin bag.

Lavender oil is effective though too strong to use as it is; make a lavender water to dab on or smooth over particular problem areas.

3 drops lavender oil
1 lump sugar (or 1 tablespoon)
1 pint (6 dl.) distilled water
Leave for two weeks before use; always shake beforehand.

Other herbs that help control body odour are: cloves, leaves of chrysanthemum, camphor and patchouli. Make infusions or pouchettes either for body application or for adding to the bath.

BATH EXERCISES

The time spent enjoying the benefits of a bath, can be usefully and easily employed for a few basic exercises that will tone muscles and keep the main trouble areas in trim.

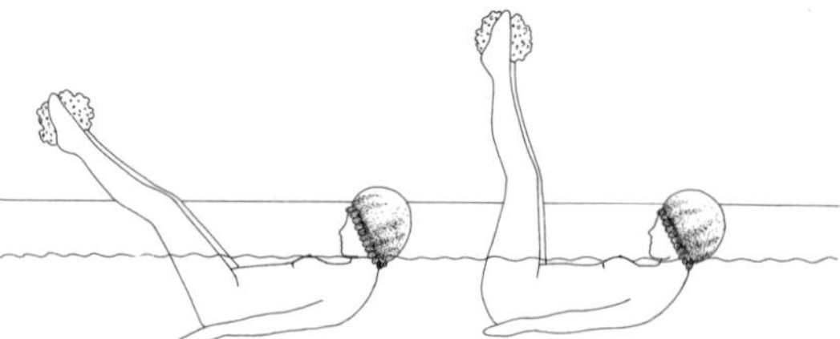

1. *Sponge grip:* Lie almost supine in bath, grip sponge between feet and slowly raise legs as high as possible; hold at zenith to count of three, lower slowly. Repeat six times. Good for the hips.

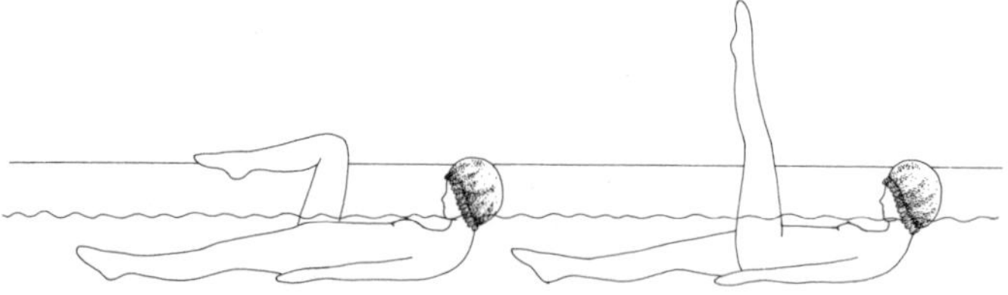

2. *Leg kick:* Lying in bath, put legs up, bent at right-angles at the knees; kick one leg up straight, toes pointed, foot arched; alternate with other leg. Do twenty kicks. Helps shape legs.

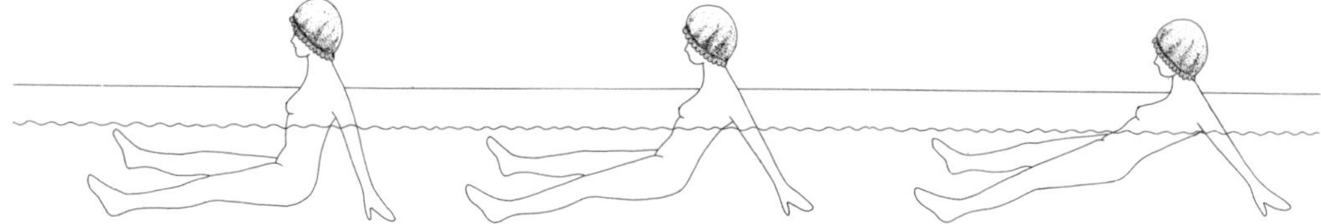

3. *Stomach pull:* Sit with legs straight out in front, a little apart, supporting body with arms behind torso; move torso slowly to a backward slant, using stomach muscles and shifting arm support backwards too; return equally slowly. Do six times.

4. *Shoulder circle:* Using sponge, make wide circles with hand in the centre shoulder area. Do six circles with each hand, going from left to right with right hand, right to left with left hand; for breast and upper arm muscles.

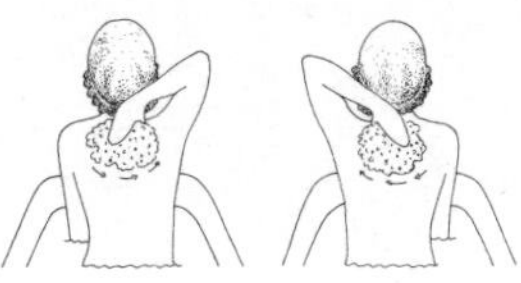

SALON BATH TREATMENTS

Sauna – A special type of dry heat. A sauna is taken in a small room built entirely of pine logs with slatted timber platforms at different levels. A central stove, sometimes wood-burning, sometimes electric, is covered with heat-resisting stones. The temperature is high – around 200° F (93°C) and if water is ladled onto the hot stones it produces a sudden burst of heat. The object is to perspire and through perspiration lose weight, open the pores, clear the skin, stimulate circulation and relieve aching muscles. Tension is helped too. To stimulate sweating, the real enthusiast hits the body with birch brooms. At first it is not advisable to stay in for more than 10 minutes; then 5 minutes or so outside – a quick cold shower is suggested – then back in the sauna for another 10 minutes. In many salons a sauna cabinet is used, an encasement where only your head is exposed – with dry or steam heat inside.

Wax – Paraffin wax is particularly good for the treatment of stiffness; it also helps get rid of excess fluid and improves skin texture and colour. The wax is solid and cloudy white; it has a low melting point and when heated becomes clear and completely fluid. It is painted onto the body and forms a second skin of wax. The body is usually wrapped with towels or linen. Heat is built up inducing perspiration; afterwards the wax is sponged off. The treatment usually takes about an hour and is often followed by a massage.

Mud – Volcanic mud contains therapeutic minerals and when it covers the body it induces perspiration, drawing out impurities. You can either soak in a mud-filled tub for about 15 minutes or be layered with the mud.

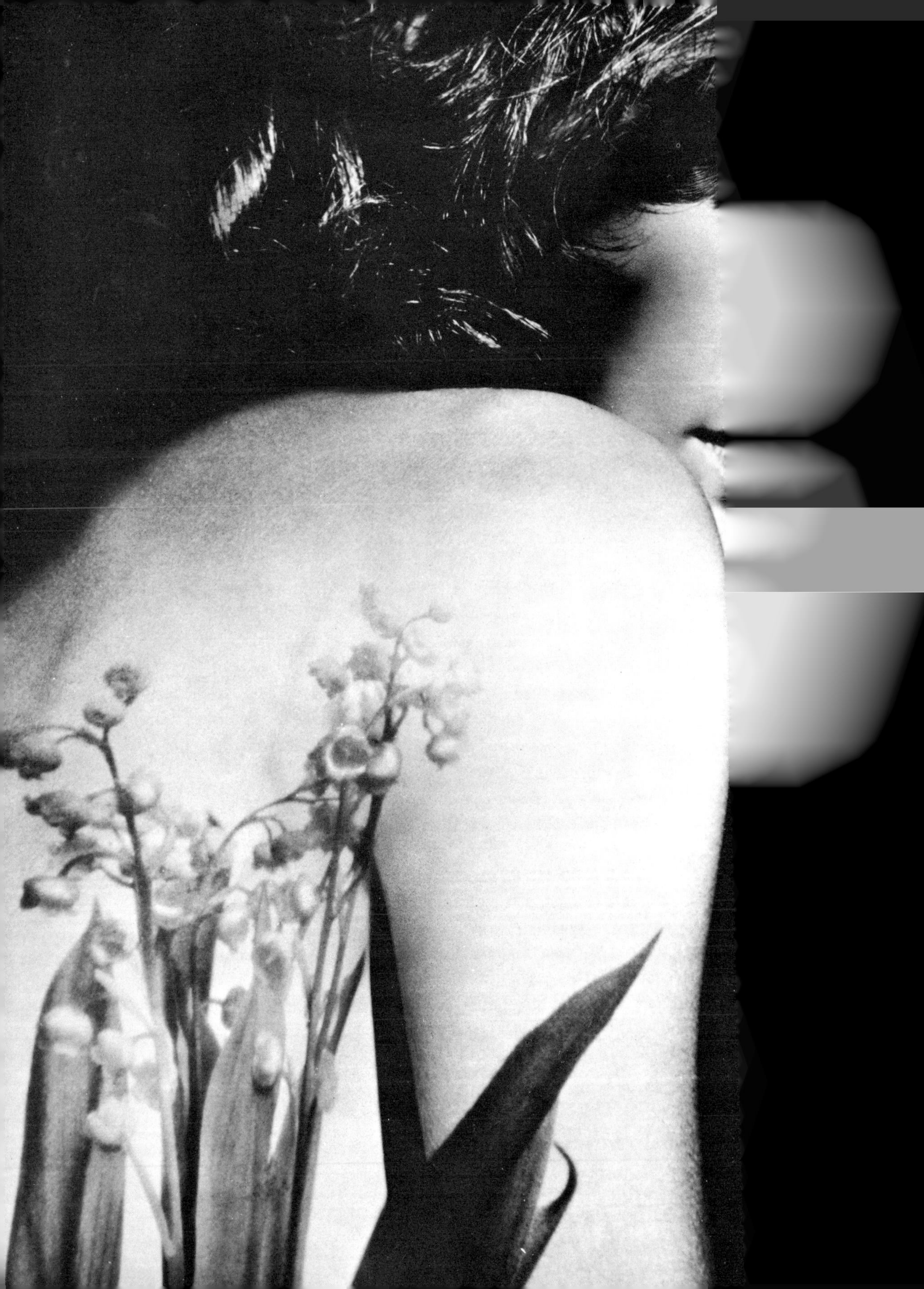

5

PERFUME

Scents trigger emotions in all animal life, and though our primary sense of smell may be less acute than that of animals, it is now believed to be a great deal keener than we have supposed. We have all but suppressed any natural odour instincts and we have little practical use for smelling, but odour is still very much part of our instinctive lives and memories.

Scientists are puzzled by our sense of smell and particularly by body odours that could affect behaviour. These are called pheromones, and are clearly evident in the animal world where they attract, repel, warn or reassure. Do they function in people? There is no evidence that they do not, and some indication that they do, particularly in sexual situations. We produce pheromones in abundance, but are very busy suppressing them or covering them up. And yet perfume can act like a pheromone, as the habitual use of the same fragrance registers on the subconscious and is immediately associated with a particular place or individual. This emphasizes the unique property of perfume: under its influence we recall and relive.

The brain transmits thoughts and memories, but the olfactory cells are responsible for our sense of smell. These are assembled in a membranous tissue high in the nose and receive the odour messages through the nose or through the rear of the mouth (during eating taste and smell are closely related). From here, via the olfactory nerves, information is directed to the brain. Natural odours produce instinctive reactions; perfume aromas stimulate the senses in a more excessive, more varied and more subtle way.

It is impossible to give a scientific analysis of the sense of smell. What smells nice is tied to the psychology of association which varies from person to person.

Perfumes did not originate in France, though they have been perfected there, and now the world centre of the industry is at Grasse, a hillside town just inland from the Côte d'Azur. Perfumes were already used more than three thousand years ago in Egypt as aphrodisiacs, medicines, and cosmetics. The name comes from the Latin *per fumam* (through smoke) which indicates its extensive use as incense at that time. Perfumery is an art as well as a science; the master perfumier is known as a 'nose' because although he may be mostly chemist, he is an artist too and with one whiff he can discern if a perfume will be successful or not. No computer has been found to replace him. The language of perfume is artistic too; perfumiers use analogies of other arts, notably music, and borrow acoustic terms to register effect. So we hear of 'high or top notes', 'low or base notes' and middle notes. A perfumier's 'top note' is the first heady fleeting impression received as the bottle is opened. It lingers briefly to give way to the 'middle note' which is the heart of the perfume portraying its character and richness. This can last several hours and the better the perfume, the longer the time. Finally comes the 'base note' composed of the longest lasting elements usually known as 'fixatives'. These are the odours of low volatility that cling and could be unpleasant if used alone, but as part of a total composition add a warm, permanent glow to a fragrance.

Most perfumes are complex intertwinings in which each accent sets off another. There can be dozens, even hundreds, of ingredients artfully blended to produce one distinct smell. Each component has its separate identity, but loses it as it is blended. A professional 'nose' can identify most aromas in turn, but the end result depends on two autonomous things: the touch of a particular perfumier and the woman who wears the perfume. The same ingredients with slight adjustment can result in something quite different, and no two 'noses' are alike. Also, perfumes react differently on different skins, so one can never say that any perfume always has exactly the same odour.

The art of the perfumier as we know it is about 200 years old. Today's perfumiers have inherited the techniques and methods invented by the French in the 18th century. It can take many years to create a new scent, and it takes a rare power of discrimination to balance the formula. There are three stages in the making of a perfume: the selection of raw materials, their preparation and blending, then the formulation. Raw materials are in two categories – natural and synthetic. The natural components come from all over the world. They have been the traditional sources of perfume since earliest times and are both botanical and animal in origin. Synthetic ingredients – called aldehydes – have been developed over the last thirty years. They have strong characteristic odours reminiscent of natural essences; sometimes they are more real than the real thing. They lend force and character to a perfume, but rarely contribute subtlety. As a rule, the higher the price of perfume, the more expensive its raw materials and the more effective the aroma.

'Enfleurage' is the French term for the old and tedious method of extracting the scent from flowers. Enormous quantities of the natural source are required to produce a fraction of concentrated oil. To obtain 1 pound (½ k.) of concentrated jasmine oil, about 300 lb (150 k.) of flowers (or 2½ million flowers) are needed. These are soaked and softened in purified cold fat. In time the flowers will yield their essential fragrant oils to the fat, then an alcohol wash is used to remove the scent. In turn the scent is separated from the alcohol by distillation. It is these floral essences that provide the top and middle notes of a perfume. The low notes are established by a 'fixative' which adds staying power. This is a misnomer as such ingredients (often animal in origin or from green or bark sources) don't 'fix' the components. They are more the tenacious lasting notes of a perfume.

Animal ingredients are as expensive as floral ones. In their concentrated state, they smell pretty awful, but in minute quantities they are an enticing and humanizing element. No good perfume can do without them; they give a distinguished air to a fragrance, but because they have an aphrodisiac quality, they must not be overdone. Can a perfume be an aphrodisiac? Technically the answer is 'no', but any good perfume is sexy and any skin smelling of jasmine, Bulgarian rose or whatever is infinitely more erotic than the same skin smelling of nothing in particular. For the practical, there is this information: it has been established that in a person who is unable to smell, sex interest is less pronounced.

The effect of a perfume depends upon its category, and fragrances are divided into groups. The type of fragrance not only indicates its components, but also its impression. For example, light floral perfumes refresh, citrus, greens and moderns revive and stimulate, spicy, sweet florals and oriental musky perfumes lull. There are general categories, but nothing is straightforward about fragrance: just as no one scent is made up of a single essence, sometimes no one overall sensation comes through. Underlying notes of sweetness can penetrate a sharp perfume, or tangy overtones give clarity to a warm sweet scent. The following categories are a guide:

Floral

Single florals are one-note perfumes that give the essence of a single blossom. This does not necessarily mean that the essential oil used is only from that particular flower. Usually when the perfumier wants to copy a natural flower fragrance, he blends together a number of different essences which produce the effect of the flower.

Then there are the floral bouquets where various flowers, often represented by aromatic or synthetic essences, are harmoniously blended. Sometimes one note predominates, but there are other notes as well. Usually specific flowers are not readily recognizable. Floral perfumes are frequently light and refreshing; some however can be very sweet (see category below) though not as overpowering as the orientals.

Citrus

These are perfumes dominated by lemon, orange and bergamot notes. They are particularly sharp, fresh, and stimulating to others as well as to the wearer. They are ideal for 'cooling' the body and perfect for those who turn perfume very sweet – people with oily skins for instance.

Green

As the name implies these fragrances are essentially fresh and woody, crisp, clean, and dry. Aromatic sharp woods from temperate climates – such as pine and cedar – are blended with mosses, ferns, grasses, and flower stems.

Modern

These have been developed over the last thirty years and primarily use synthetic oils. They are highly complex products of the chemical laboratory and the professional 'nose'. Individualistic and distinctive creations rather than duplications of nature, they are characterized by brilliant top notes, a rich middle section, and often provide a depth and emphasis that natural perfumes alone cannot achieve. Many contain notes from several fragrance categories, but on the whole they are bright, cheery, and cool, ideally suited to an active modern life, pleasant and uncomplicated. This modern group has been the most popular category in recent years, and has had the most additions. Modern florals are sparkling with specific flower notes not easily identifiable. Modern green and woody florals are drier blends – grassy and fresh, but not as dry as the modern greens which are noticeably tangy with the zest of the outdoors. Modern mossy and herbal blends are sharp and run from light to resinous. They are very bracing and said to have a 'sexy dry-out' which in the language of the perfumier means that once the distinct high notes have evaporated, you are left with a clean fleshy scent which is more human than botanical. This green-moss-herb group is cited as the trend of the future.

Spicy

These are heavier in character than the florals and can be quite pungent. The blends combine essences of cinnamon, cloves, vanilla – and sometimes ginger – with the more exotic flowers.

Sweet

Mostly floral combinations made from the more penetrating of the fragrant blossoms – jasmine, tuberose, and gardenia. They can be very sweet and need to be used carefully as they are likely to become overpowering after a very short while, particularly if the metabolism of one's skin is such that it turns a perfume sweeter. Many skins react this way and another person is usually more aware of it than the wearer.

Oriental

Very rich and full-bodied fragrances, based on the more aromatic of the eastern woods and grasses (like sandalwood) and heavy with the scent of musk, ambergris and civet. The most sultry perfumes, their appeal is very much an individual reaction. They may be exotic to one person, and too much for another.

Whatever category a perfume may fall in, most come in three strengths: perfume, toilet water, and cologne. Today the terms toilet water and cologne have become interchangeable, though the former is considered a little stronger. Both are diluted perfumes containing a higher percentage of alcohol which accounts for their cooling and refreshing quality: the result of the rapid evaporation of spirit. The fragrance lingers on though not as potently as that of the concentrated perfume. This lasting power is particularly true of modern blends, where the synthetic aromatics provide a forceful middle note. Scent permeates all beauty products and frequently the same one is found in a series of preparations: soap, bath oils, and foams, body lotions and powders, hand lotions, towelettes, solid perfume sticks and cream sachets. All are soothing and economical ways to extend fragrance enjoyment.

How do you set about selecting a perfume? There is really only one way: with authority, tenacity, and leisure. Perfume is expensive; perfume is an investment in personality and mood; perfume is complex and individual; perfume is hundreds of different fragrances. You have to sniff, to sample, to sniff again. It is a matter of trial, error and eventual success. You are not expected to buy the whole bottle to find out if you like a perfume or if it likes you. Tester bottles are there for testing. Use them; the more you try, the more discriminating you become.

Scent must reflect mood and occasion as well as personality. Women are experimenting with different fragrances more than before. The idea of finding one perfect perfume and sticking with it forever is now considered too restricting. Some women find two and stop there – one fresh scent for day, a more brilliant one for evening. Others use several and choose the one that strikes the right note at the right time. No perfume evokes the same mental image to any two women. Find the one that makes you feel fresh and lively, the one that stimulates your mind, evokes your sensuality.

Professional noses evaluate perfume by testing it in its most diluted state – as a cologne or toilet water. A drop of perfume is a potent thing, and it can overstimulate the nose to a state of numbness. The best way is to spray a cologne on your left wrist and another on your right. Sniff it right away to get the impression of the top notes, but don't make a decision for about an hour. Within that time it will have reached the final drying out stage, when the top note has given away to the main body of the perfume. Keep checking your reaction throughout the day, but don't try any new scents. You could sample a third fragrance on the back of one hand at the same time as spraying your wrists but usually more than two is confusing, particularly for beginners. Another point: it has been shown that your sense of smell is least acute in the morning and early afternoon, so it is better to test later in the day.

What affects fragrance? The chemistry of the skin can change a perfume. For instance, a woman with fair skin will get better results with a delicate fragrance than a woman with darker skin because of her type of sebum (oily substances). Perfume lasts longer on an oily skin but tends to become sweeter. If you smoke you lessen the effectiveness of fragrance, not only because the smell of tobacco pervades body and clothing, but also because the nicotine is apt to alter the chemistry of the skin, reducing the staying power of a perfume. Medications, including the Pill, can affect your fragrance as they intentionally interfere with the body's metabolism and consequently change the skin's reaction to a scent. This can also happen if one's diet is suddenly switched from its usual pattern. If perfume is subject to even a minor odour deviation the end result will be different. During menstruation natural body odour doesn't alter but your perception of smell is not the same. This explains why a woman may think her perfume is going 'off' – but to others she smells the same. Climate and environment can also affect fragrance: in a warm climate perfume evaporates quicker and tends to bring out the base notes earlier, which explains why so many perfumes seem sweeter and heavier in tropical conditions. In cities air pollution seems to strangle some perfumes, which means you have to re-apply scent more often than in the country.

The ultimate effect of perfume is in the way you use it. Don't think of it as the last thing you put on before leaving the house. That is the wrong method and the wrong psychology. Perfume should put you in a certain mood. It is for your benefit first, so apply fragrance directly after a bath or shower, before getting dressed. Learn to layer it. Begin with scented soap, bath oil, and powder. Splash on a cologne or toilet water – all over and generously. Then follow with dabs and strokes of perfume essence, used sparingly. The best way is to emphasize the pulse points from the toes up; these warm spots of the body bring out the true note of the perfume and accent the general impression given by the cologne. The spots for dabbing are: ankles, behind the knees, between thighs, bosom, throat, back of neck, wrists, and crook of the elbow. Behind the ears is not such a good place as the oil secretions there are often different from the rest of the body.

Whether to put perfume on clothes is mainly a matter of taste. Perfume does stain, so it should be sprayed under hems, under collars etc. and remember that essence not in contact with your skin doesn't take on its individual character. Don't use perfume as an antidote for sweat – the chemical reaction is invariably fatal. Perfume must be refreshed during the day. When the heart of the perfume gives way to the base notes, it is time to renew it, not only because the best part of the perfume has gone, but also because the last lingering tones can be unpleasant. A good perfume lasts from four to six hours.

Once a bottle of perfume is open, it is uneconomical not to use it. Keep it in the cool and dark because it oxidizes when exposed to heat and light. Once the seal is broken, slow evaporation means a less perfect, less balanced perfume. For travelling, a spray container is best, or a small securely sealed bottle. Avoid plastic, scent tends to evaporate through it.

What finally ends up in a bottle has taken years of judgement and preparation. This is one reason why perfume is expensive. The perfumier puts his heart, his expertise, his nose, endless time and different kinds of flowers, grasses, barks, roots, leaves, and fixatives into a single creation. Listed below are the more important of these ingredients – all from natural sources. The synthetic aromatics (with formulas and names only a chemist can digest) follow parallel lines in smell and use. But here are the more important and most commonly used basics, the elements that have gone into perfume making over the centuries.

Botanical Sources

BERGAMOT: Small, fragrant member of the citrus family that looks like a green orange; it is inedible but filled with an oil that has a clean, tangy scent. It grows only in Calabria in Southern Italy. In some countries natural bergamot is no longer used in perfume as it can cause dark splotching of the skin but the chemical synthesis is extremely good.

CEDARWOOD: This tree gives an oil which provides a woody undertone to a perfume; it is also valuable as a fixative. The best cedars are found in Morocco.

CLOVE: Best known as a spice, but the buds provide attar of cloves, a useful component in the spicy and oriental scents.

CYPRINUM: An essence that comes from the flower of the henna; heavy and long-lasting, particularly sweet scented.

JASMINE: Possibly the most precious of floral ingredients. White jasmine provides the fragrance and reaches its peak of intense perfume at dawn. Almost every perfume contains some jasmine and although chemists have been able to isolate all the essentials of the essence, no one has been able to synthesize its fragrance – very close, but not its equal. The flower is a native of Persia and Kashmir, but today is grown commercially in Mediterranean countries, particularly around Grasse in France.

LAVENDER: Used when a delicate fresh fragrance is required; grown mostly in the hills behind the Côte d'Azur, at times the scent is so strong that it permeates the whole area.

ORANGE FLOWER: Often added to a floral bouquet to give fullness and a tinge of intoxication; if too much is used, the effect can be rather sweet.

PATCHOULI: A member of the lavender family and a native of Bengal; the essence is obtained from the leaves and stem of the herb, and because of its wild, haunting odour it is used mainly for the musky and oriental perfumes.

ROSE: First of the natural perfume oils, the most pleasantly fragrant of blossoms and the most versatile. It can be used alone or incorporated into fragrances. The species used for perfume is *Rosa Centifolia*, and vast fields are cultivated near Grasse. Flowers are hand-picked at night when their scent is at its zenith. A more opulent version is the Bulgarian rose which has a more voluptuous scent and is also a favourite with perfumiers.

SANDALWOOD: Comes from the white wood of *Santalum Album*, a parasitic tree found in India and Australia. It is a seasoned, exotic scent and because of its density and capacity to provide long-lasting base notes it is used as a fixative.

VETIVER: This is extracted from the roots of a grass that grows in the Far East and parts of Central and South America. Eastern in quality, it provides a heavy aroma and is used mostly as a fixative.

VIOLET: One of the enigmas of perfumery, this flower which would seem such an obvious choice for an essence inhibits our sense of smell. When we sniff a violet for more than a certain length of time, the flower seemingly loses its fragrance – in fact we lose our ability to smell it. Perfumiers have discovered that the root of the Italian iris produces the best approximation to the fragrance of violets.

YLANG YLANG: The blossom this essence comes from is pale green. It is oriental and the fragrance wildly sweet, yet when woven into musky blends it makes them subtle and rich.

Animal Sources

AMBERGRIS: The most unlikely of all perfume ingredients, this grey, odourless, porous, fatty substance is the spew of the sperm whale. It is found floating on the sea (it dissolves in alcohol but not in water) and is a perfume fixative of the highest order. A perfume infused with ambergris is sexy as it gives a fragrance of an erogenous animal note. It is rare and expensive simply because it is difficult to find, and likely to become rarer and more costly as whales are an endangered species.

CASTOREUM: An oily brown substance produced by the lymph glands of the Canadian beaver – like all animal derivatives, it is used to give a sexual, lasting quality to perfume. It is the strongest of all animal fixatives, and so blatant is its scent that it is used sparingly and, in modern fragrances, hardly at all.

CIVET: The secretion from a gland under the tail of a civet cat. It is useful as a fixative, but rather strong, so must be used discreetly.

MUSK: A glandular secretion of the male musk deer whose habitat is the Himalayas. As with all animal elements in perfume, it is strongly erotic and used as a fixative. At one time, it was used on its own as a one-tone natural aphrodisiac. Now, on a more restrained level, it is added to floral blends. The musk deer is in danger of becoming extinct, so rather than forgo the obvious advantages and appeal of musk, chemists are now producing synthetic versions which are considered as effective.

Despite the various basic natures of ingredients, perfume is the most intangible of beauty sources. It will not help looks in any way but it can uncannily provide an aura, change an attitude, create a mood and stir up emotions to a remarkable degree. Perfume is not necessarily a mere beauty agent, but is a way of soothing one's own physical and emotional state. The heavier perfumes, those with more animal elements or with a heavy scented floral base, have a drowsy effect that puts the mind at rest and so chases away mental distraction. This mysterious curative power is also seen in the way a fresh sharp scent can stimulate our sense of smell; we breathe in deeply, nasal passages are cleared, the head is relieved of tension and we feel refreshed. Such a scent is the classic eau-de-cologne. And surely, the fact that for centuries perfume has been closely associated with seduction must be based on more than hearsay. Indeed, because of this, perfume is often regarded with suspicion. Perfume is certainly complex as much is unknown and much is contradictory. But there are facts that establish its realities and possibilities and facts that help define the human reaction.

THE HAIR

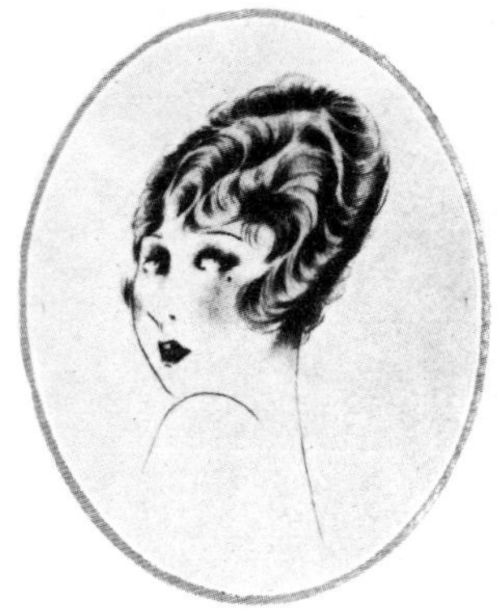

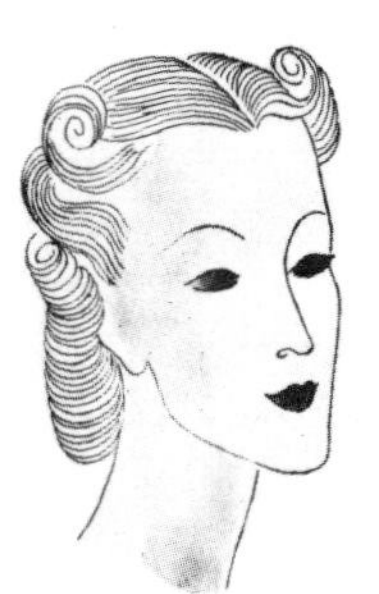

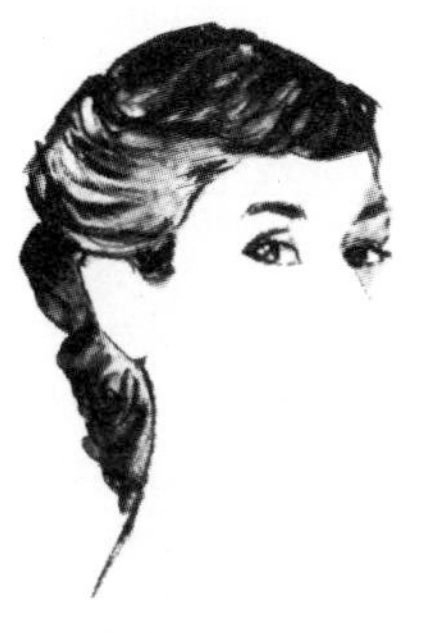

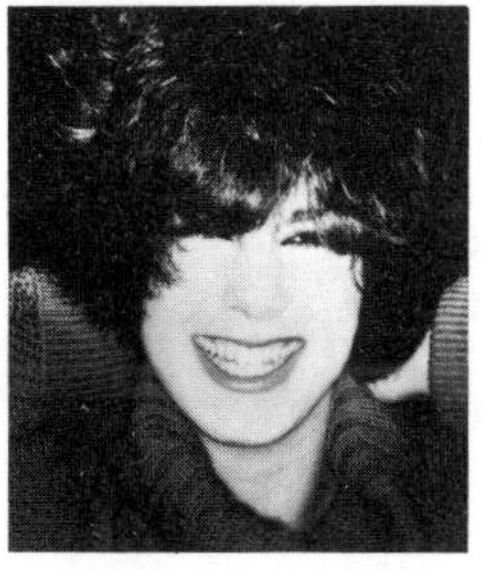

Nestlé's wonder machine for 'perming', although invented in 1906, only really hit the masses in the 1920s, changing the manes of nations. In London Eugène claimed to be the 'ablest and most renowned permanent Hair Waver of Paris & London' . . . the Mason Pearson hairbrush was 'enjoyed by all' . . . and Inecto-Rapid was 'used by ROYALTY, endorsed by 5,000 leading hairdressers' and 'permanently restored colour to Grey Hair in 15 minutes. Vogue *warned: 'Ill-kept hair spoils all possibilities of good looks and smartness.' By 1929 the shingle had succeeded the bob and the Eton crop was soon to come. With the 1930s came a 'new sense of individuality'. 'Curls must never appear untidy and so, to hold them in perfect control, some of the smartest women are adding to their coiffures decorative details that are practical, smart and becoming.' You could keep your hair in 'perfect order' with a Lady Jayne Slumbernet and 'science' discovered a way to bring back colour and gloss to faded hair 'by natural methods' – the only method 'endorsed by the Press'. But just in case that didn't work you could buy a bobbed head-dress for eighteen guineas. There was increasing interest in hair care and* Vogue *advised 'a good shampoo every two, or perhaps three weeks'. In the 1940s hair fashion was dictated by the war: girls working in factories had to wear turbans and snoods to stop their long hair getting into the machinery and servicewomen had to wear their hair above the collar.* Vogue *asked: 'Why does that shoulder-mane seem so out of date?' With the 1950s the teenagers took over, first with the ponytail, later with the loose hair cult and the Carita sisters in Paris made the first fashion wigs – to match Givenchy dresses. The accent was on you. André Bernard's 'creations moulded to suit your individual charms'; French's creations 'for you alone'; Riché's 'short-styled softly waving coiffure – the fashion follows you'. The wig boom began in 1960, Harrods – like other big stores – opened a wig counter and by the end of the decade the State was supplying human hair on the N.H.S. In 1963 Vidal Sassoon created his revolutionary new haircut – hard, architectural, thick chopped bob – and later came Jean Shrimpton's 'tiger mane', pre-Raphaelite 'ripple waves' and the first 'afro' styles. With the 1970s hair health became a fetish; henna brightened the colour, added shine and weight. 'With less backcombing, less lacquer, more brushing, more shine, there's a new deal in hair health.'*

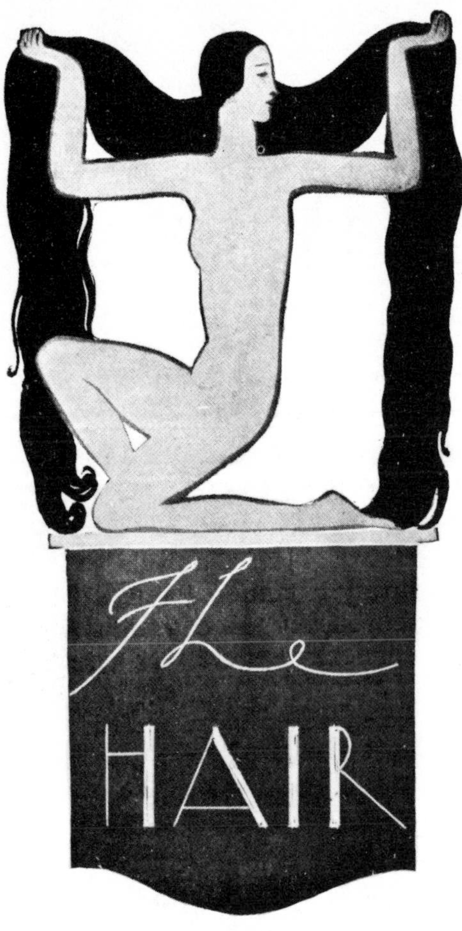

THE GRACIOUSNESS OF GREY HAIR

By a Sophisticated Charm, a Fitting Choice of Costume, and Exquisite Grooming, the Wearer of Grey Locks Becomes a Personage.

'Alas, poor might-have-been, who mourned her raven hair and failed to see that grey was vastly more distinctive. Too soon, the dye-pot did its work – and robbed her.'

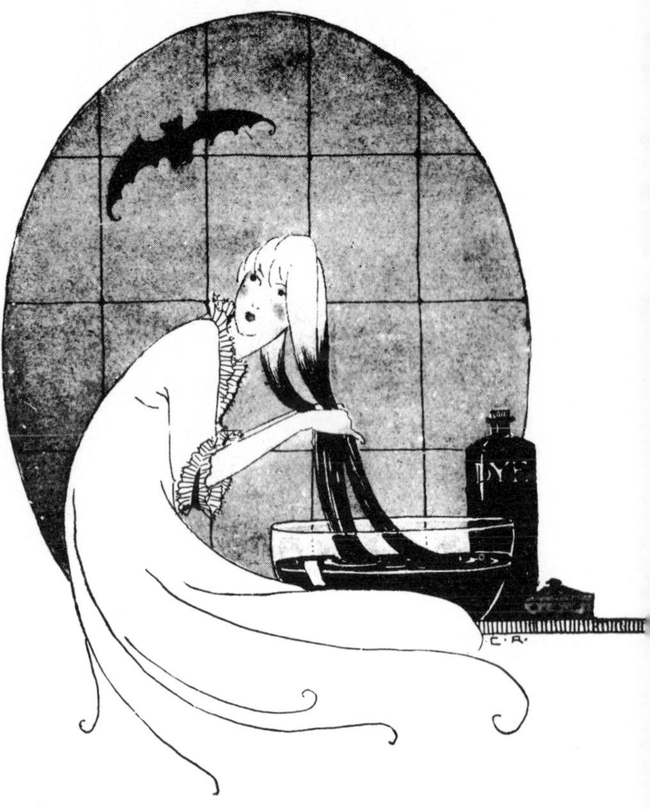

PARIS MAKES AMAZING EXPERIMENTS IN COIFFURES

No Two Heads – No Head on Two Days – May be Coifed the Same

'The return of the gowns of the Princesse de Clèves is, naturally, the occasion for the return of her coiffure, and this, too, makes novel and striking use of braids.'

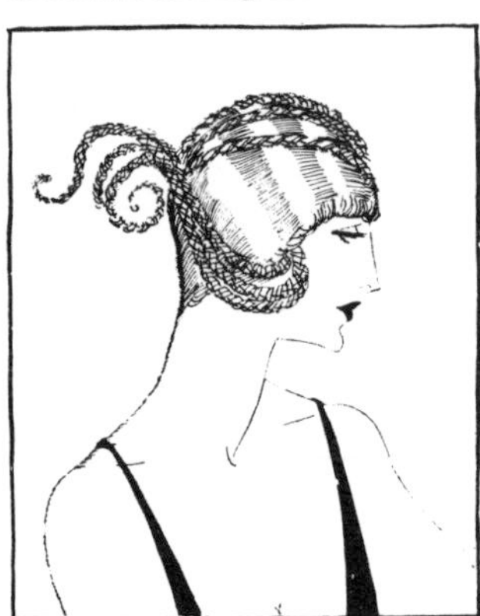

'So great an aid to the toilette is that newest invention, the electric wave, that even the woman of soft and silky hair occasionally attains such coiffures as this, although, in time, she will doubtless decide not to.'

'With the high collar, one may expect the high coiffure which lifts the hair away from the neck. Less readily will woman part from the puffs about the ear.'

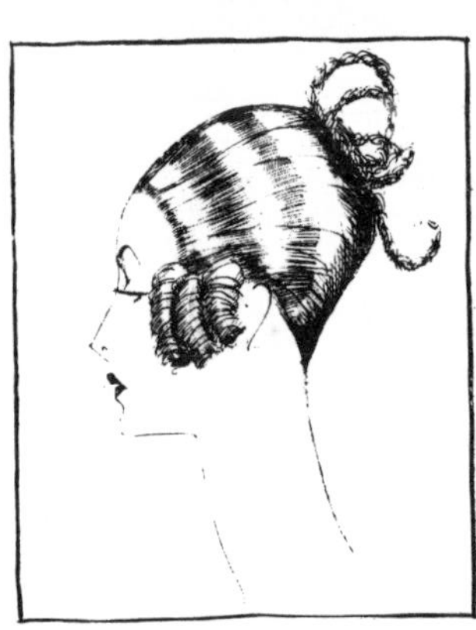

1920

Mr. Eugène has personally given, in his Paris Salons, a demonstration of his famous Patented Appliances to the well-known film producers, Messrs. Gaumont. This series of cinema demonstrations may be seen throughout Great Britain during September, and show how Eugène's wonderful process can transform the lankiest hair into soft becoming waves.

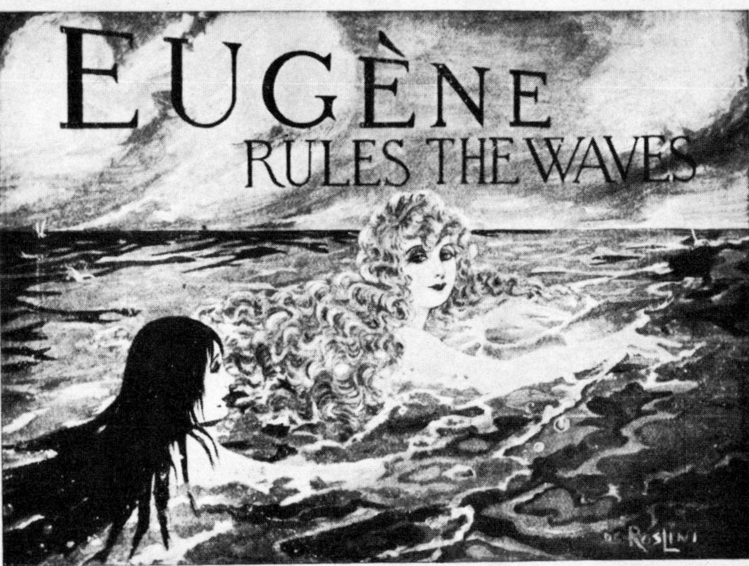

Inventors and Patentees of the world renowned EUGÈNE *APPLIANCES for Permanent Hairwaving*

Eugène Ltd.

LONDON
23 GRAFTON ST. W. 1
Telephone: Gerrard 4607
178 New Bond St. W. 1.

MANCHESTER
2 St. Anne's Place
Telephone: Central 2803

PARIS: 265 Rue St. Honoré

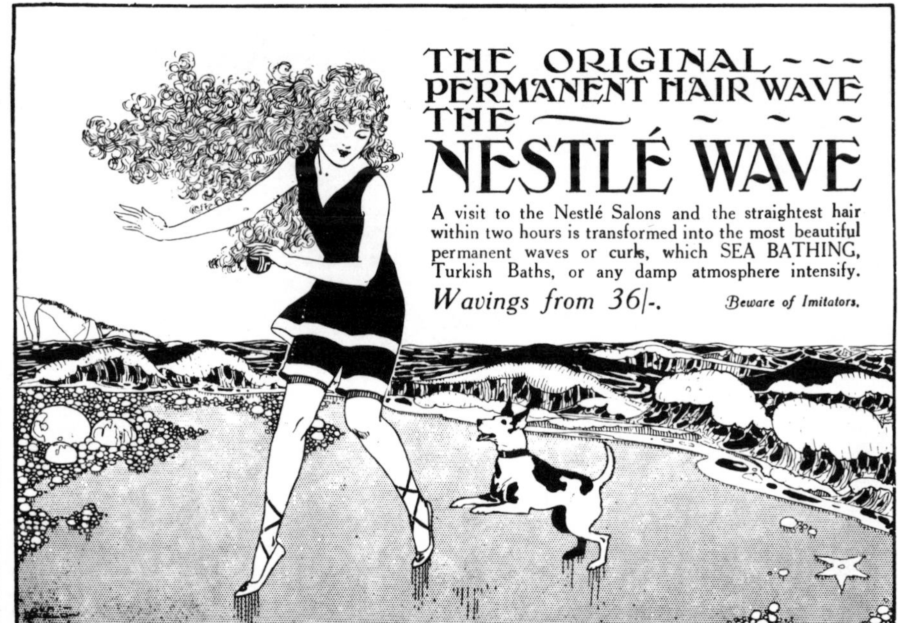

THE ORIGINAL
PERMANENT HAIR WAVE
THE
NESTLÉ WAVE
A visit to the Nestlé Salons and the straightest hair within two hours is transformed into the most beautiful permanent waves or curls, which SEA BATHING, Turkish Baths, or any damp atmosphere intensify.
Wavings from 36/-.
Beware of Imitators.

NESTLÉ LICENSEES THE PROVINCES

The following firms are licensed to carry out the Nestlé Wave:

BATH.—Mills & Watkins, 3 Georg Street.
BEDFORD.—W. J. Wilkinson, 41, Tavistock Street.
BOURNEMOUTH. — S. A. Thomson, 92, Poole Road.
DUNDEE.—Miss Hill Rennie, 7 Union Street.
EDINBURGH.—John King, 52 Princes Street.
EXETER. — D. Theuwissen & Co., The Arcade.
N. FINCHLEY.—Mrs. H. Norris, 79a, High Street, N.
GLASGOW.—Maison Lewis 140, Douglas Street.
HARROGATE.—J. Kasper, 19, Parliament Street.
HULL.—Swallow & Barry, 24, George Street.
ILFORD.—Madame Seabrook, Cranbrook Buildings.
LEEDS.—Miss Manning, 27 County Arcade.
LEICESTER.—Alfred E. Bird, 77, Queen's Road.
MANCHESTER.—Maison Taylor, 26-28, King Street; 131, Oxford Road, All Saints.
NEWCASTLE.—Marguerite Joyce, 1, St. Mary's Place.
WOLVERHAMPTON—Madame Elizabeth Hewart, 152, Tettenhall Road.
YORK.—Swallow & Barry, 26 Stone Gate.

THERE IS NO DIFFERENCE BETWEEN NATURE'S WAVE AND THE NESTLÉ WAVE.

WRITE FOR NEW ILLUSTRATED BOOKLET.

C. NESTLÉ & CO., LTD.
Directors: Alfred Harris, George Aldworth.
Telegrams: "Kantist, Wesdo, London."

48, South Molton Street
Phone: Mayfair 2986.
43, Dover Street, Piccadilly
Phone: Regent 1134

LONDON, W.1

1920

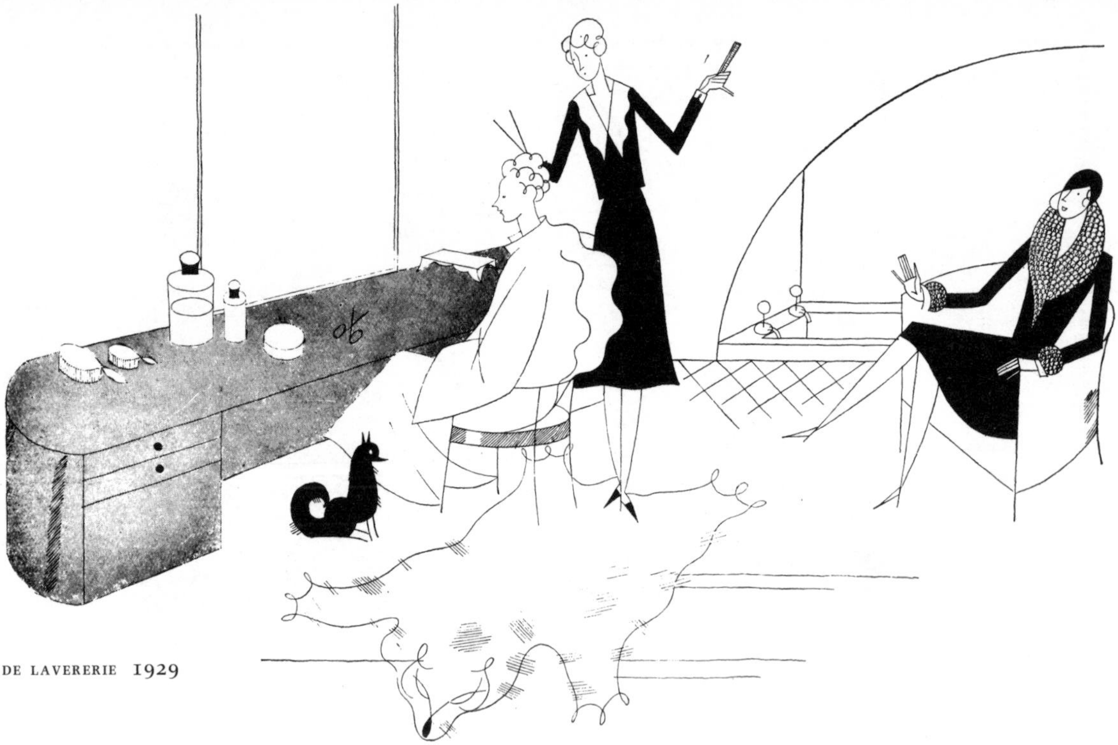

DE LAVERERIE 1929

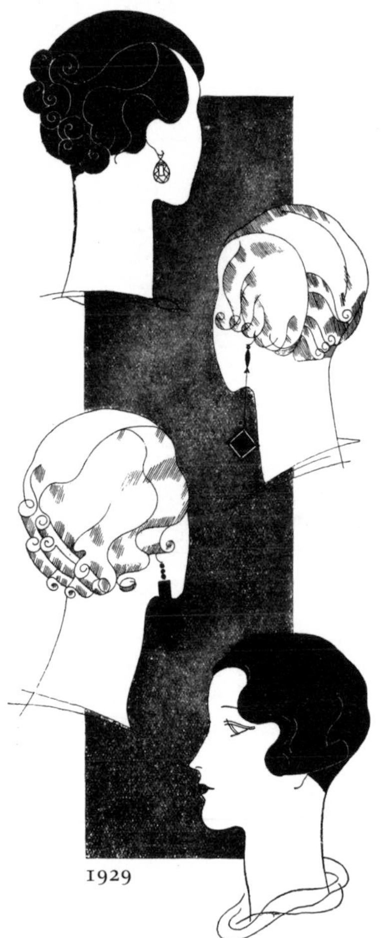

1929

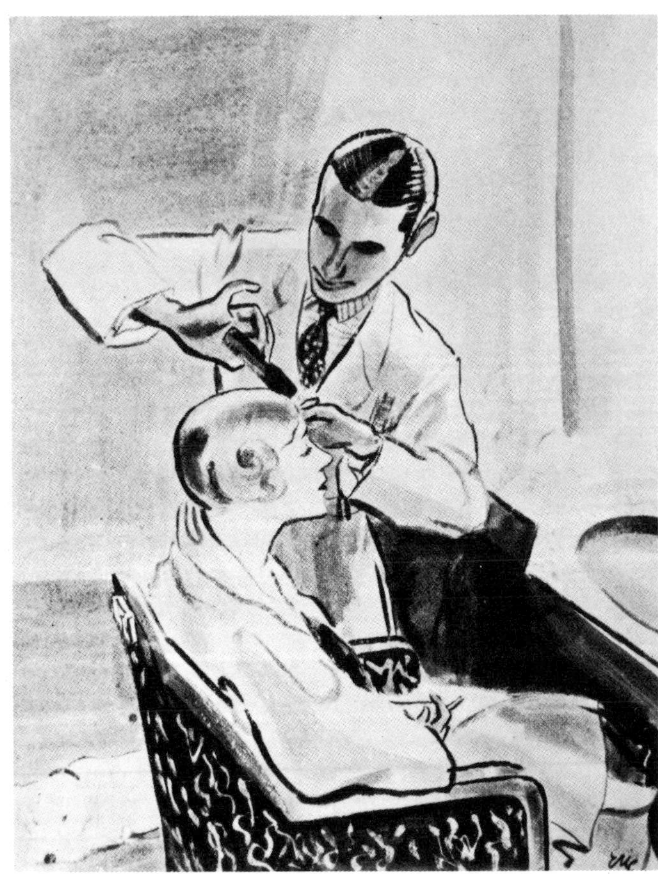

1930

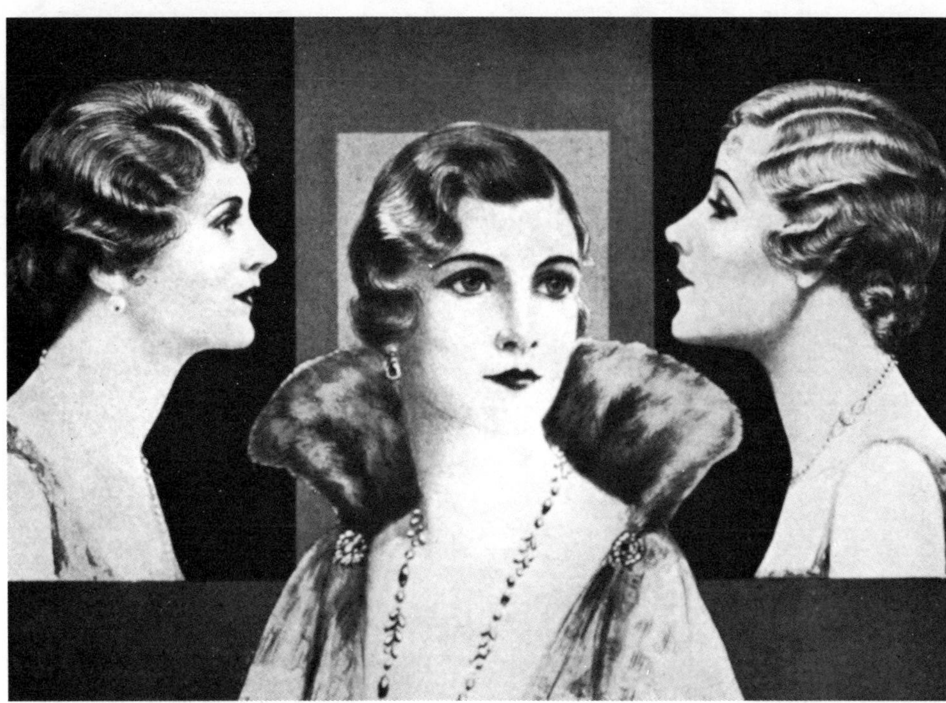

The Triumph of Maison Georges 1930

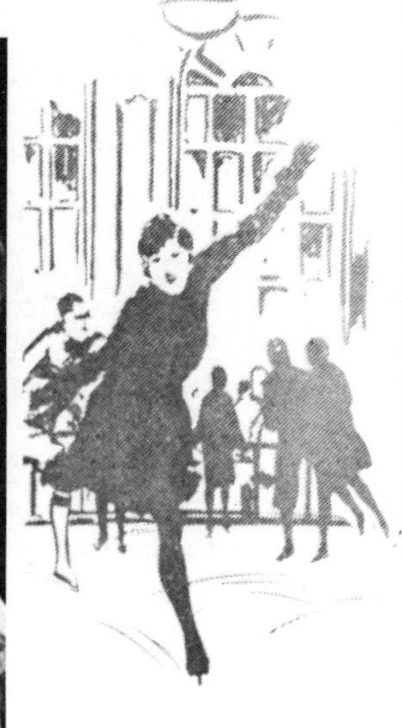

'Your choice will provide you with the PERFECT COIFFURE.'

'Up aloft does Guillaume dress their hair: the Princesse Jean Poniatowski and Madame Pol Roger. Ear-revealing, forehead-revealing, nape-revealing – these two coiffures call for a good natural hairline and clear-cut features. But if you can't boast these assets, there are many modified versions of the up-and-up line, including at least one which is sure to suit you: study the sketches given here.'

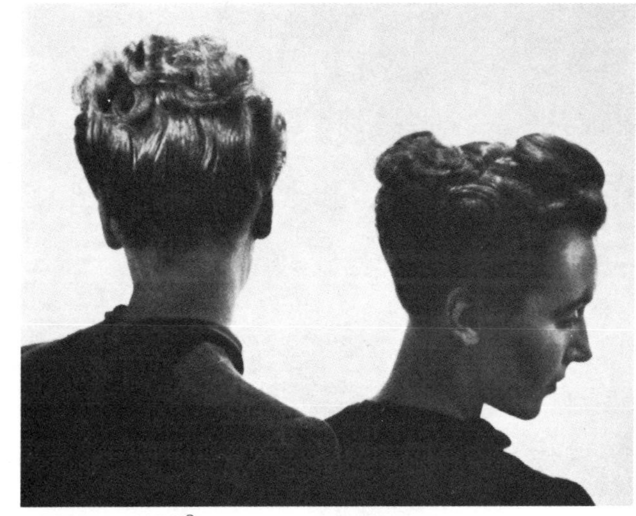

ANDRE DURST 1938

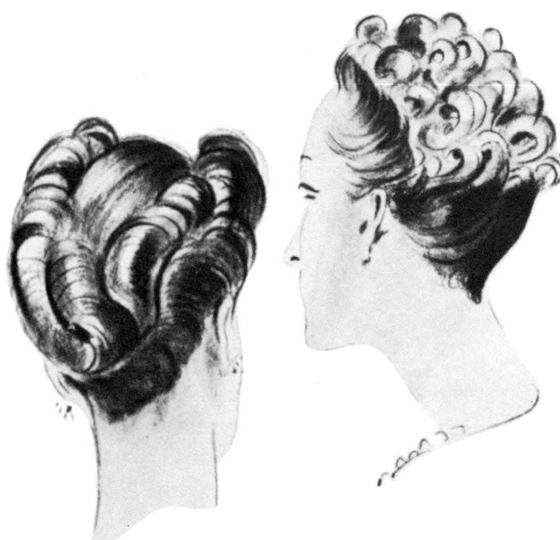

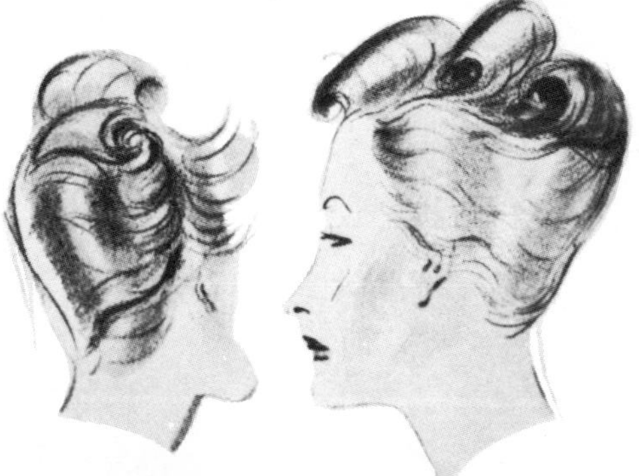

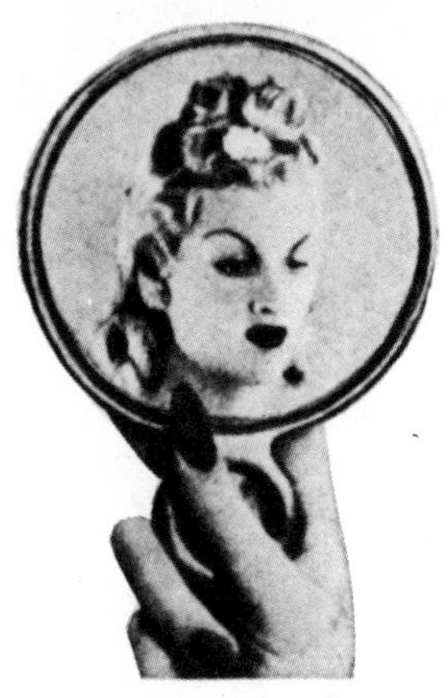

1939: Plucked eyebrows

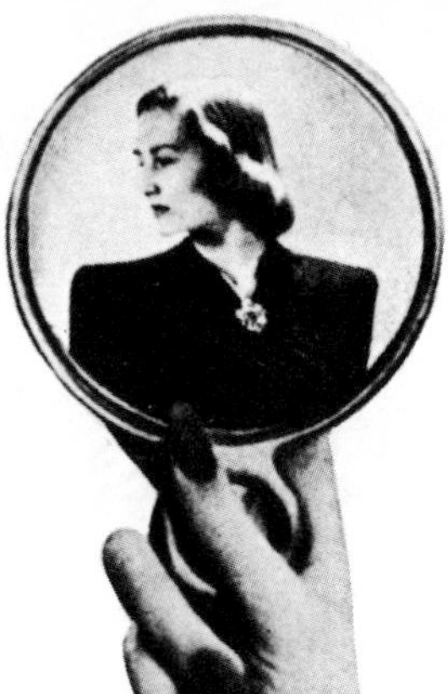

1943: Page-boy cut

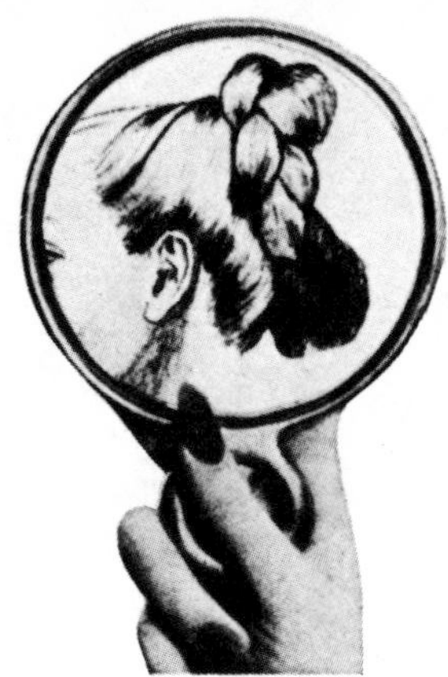

1946: Pinned-on plaits

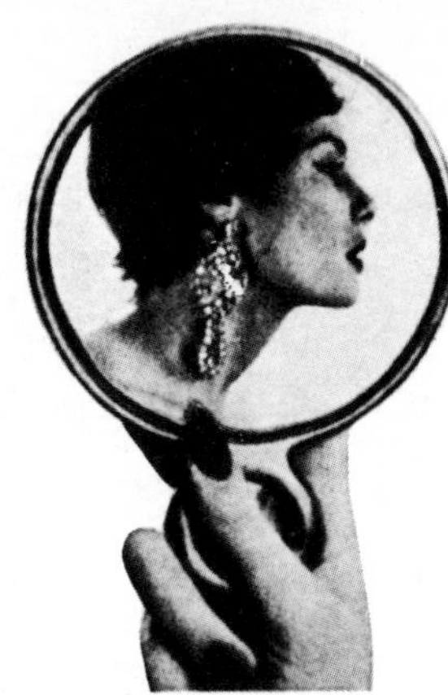

1949: Gamine style

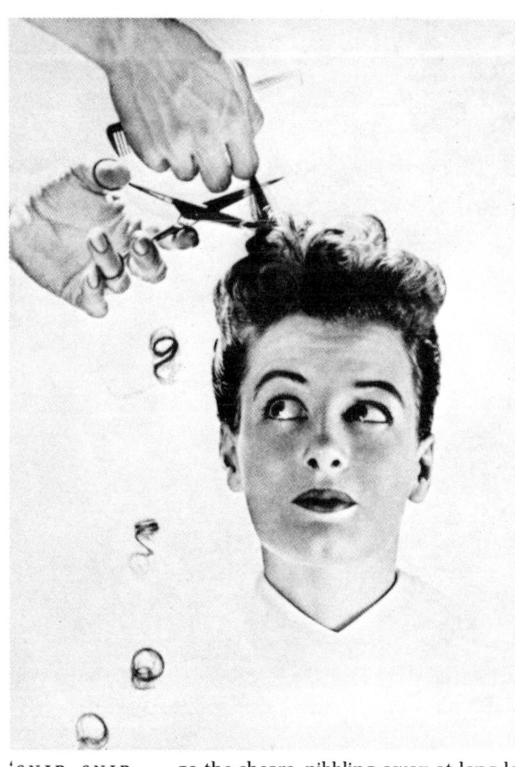

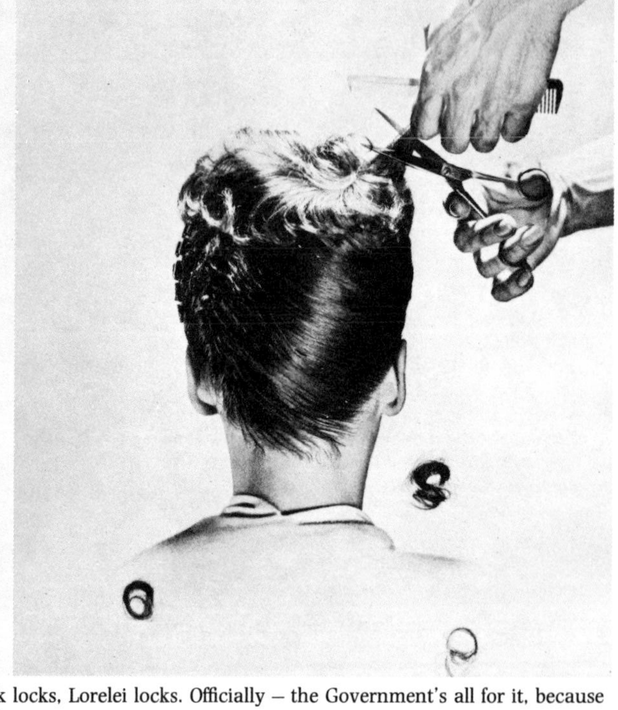

'SNIP, SNIP . . . go the shears, nibbling away at long locks, lank locks, Lorelei locks. Officially – the Government's all for it, because short hair can't get in the way of war work, takes little precious time. RAWLINGS 1943

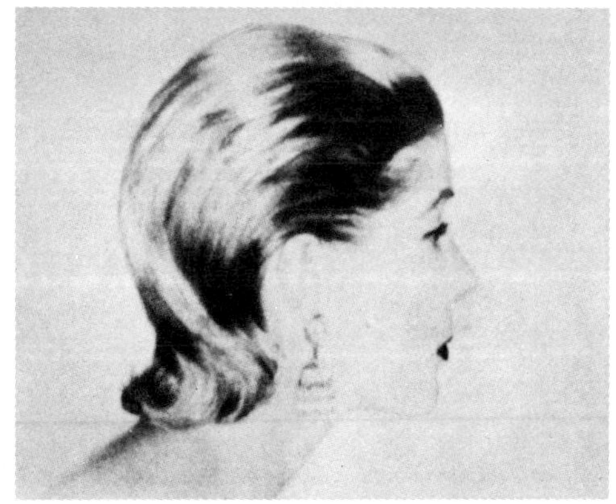

New York

KLEIN 1955

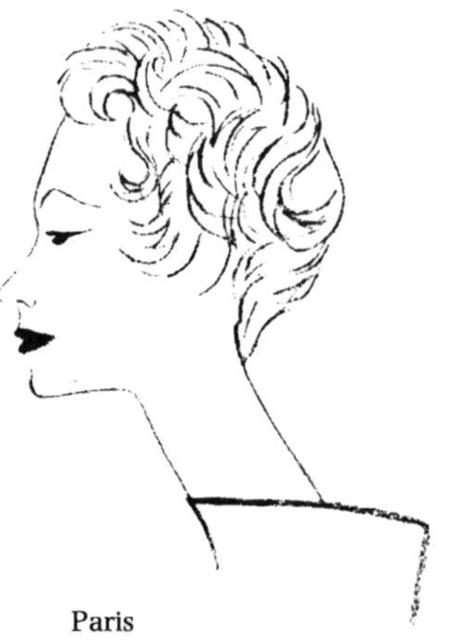

Paris

BOURET 1955

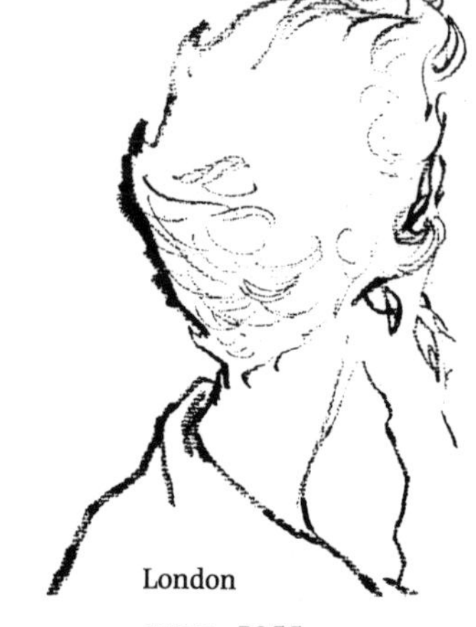

London

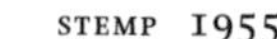

STEMP 1955

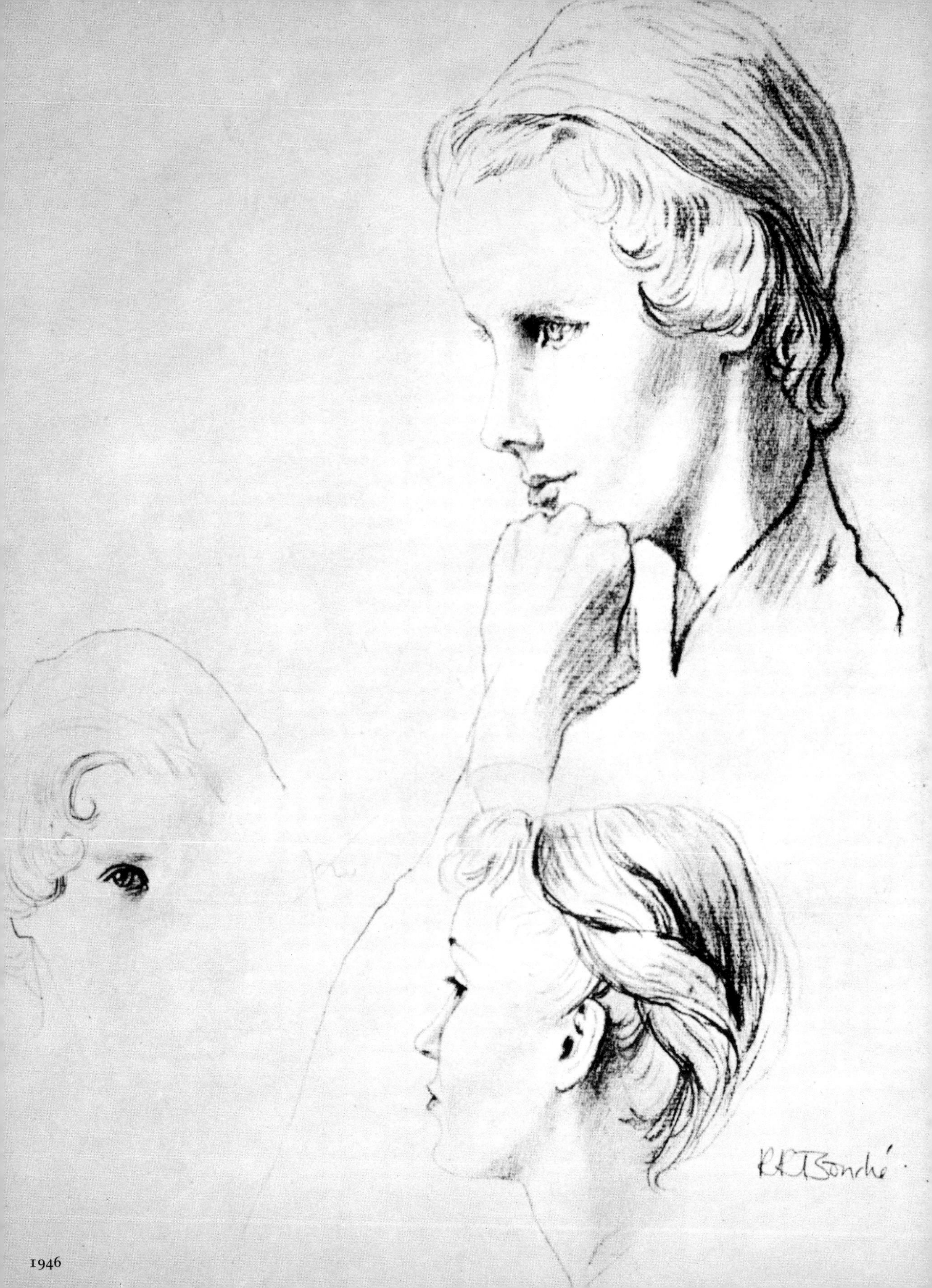

1946

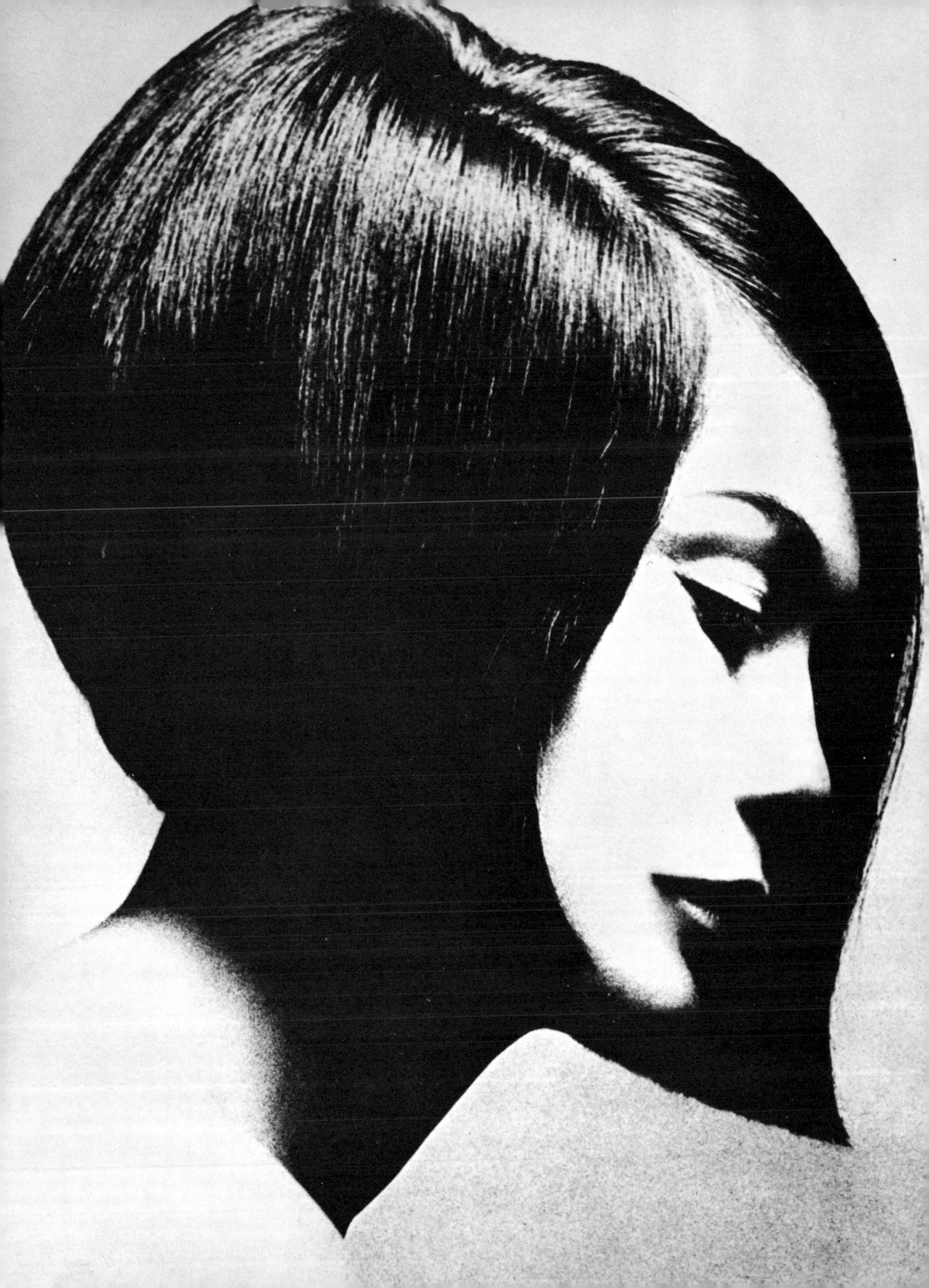

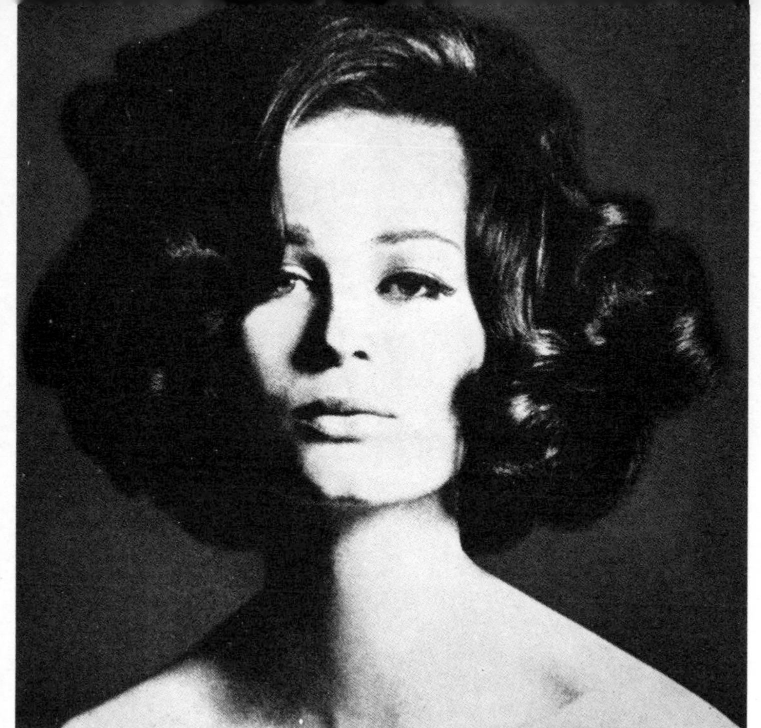
DAVID BAILEY 1962

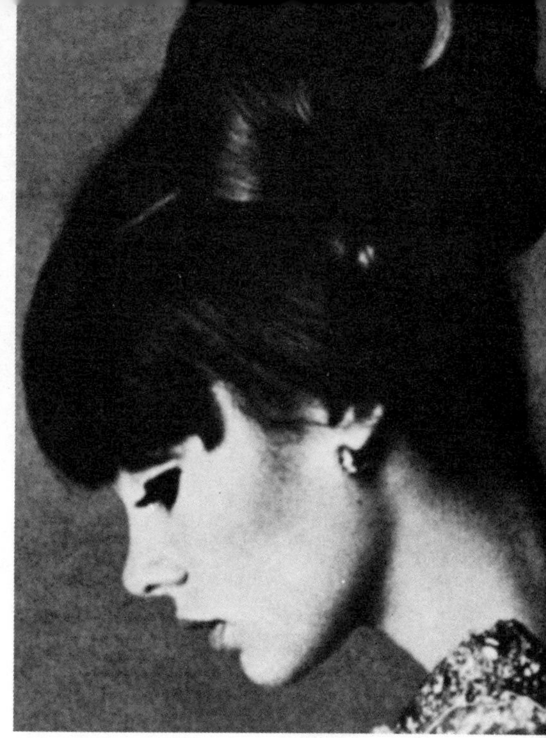
DAVID BAILEY 1963

LEOMBRUNO-BODI 1964
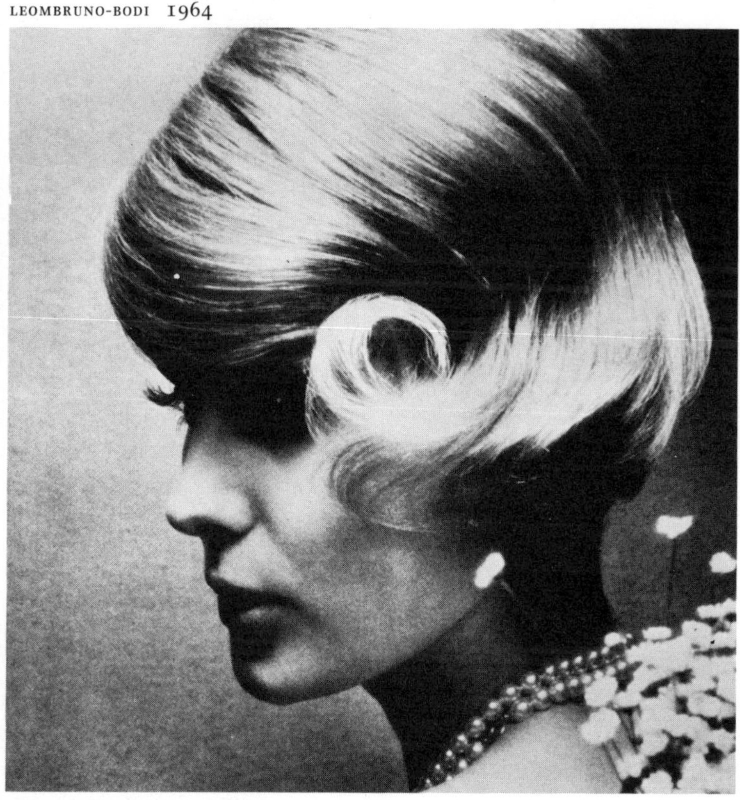

DAVID BAILEY 1964
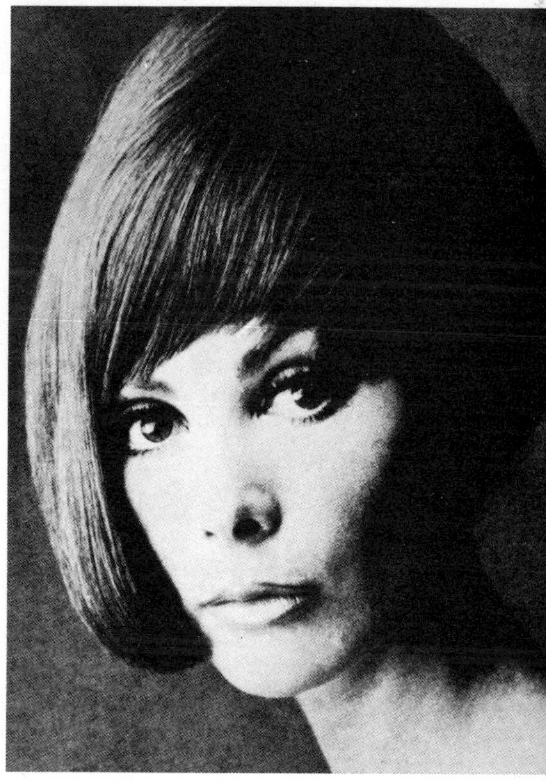

Opposite: The Vidal Sassoon cut. DONOVAN 1962

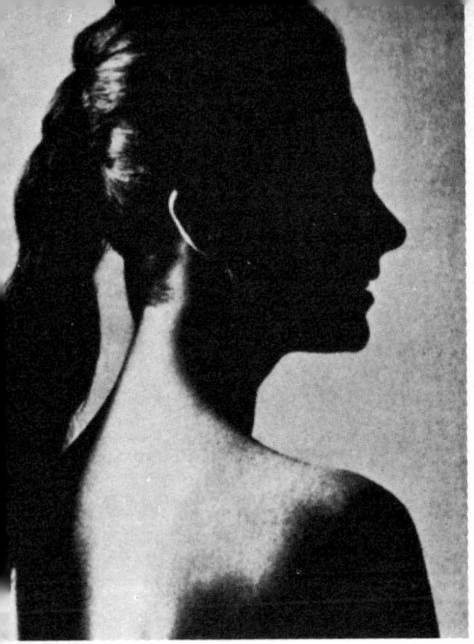

LEOMBRUNO-BODI 1964

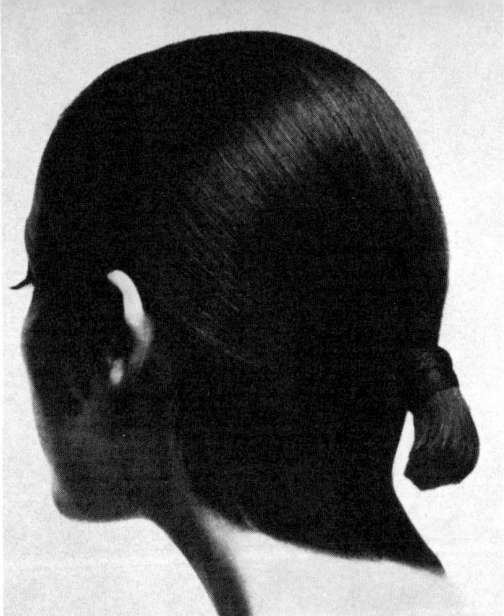

STEPHEN BOBROFF 1968

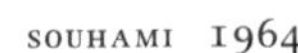

SOUHAMI 1964

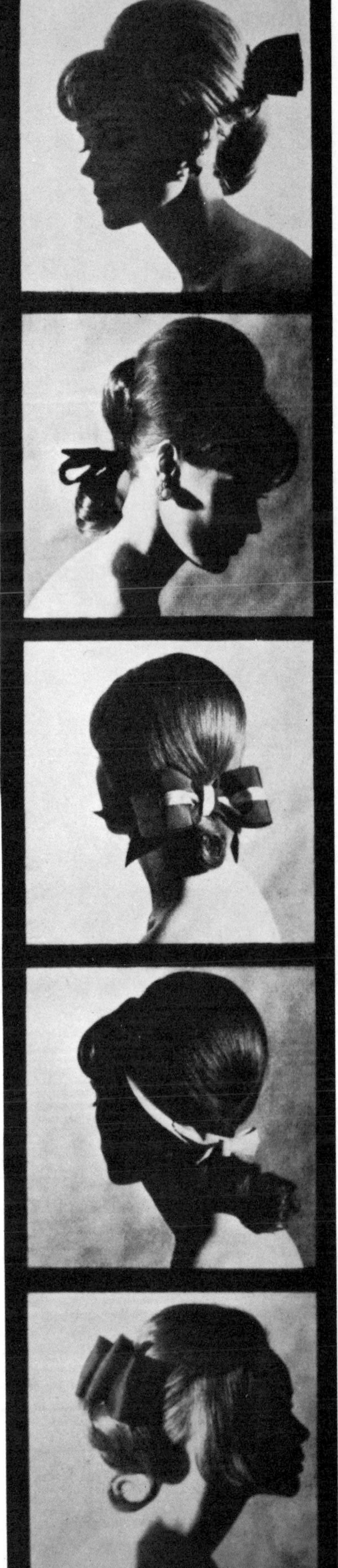

PETER RAND 1964

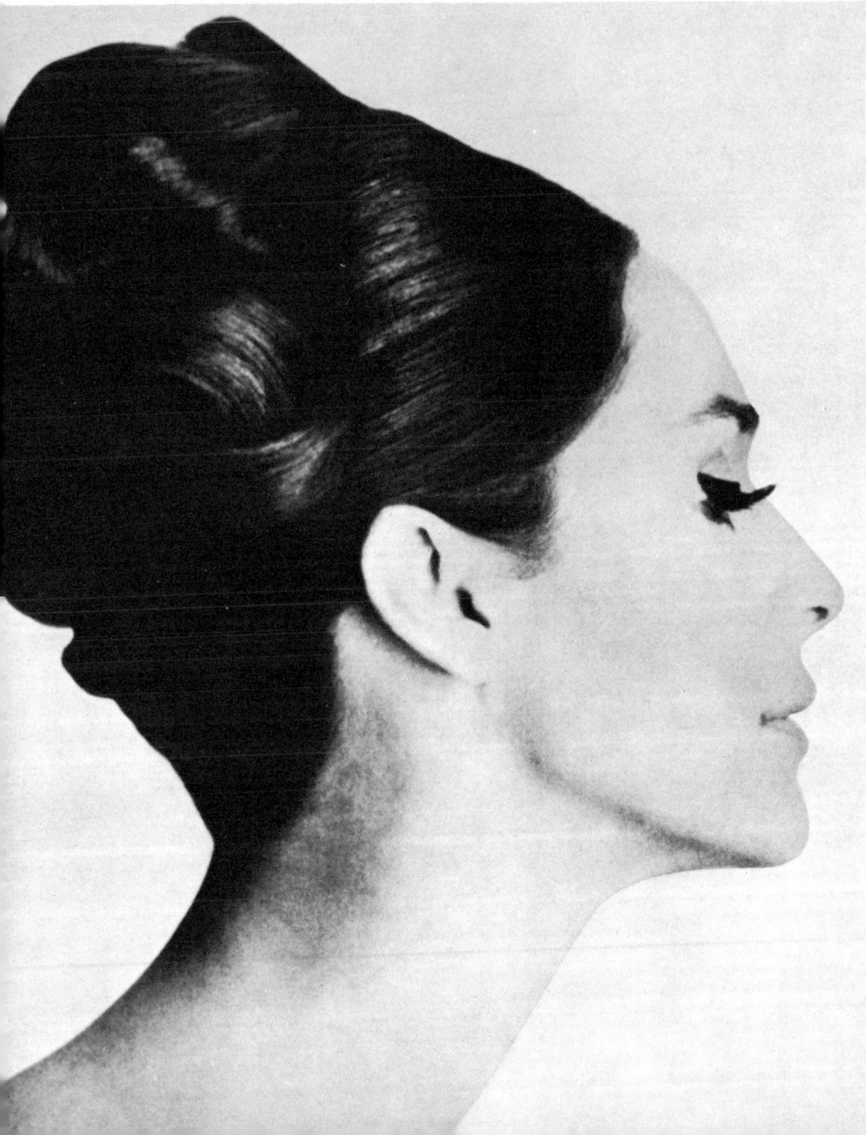

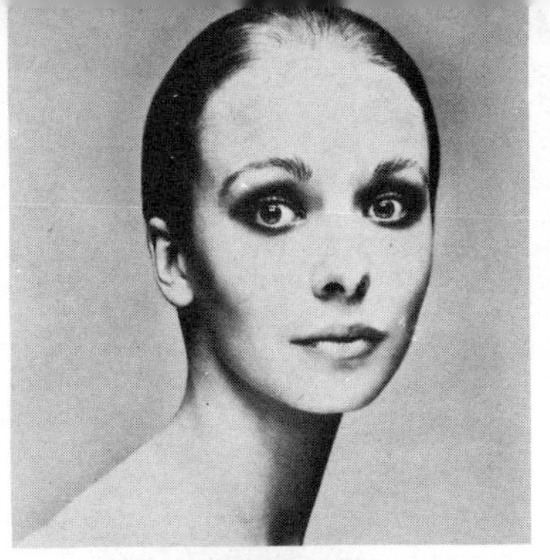

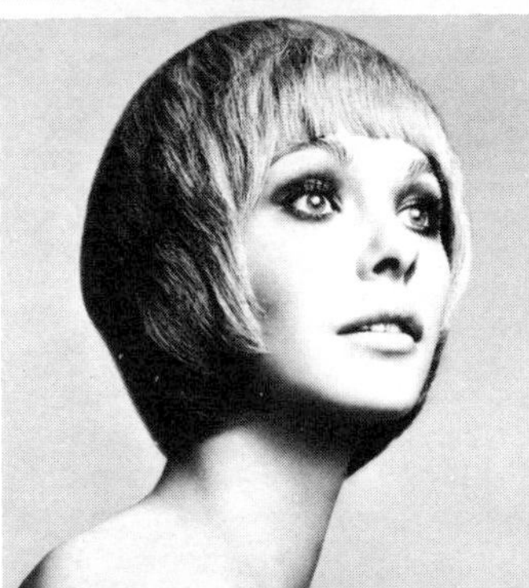

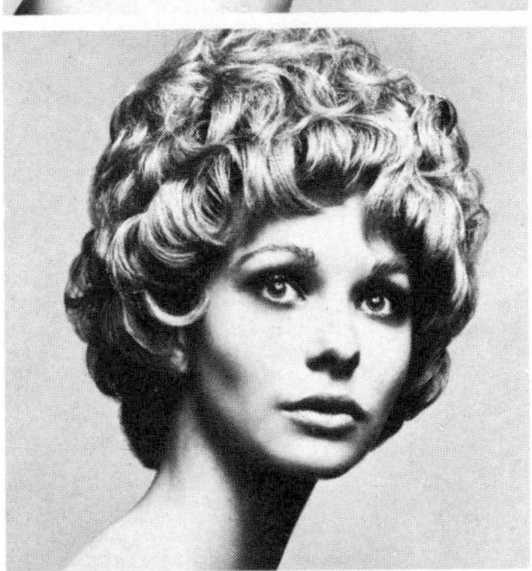

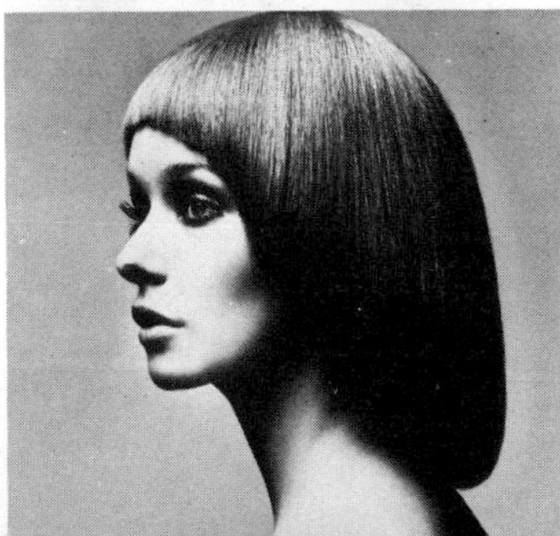

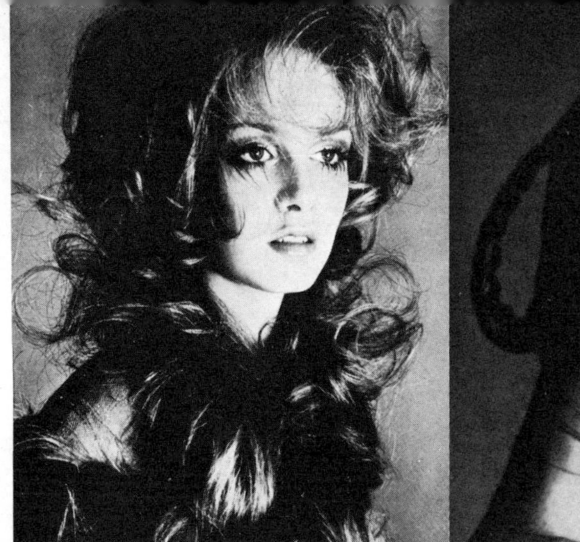

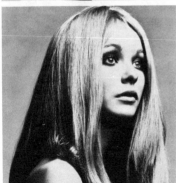

AVEDON 1968

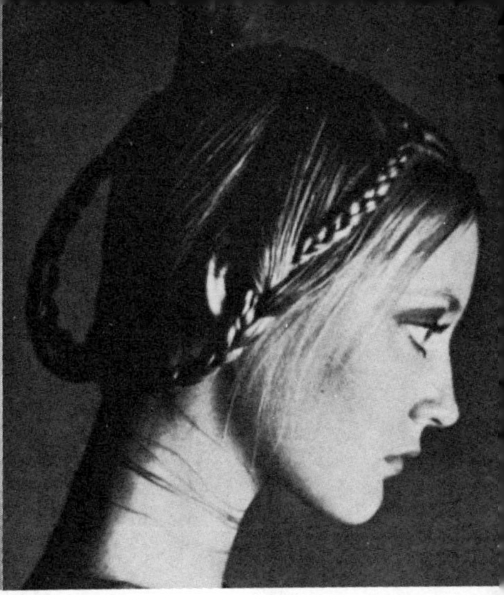

AVEDON 1969

Left: 'One face, four new looks with four new hairpieces.' PATRICK HUNT 1969

PATRICK LICHFIELD 1969

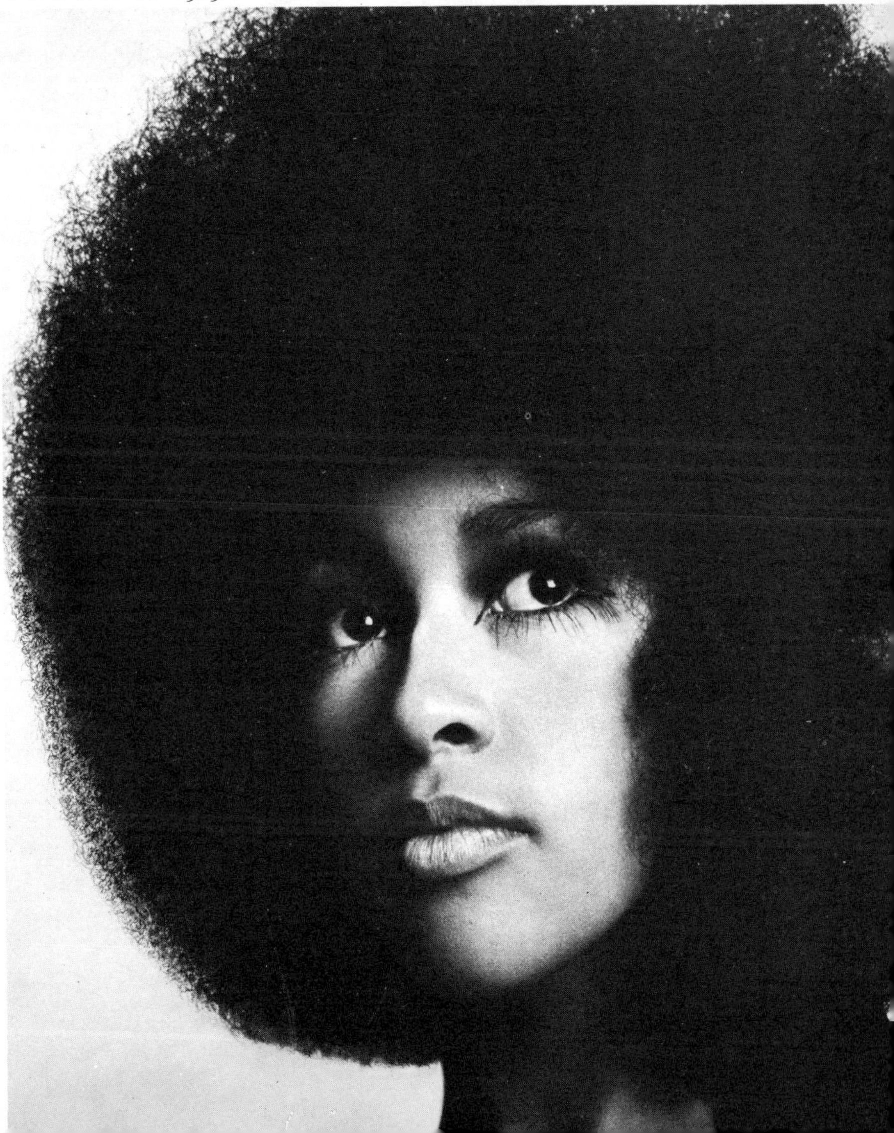

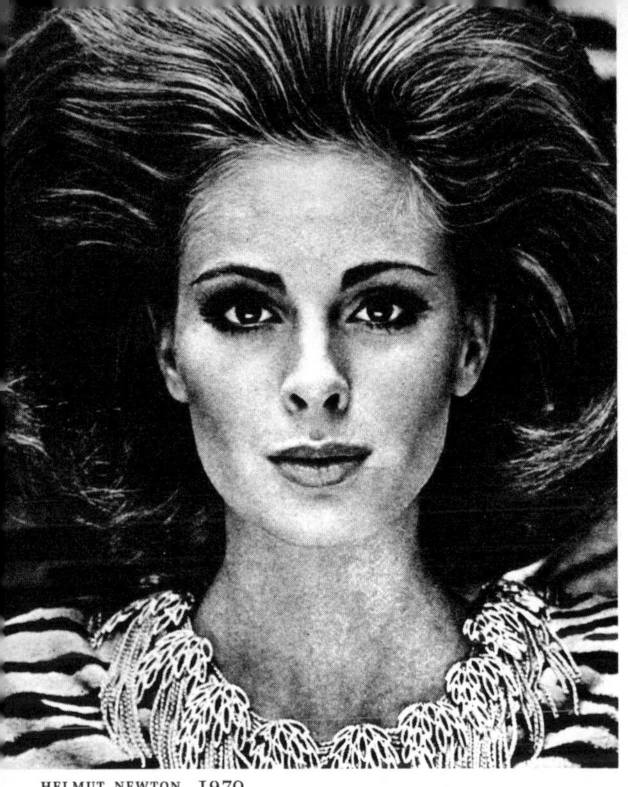

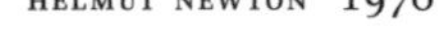

HELMUT NEWTON 1970

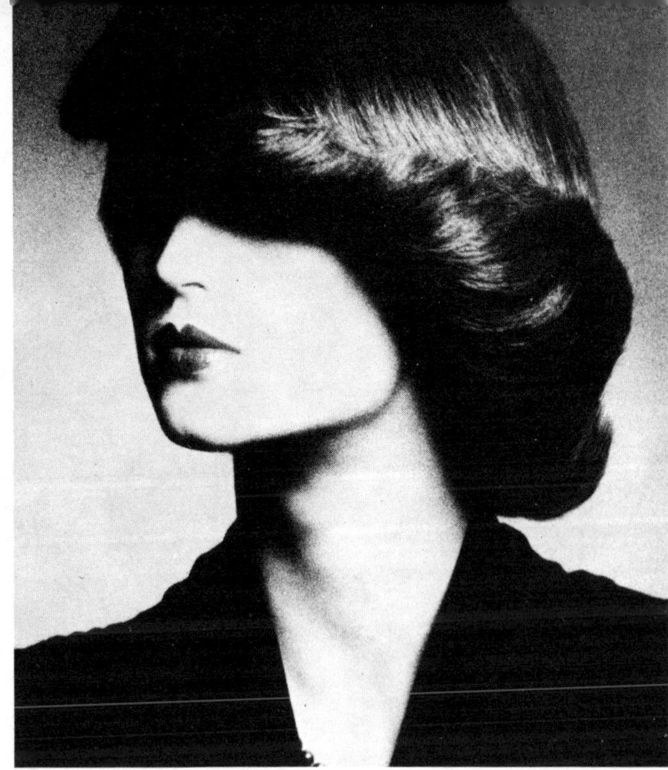

SARAH MOON 1973

Opposite: JOHN SWANNELL 1976

STUART MACLEOD 1975

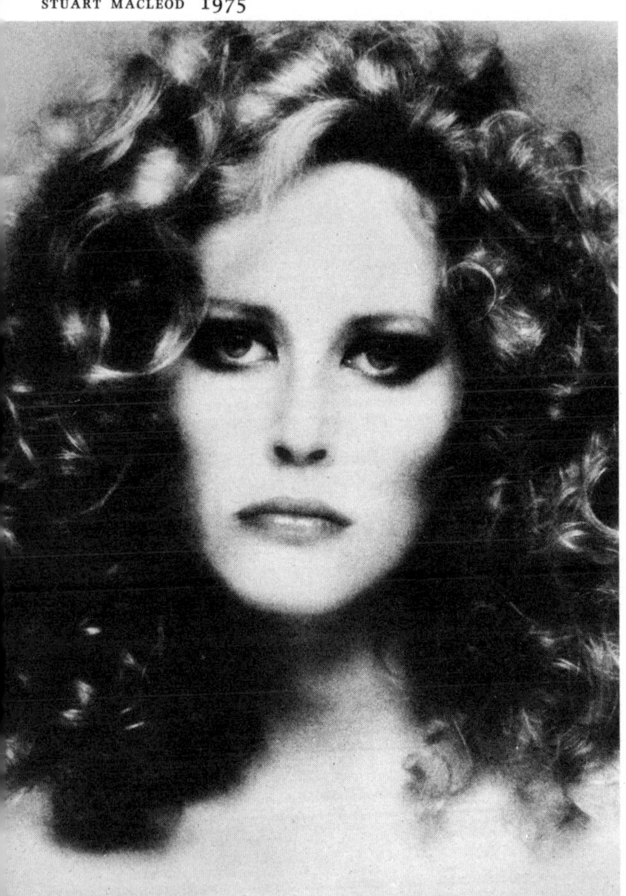

DAVID BAILEY 1976

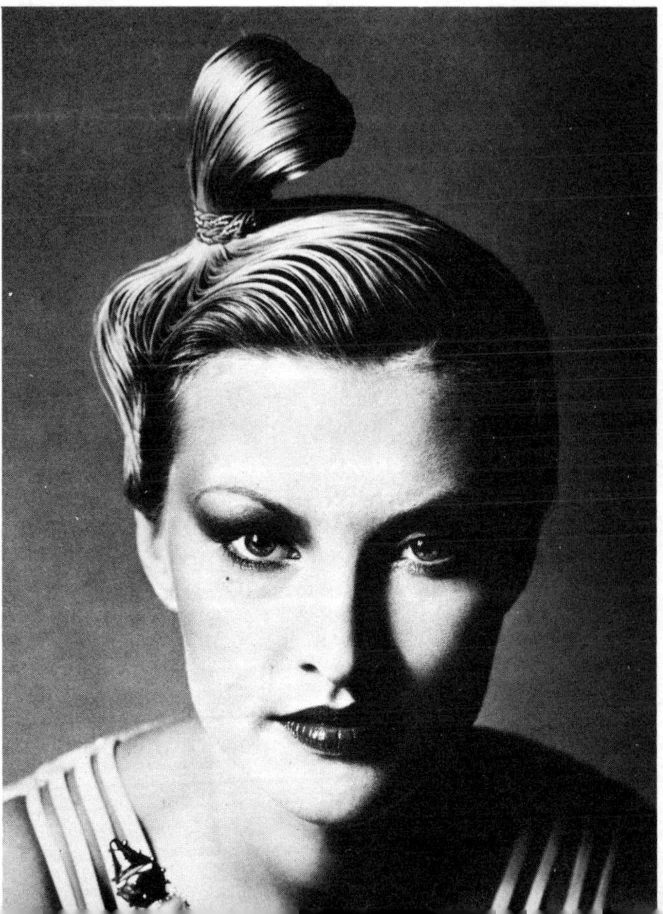

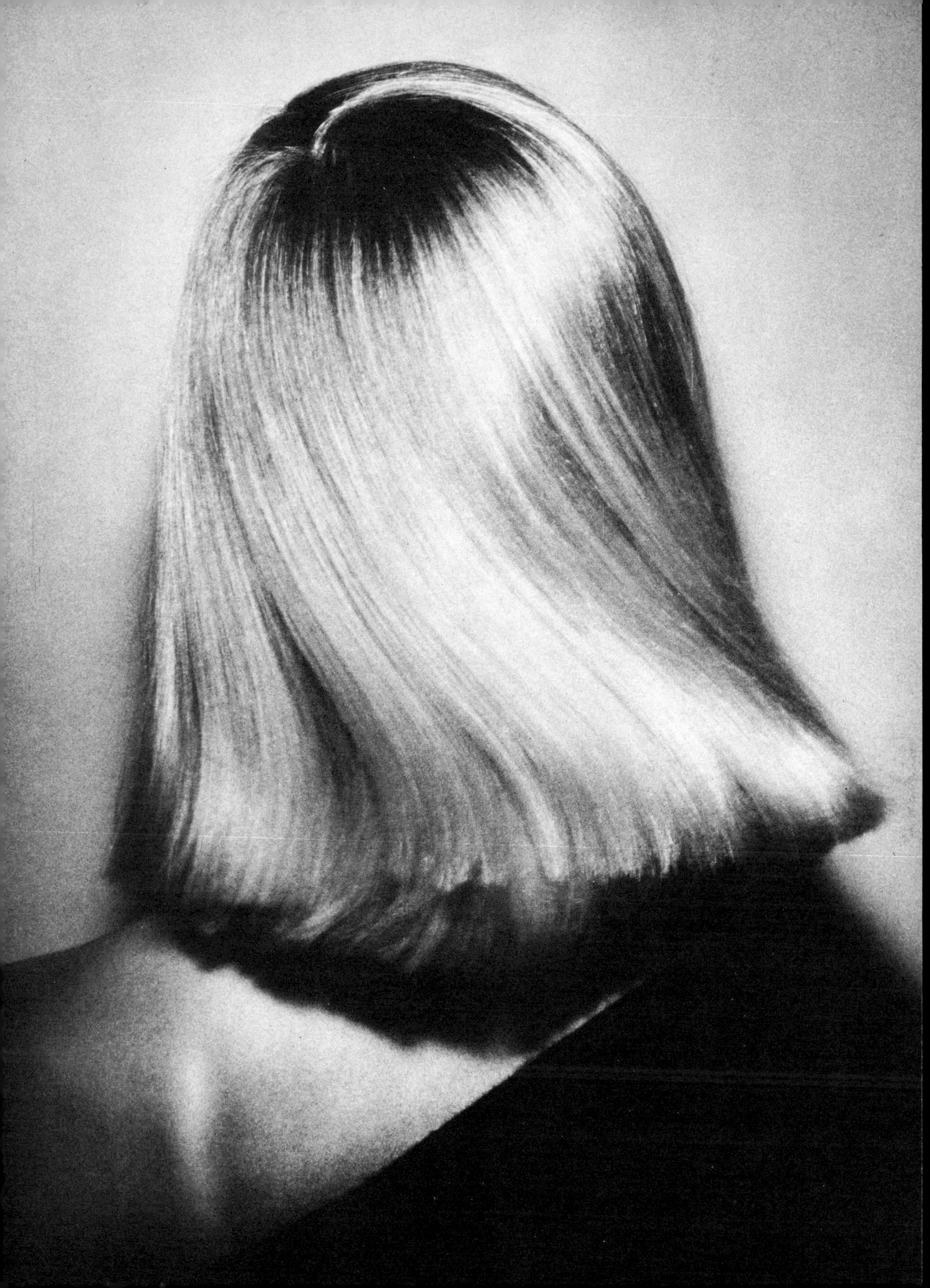

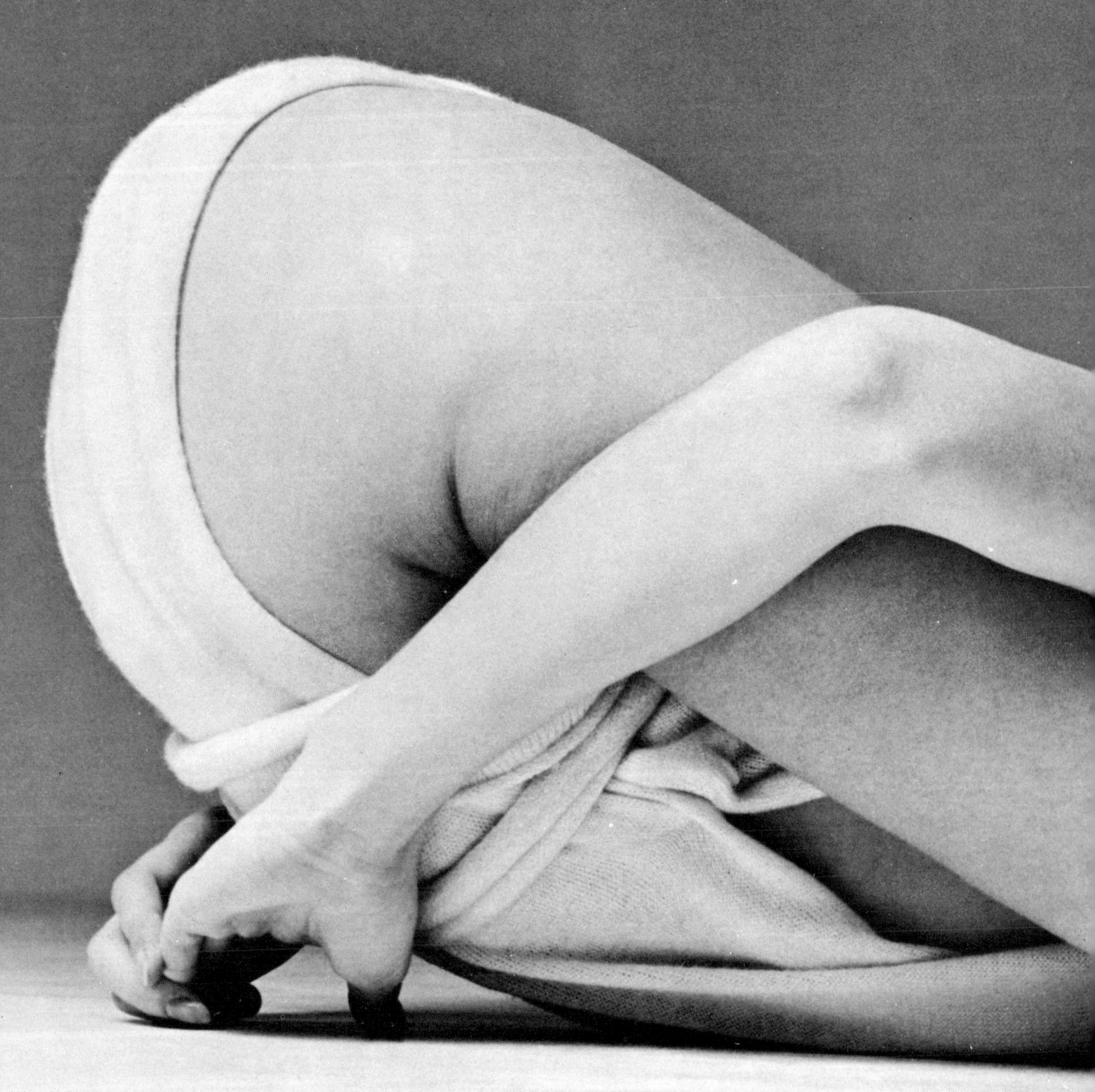

AVEDON

PART III THE SCIENCES

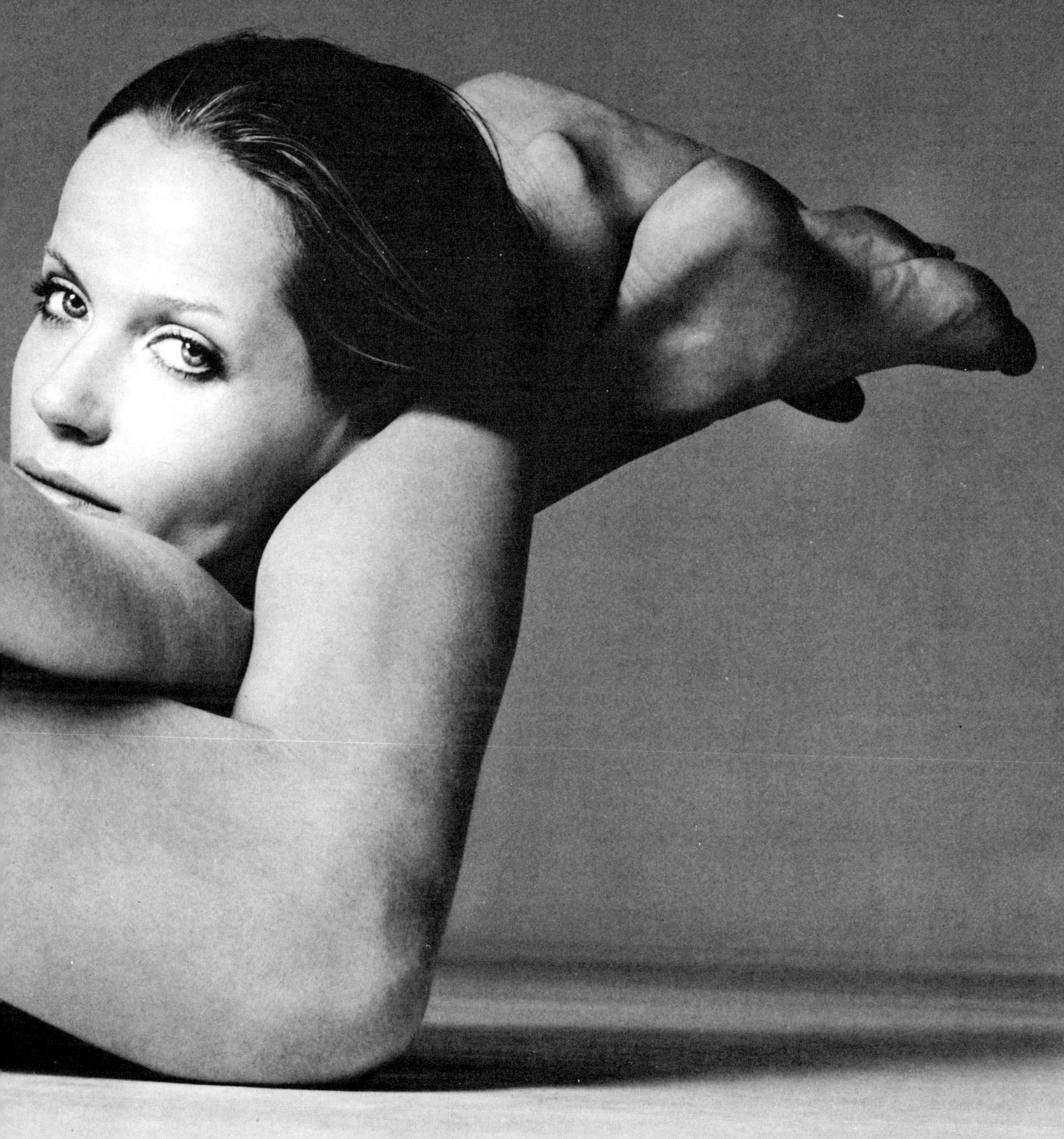

1

NATURAL AIDS

Experiments have shown that the breaking down and building up of cells – the essential body metabolism – is helped by the consumption of plants and their juices. This vegetable matter has an influence on gland activity. Juice and human blood are closely associated in their metabolic function, and roots, barks, foliage, and herbs are restorative in building up health and resistance to disease. They are used in various ways – eaten raw or cooked, infused, distilled, and applied externally.

VEGETABLES

A knowledgeable use of vegetables is a preventive measure, and if some minor trouble should interfere with organic function, certain vegetables can often correct the problem and help restore the body's equilibrium.

Artichoke: Particularly beneficial for the liver; it can purify the blood and act as a diuretic (an increased flow of urine). It can provide protection against urea, cholesterol, arthritis, and certain intestinal viruses. It is bitter when not cooked or as a juice but it is certainly worthwhile taking. Press the juice from stem and leaves, or steep the root in wine. Either liquid will help keep away rheumatism if two or three teaspoons are taken before meals – perhaps in a glass of wine to improve the taste. A tea brewed from the fresh leaves is good for a liver attack.

Asparagus: Can improve a sluggish liver and help diabetes; kidney ailments and bladder stones often benefit. Its tonic properties are said to affect the brain, heightening both mental and emotional faculties, while it has a calming effect on heart ailments and palpitations.

Cabbage: When boiled, it is sometimes difficult for delicate stomachs to digest, so steam it or eat it raw. It can be put through a juicer, and, if lemon is added, makes an appealing and nutritious drink. Valuable for cirrhosis of the liver, especially when caused by alcoholism, and a preventive against arthritis and gout. Cabbage water brewed as a tea with sage is a soothing night cap, and gargle with it for a sore throat. Externally, a hot compress – cabbage leaves, finely chopped and sandwiched between muslin – can relieve various muscular aches and pains, neuralgia, sciatica, and rheumatism. It can be placed on any painful area to help alleviate liver attacks, intestinal pains and period pains. On the head it can reduce a migraine; on the chest and throat it helps colds and asthma. It is a first-aid item; for a burn or insect bite, a crushed cabbage leaf will reduce the pain and facilitate healing. It will help to heal any cuts or sores, lesions, pimples, abscesses, boils, skin eruptions, and superficial infections and swellings.

Celery: Helps to purify the blood, and said to be useful in cases of diabetes, gout, and rheumatism. During a rheumatic attack a small glass of pure celery juice can work wonders. It is a good tonic, produces perspiration and is a diuretic, therefore often included in slimming diets.

Cucumber: Has the ability to get rid of excess fluid and is highly valued for cleansing the body of its toxic matter, and for slimming. The juice, or merely the vegetable cut in fine slices, is soothing for burns and sunburn.

Dandelion: The most superlative diuretic; it purifies the blood by destroying excess acid; it increases the activity of the liver as well as that of the pancreas and spleen. It is beneficial for anaemia, diabetes, skin troubles, gout, and rheumatism. The leaves can be used in a salad; the root makes a good tisane when simmered for not less than half an hour in water; juice pressed from the roots is a tonic for the entire body. The white sap from the stalk can be used to dry out warts, and as an eye wash – one drop in each eye is recommended for minor infections.

Fennel: Soothes the stomach and is a mild laxative. Its principal asset is as an aid to the reproductive system. It helps to regularize menstrual periods, particularly normalizing an insufficient flow. It is said to increase the milk supply of nursing mothers, particularly if boiled with barley. Made as a tisane, it is a fine eye wash.

Garlic: Has become synonymous with good health, vitality and longevity. It contains powerful antibiotic elements, keeps germs at bay, is antiseptic, antibacterial, a laxative, and a diuretic. The smell of garlic puts many people off, but the more you eat, the less it seems to show and it is simple to counteract the odour by chewing fresh parsley or coffee beans. Garlic tonics are old folk lore – here are two: 1) mince a couple of cloves and steep in a glass of white wine for a few days; take a teaspoon on rising every morning. 2) steep chopped garlic in alcohol in the ratio of one part garlic to two of alcohol; allow to steep in warmth, preferably in sunlight, for two weeks; strain; begin by taking two drops in a glass of warm water before lunch or dinner, each successive day increase the dose by one drop until a maximum of twenty-five is added, then reverse the procedure, returning drop by drop to one. It is a tonic that can be taken several times a year, but allow an interval of six weeks between treatments.

Lettuce: Very calming, so much so that as a sedative it can have a hypnotic effect. It should be taken by those suffering from insomnia as a tea (simply boiled), or braised and eaten late in the evening. Better than any sleeping pill, say sufferers.

Onion: This close relative to garlic has much the same powers but to a lesser degree, and they are not lost in cooking. Raw onion is especially recommended for rheumatic patients. It is a good diuretic, acting not only against retention of fluids, but also helping to get rid of urea and sodium and is a particularly good tonic; helpful in combating colds and tonsillitis. A recipe for a tonic onion wine is: 5 oz. (150 g.) grated onion, 3½ oz. (100 g.) honey; mix together and add a quart (1 l.) of good white wine, cover and steep for two weeks; strain; take four teaspoons a day – it may taste strange, but it is very strengthening.

Radish: In small quantities stimulates digestion, but in large doses can produce violent contractions. Good for anaemia. The mucous tissues of the throat and lungs react to its sting, so it can be helpful in cases of respiratory infections. For bronchitis a teaspoon of a mixture of one part radish juice to two parts honey will help clear away phlegm and a sore throat, if taken before every meal and before sleeping. For a hangover: a plate of sliced radishes lightly sprinkled with salt and olive oil. As a poultice it can help aches – if you have rheumatism try it.

Watercress: Good for circulation and the liver; a glass of watercress juice first thing every morning is really bracing. It can help clear the lungs and relieves catarrh and congestion of the bronchi.

HERBS

Our ancestors profited from the secrets of herbal medicine, and now we are simply rediscovering the healing teas, infusions, gargles and poultices that were used to treat the minor illnesses in the family. Certain herbs have certain curative effects, and there are many of them. However, it is not necessary, nor is there usually the time, to become an expert on the subject before you start. Do it gradually, build up your botanical knowledge slowly and surely.

Begin by limiting your selection to familiar herbs, to the garden and field varieties that flourish locally. Garden herbs are aromatic and can be used in cooking as well as for medicine. Field and floral herbs are almost always purely for medicinal purposes.

Herb gathering is an art; not only do you have to know what part of the plant to gather, but the time of day and the time of year for the best results. The best hours are usually in the early morning or late afternoon, as the foliage should be dry but not scorched by the sun. It is useless to gather wet plants, for instead of drying out they are apt to mildew. Roots should be pulled in the spring or autumn when they are most juicy. Stalks are particularly full of goodness in the autumn when the rest of the plant has dried out or become inactive. Leaves are generally picked before the flowers appear, exceptions being the aromatic garden herbs, as their active essences do not diminish during flowering. Flowers are better gathered immediately they appear and certainly before pollination.

When drying herbs be absolutely sure they are put in a dry and airy place: the top of a cupboard, a shelf, a table in the attic. Clean them carefully first; usually leaves and flowers are dirt free, but roots need washing and patting dry. Put the herbs on paper, separate the varieties and turn them from time to time.

If not used in cooking or applied externally in natural form, herbs give off their active elements in water or in alcohol. For healing purposes, water is usually used, alcohol compounds being for external use only. There are two techniques, known as infusion and decoction.

Infusion – made as tea. Basic recipe: 1 oz. (30 g.) of the essential ingredient to a pint (6 dl.) of boiling water. Leaves and flowers should not be boiled, so pour the boiling water over them. The herb should be steeped for a minimum of half an hour and a maximum of 3 hours. For a simple tea, leave the pot or cup covered with a cosy for 10 to 15 minutes depending on the strength you prefer. Use only china, glass, or ceramic pots, stainless steel or unchipped enamel pans – never aluminium or copper. The container must be kept covered during steeping; afterwards strain the liquid into a jar or bottle. A herb can also be infused with milk: cold milk absorbs the essences of most herbs without heat. The general recipe is one tablespoon of the herb to every cup of milk; steep for several hours.

Decoction – simply boiling and usually necessary with seeds, wood, bark or root of a herb. Put 1 oz. (30 g.) into a saucepan with a quart (1 l.) of cold water. Bring to the boil slowly, then simmer until the water has been reduced by about half – this usually takes about half an hour. Keep the lid on during boiling, and use only stainless steel, earthenware or glass containers. Remove from heat, stir well and allow to cool before straining.

GARDEN HERBS

Basil: Soothing, helps calm the nerves. An infusion of basil taken hot at night encourages perspiration and stops a cold in its early stages. It will help relieve menstrual pains and fend off intestinal infections. The leaves can be effective when applied to snake bites and insect stings.

Bay Leaf: Antiseptic qualities, hence its wide use in marination and pickling of food; also stimulates the digestion.

Marjoram (or oregano): An excellent tranquillizer. Good as a tonic and particularly recommended for loss of appetite. Helps cure a headache and hepatitis. People with rheumatism should apply marjoram compresses to the painful areas. For a cold, boil marjoram in water and inhale the vapours. For toothache, drop oil of marjoram on the tooth.

Mint: A very strong antiseptic – even the smell of mint keeps away flies and mosquitoes. Beneficial for the entire digestive system, liver, gall bladder and intestines. Mint can stimulate the heart and the nervous system – it can revive the mind and counteract the enervation of hot weather. Its antiseptic properties make it a good respiratory medicine. At the start of a cold, inhale the vapours from a boiling infusion.

For asthma sufferers and other diseases where shortness of breath is involved, put a few drops of essence of mint in a cup of warm water, mix thoroughly then bottle and tightly cork. When breath becomes strained, a few drops sprinkled on a handkerchief and held to the mouth and nose, will give relief. Mint is a marvellous remedy for headaches – just placing freshly gathered leaves on the forehead can help. Mint tea can help to cure a headache, and if accompanied by stomach aches, as during menstruation, add half a teaspoon of ground ginger and a pinch of bicarbonate of soda before pouring on the water. Also for the head – a warm compress of mint infusion placed on the brow. A drop of essence of mint on the sensitive spot can soothe toothache.

Parsley: One of the easiest herbs to grow and should be used liberally. Apart from being rich in vitamin C, it has stimulating properties and is valuable in all liver ailments, particularly jaundice. It makes a pleasant tea, and is good steeped in warm milk. An infusion helps eye ailments. It is known to relieve gout and rheumatism and this recipe for parsley jelly will help those aches and also purify the blood: wash a large bunch of parsley, press it down firmly in a stainless steel or earthenware pot, cover with water. Bring to the boil then simmer with lid on for two hours. Strain. To each pint (6 dl.) of the liquid add a pound (½ k.) of sugar and the rind of a lemon. Bring to the boil and simmer until it sets.

Rosemary: Can alleviate nervous conditions, quicken the senses, clear the vision and help a weak memory. It is helpful in cases of malfunction of the liver and gall bladder; an infusion is a good mouth wash for gums, bad breath, and a sore throat. A hot tea morning and night is recommended for rheumatism and arthritis and a handful of rosemary boiled for 15 minutes in a quart (1 l.) of water, makes a good poultice for rheumatism. Rosemary wine is a marvellous tonic for the entire system. Steep 1¾ oz. (50 g.) in any Bordeaux for a few days – have a glass with every meal.

Sage: Strong antiseptic properties. Wounds heal rapidly when washed with sage tea and an infusion can be used as a gargle or a vaginal douche. Effective for fevers as it reduces night sweating and will help prevent flu developing. It has a regulating effect on the hormones, so it is considered important for pregnant women and during the menopause. A mild tea is useful for girls during puberty. Above all sage will enrich the blood and tone up the system. An after-dinner drink can be made by steeping 1¾ oz. (50 g.) of sage in a pint (6 dl.) of wine; leave for a week; take a small glass after meals – it is great for the digestion. Sage is well known for its anti-flatulent properties and can counteract any ill effects foods might have, particularly rich and fatty ones. A cup of sage tea is as effective as any pill, and if you are inclined to feel a little sick, add a quarter of a teaspoon of ground ginger; drink boiling hot.

Sage wine is particularly good for those suffering from anaemia and other blood disorders. Make it this way: take half a peck of freshly picked sage leaves, 3 lbs (1·5 k.) seedless raisins, finely chopped, 3 lbs (1·5 k.)

brown sugar; put these ingredients into a large earthenware pot and cover with 8 pints (4 l.) warm water; stir until sugar is dissolved then add $\frac{1}{4}$ oz. (7 g.) yeast. Let it stand for a week, stirring each day. Strain and, when fermentation is completed, bottle.

Thyme: Very strong antibacterial qualities and is a protection against catching colds and flu. Its tonic properties are considerable and it is recommended to sufferers from catarrh or a sore throat. Here's a recipe for a cough medicine: boil 1 tablespoon whole linseed in a quart (1 l.) of water, while boiling pour this over 1 oz. (30 g.) thyme and a finely sliced lemon; sweeten with honey; stir well and strain when cold. The dose is a tablespoonful five or six times a day. Externally it is a dependable disinfectant; cuts and gashes don't fester if washed with an infusion of thyme. It helps rheumatism and arthritis, particularly as an oil essence in a warm bath. Chopped thyme makes a good poultice for rheumatism; warm a mash of it and apply.

FIELD HERBS

At first it is not easy to recognize field herbs. Check in an illustrated guide. The most common for medicinal purposes are:

Borage: One of its more peculiar properties is that it banishes melancholy and comforts a heart saddened with grief; in today's terms, this means depression. Make a borage tea from both flowers and leaves and use for sudden fevers due to measles, scarlet fever, bronchitis or flu. It is rich in calcium and potassium and influences the entire glandular system. The juice of fresh borage is a good purifier, and is claimed to thoroughly revive the kidneys. Seeds and leaves are said to increase mother's milk.

Celandine: Limit this to external use, because it can be poisonous. If you break the stem, an orange juice trickles out, and if you put this on a wart – three or four applications – it will dry out, discolour and finally drop off. It is equally effective against corns and callouses. The sap, diluted with water, can be used as an eye wash against conjunctivitis.

Camomile: An infusion taken in doses of one or two tablespoons three times a day is excellent for most nervous conditions and if added to hot water and drunk before retiring, will induce sleep. It strengthens digestion and is recommended to sufferers of spasmodic coughs due to indigestion. As a lotion it can soothe toothache or neuralgia – make an infusion of equal parts of camomile flowers and poppy heads (altogether about 1 oz. [30 g.]) with a pint (6 dl.) of boiling water. A poultice of camomile is said to prevent gangrene and remove it when present. If you sponge a weak infusion all over the body, it prevents any type of insect from biting you.

Comfrey: A powerful remedy for coughs, sinusitis, lung trouble, asthma, ulceration of the kidneys, stomach or bowels. Boil 1 oz. (30 g.) of crushed root in a pint (6 dl.) of water for 10 minutes, add an equal quantity of milk, simmer for a quarter of an hour. A wineglassful should be taken every 3 hours. An infusion of the leaves is also good, sometimes flavoured with lemon juice to improve the taste. Poultices of muslin or cloth wrung out in a strong infusion relieve the pain of bruises, sprains, and fractures. Poultices of fresh leaves are excellent for ruptures, flesh wounds, burns, and moist ulcers. A poultice can relieve pain in the joints.

Nettle: Contains iron, sulphur, potassium and sodium and is helpful for kidney trouble. A poultice of the green leaves can relieve pain; the boiled leaves applied externally will stop bleeding almost at once. Nettle tea is good for rheumatism and directly affects the circulatory system, helping to arrest haemorrhages, nosebleed and reducing a heavy menstruation. An infusion of the leaves can be used as a gargle for a sore throat, and as a wash for such skin conditions as eczema, acne, and herpes.

Shepherd's Purse: Rather like a cress. The whole plant can be picked and dried, though it can also be put directly through a juicer – in this form it is most beneficial for all disorders of the blood. It can help to check haemorrhages, spitting of blood and nosebleed; it eases excessive menstrual flow of girls during puberty or women at the menopause. Poultices of Shepherd's Purse affect both varicose veins and haemorrhoids.

Yarrow: If the tea is taken freely at the beginning of a cold – preferably mixed with elderberry blossoms and peppermint – it will clear it very quickly. An infusion is a very good douche for leucorrhoea. The juice of the yarrow if applied to a cut will stop bleeding and aid healing.

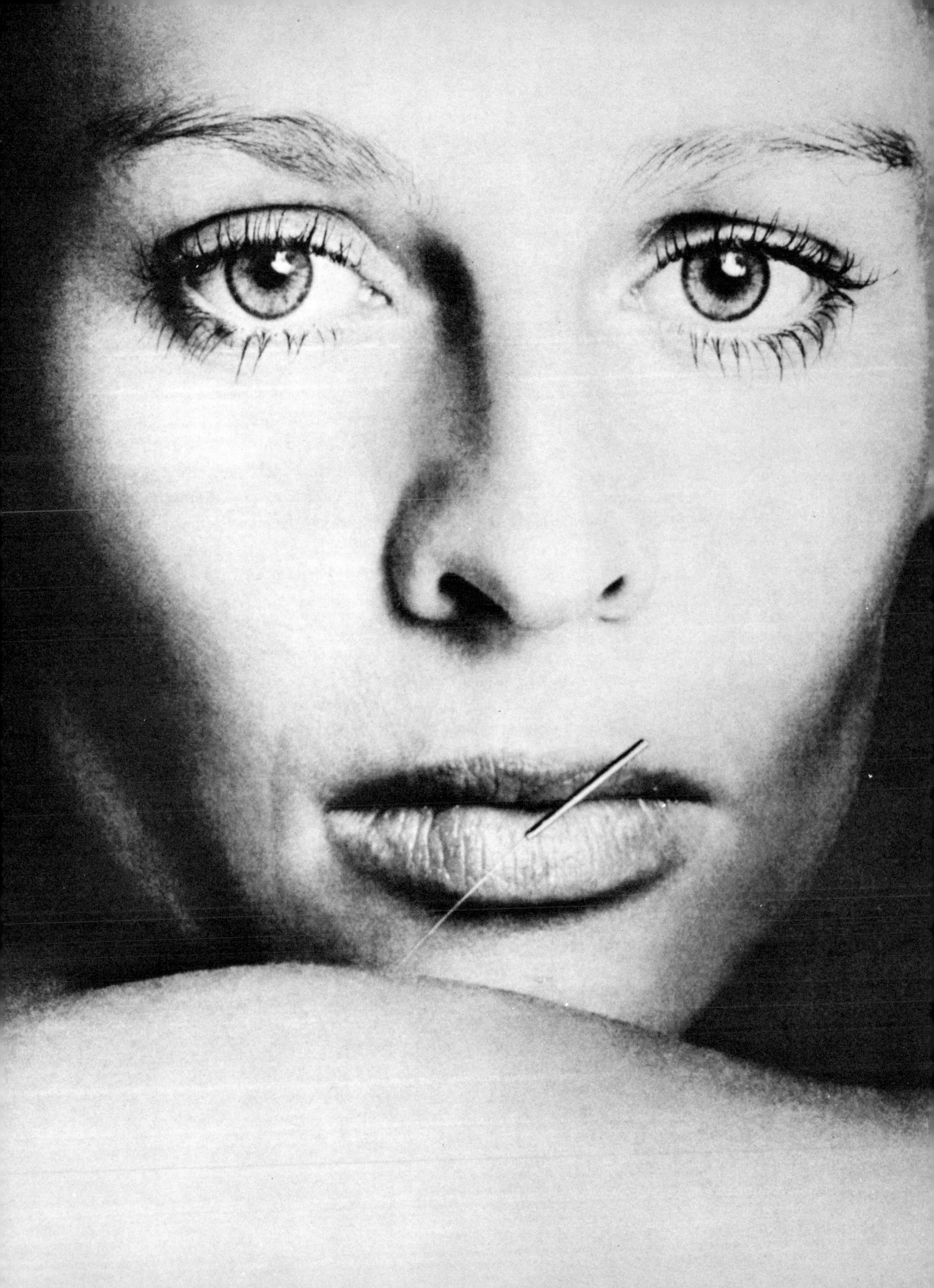

2

ALTERNATIVE MEDICINE

Fundamentally there are two distinctions between orthodox and alternative medicine. Orthodox treatment relies mainly on combating disease with the help of drugs or surgery; unorthodox treatment concentrates on encouraging the body to fight for itself, saying that it is a person's life force that determines the outcome. Orthodox medicine usually isolates a disease or a disorder and treats solely that; alternative practitioners consider the body as a whole, and treat the cause rather than the result.

The life force is a combination of the biological, mental and spiritual will to survive. The mechanism by which it works is little understood and the events that force it into action are varied and often unpredictable. Although the ideas and techniques of the alternative group vary they all rely mainly on this life force, and try to accelerate its action. We have built-in recuperative powers which can be seen at work on such a simple thing as a cut, which quickly heals into a scar, then fades.

Apart from the life force, the life of the person is taken into account. Alternative medicine deals with people, not symptoms. All systems stress the importance of detailed history, not judging by outward signs alone. Rapport between patient and doctor is of prime importance – if there is trust and confidence in a cure, it often works. One of the most effective forces is the power of suggestion. People who become fringe practitioners do so because they are convinced of their beliefs and this is contagious.

Diagnoses of the various disciplines are often quite different and specialized. A herbalist, for example, cannot work from the same type of diagnosis as an orthodox man because his conception of disease is totally different. He does not attempt to find out which germs have attacked the body, but which organs are failing in their function so they no longer can resist. Chiropractors and osteopaths make diagnoses from touch and X-rays, acupuncturists from pulse points.

ACUPUNCTURE

Acupuncture has been the standard form of medical treatment in China and other Eastern countries for 5000 years. To the Chinese the health of the body depends on the action and interaction of the invisible forces of life; their disharmony is revealed by disease, their disappearance by death.

Acupuncture aims to correct imbalance and is based on the belief that the body contains channels through which energy flows. They are called meridians and should not be confused with the physical nervous system though one affects the other. If the body is healthy the life force moves continuously through the meridians. If there is any bodily malfunction, the flow in the relevant meridian will decrease as though 'blocked', thus disturbing the body's equilibrium and causing illness, not necessarily at the place of the disturbed organ. The acupuncturist's skill lies in his ability to free the meridians for an even passage of energy.

This he does by lightly inserting needles of pure gold, silver or copper in the flesh at specific points along the lines of the meridians. The needles penetrate just below the skin and with a good therapist do not hurt at all.

The needle sets up a current of impulses along the line of the meridian which is picked up by the central nervous system, passed to the lower centres of the brain and passed out again to the stricken area. There are nerves in every part of the body controlling body processes and when stimulated some will increase or decrease the flow of digestive juices, the rate of the heart, contraction of blood vessels, secretion of hormones etc. There is little likelihood of the wrong organ being stimulated, as acupuncture is a self-regulating system and it is rare for the stimulation of an acupuncture point to produce a reaction if it is not needed.

The Chinese claim to have proved the presence of meridians by electronic aids and by a specialized form of photography. Choosing the meridian is traditionally done by following carefully detailed charts and by feeling the pulse in a special way and in specific areas.

Diagnoses are done with three fingers and the body is divided into twelve segments, each of which is checked separately.

The needle is not inserted where the pain is. For general work there are 365 points along the twelve meridian lines and it is up to the doctor himself to find the exact point – which is only a bit larger than the point of the needle. This is the factor that establishes the calibre of practitioner. Mastering such a technique cannot be learned from books, it is a combination of a sixth sense and years of experience. Some people are more sensitive and receptive than others, and they sense a small nodule of power at the exact point that needs stimulation.

Unfortunately for Western practitioners, most patients only consider acupuncture as a last resort, having found no relief in orthodox methods. But the particular value of acupuncture is in its preventive capacity. In China patients pay their doctor to keep them well and not when they are sick. Regular check-ups make it easier for symptoms and conditions to be detected and corrected before they are allowed to develop seriously.

The pulse diagnoses enable the acupuncturist to track down illness months, at times even years, before any physical manifestation appears. For such preventive measures it is necessary to check pulses every six months. Treatment at an early stage is said to maintain general health at a higher level, giving a positive feeling of well-being and increased physical and mental energy.

A patient with a disease of several years standing needs about seven treatments to be cured or given maximum relief. Acupuncturists report that some patients notice a response after the first treatment, others feel a difference minutes after the needle has been inserted.

A new development of acupuncture is the way it can be used instead of anaesthetics. Needles are inserted to numb certain areas of the body so that operations can be carried out without pain and without pain-killing drugs. It means less shock for the patients. The same method is successfully used in childbirth.

AROMATHERAPY

Oils and essences were the backbone of Egyptian medicine but aromatherapy as we know it now has only been developed in the last fifty years.

The system consists of massaging an aromatic blend, occasionally specially formulated, into the main nerve points of the body where it infuses cellular matter, acting as a stimulant to restore the body's rhythm. To know your rhythm, and maintain it, is a basic rule in aromatherapy and essential in combating the infiltration of illness. Growing old, say aromatherapists, is but a slowing down of body rhythm.

It is a safe, inoffensive and easy method to accept. It restores the defences of the body and normalizes the dominant functions. It tries to bring to the blood the sweet-smelling elements which aromatherapists believe are necessary to rectify defects.

The regeneration of tissue is seen in the fresher, livelier look of skin after treatment. Acne and eczema can be greatly helped but the capacity to rebuild cells and tissues is demonstrated most clearly when wounds are treated: scars disappear and burns leave no trace. Some orthodox surgeons have worked in cooperation with aromatherapists not only to alleviate scars, but to prepare the skin before an operation to prevent the formation of a raised scar in cases of grafting and plastic surgery. In the same way the skin can be preserved during X-ray treatments. One of the more remarkable results of restoring normal rhythm is the way it stimulates bone reconstruction.

Of particular interest is the effect of fragrance on the psychic and mental state. Scents can cause a state of relaxation, relieving tension and making it easier to dispel traumas. They can make powers of perception clearer and more acute.

Absorption takes place through the skin, so that the volatile elements work their way into the blood and come into contact with the central nervous channels. The temperature at which aromatics are applied is significant. In most cases they should have the same temperature as the skin; then, after the initial massage, a warm damp compress is applied to aid penetration. Application and massage concentrate in the spinal area.

Essential oils comprise organic molecules with free electrons – free to activate beneficially with other molecules. Essential oils are the vital elements of plants. They are extracted from the roots, stalks, leaves, flowers or fruit. The amount of essence varies, and – like wine – vintage essences exist. According to the part of the plant from which they come, the oils have a different composition and fragrance. The age of the plant affects their power. The production of the essential oil is active in young plants, increases up to the time of flowering, but then seems to stop.

The aromatherapist is interested primarily in restoring the natural rhythm of the body so it can help itself at the most efficient level; he prepares the aromatic formula from his knowledge of the physical and mental condition. He may examine reflex zones, use crystallography and blood spectography; personality and emotional patterns are as important as the physical ones.

The mixture is designed to compensate for deficiencies and reduce excesses, i.e. it is a stabilizing force. It will contain essences of various densities and variable times of evaporation. Oils evaporate in the direction of the skin and penetrate it in the order of their fluidity. Heavy resin-bearing scents and dense oils influence the quality of the tissues and the assimilation of food. Essential oils of average tonality influence function, while the very fluid oils seem directly to influence the mind.

The aromatic formula relates absolutely to the individual and might have little beneficial effect on another person. Formulation of individual mixtures is complicated; combined physical and mental conditions have to be taken into consideration. Treatment involves a series of sessions, the number and frequency depending on the diagnosis.

Some of the common essences in the aromatherapist's dispensary are: rose – this has many healing virtues and particular influence on the female sexual organs; it does not stimulate but cleanses and regulates; it also helps cardiac rhythms and blood circulation. Lemon Grass (Indian verbena) – has a preventive quality, a very important ingredient in the care of the skin, claimed to assist in arresting tumours. Palmrosa (Italian geranium) – essence acts on the intestinal flora. Benzoin – helps dispel anxiety. Sandalwood – for renal and cardiac deficiencies.

CHIROPRACTIC

This is an entirely manipulative art based on a particular approach to the spinal column and pelvis in relation to the nervous system and its influence on organic function. The chiropractor believes disease appears in the body because of interference in the nervous system at its main connective centre: the spine. Pressure, strain or tension upon the spinal cord caused by segments of the vertebral column being out of place, however slightly, affect nerve transmission and expression. Minor derangements through an accident or faulty posture can cause nerve inflammation and hinder nerve passage through the small openings of the joints. This results in an unhealthy state of the parts of the body controlled by the nerves in question. The aim of the chiropractor is to find the exact spot of joint and nerve trouble – usually with the help of X-rays – and by skilful manipulative adjustments to properly realign the joint or the spine. The nerves are then once more able to function freely; normal transmission is restored and the body's own resources restore healthy function.

To most people chiropractic is little known and only heard of in cases of 'slipped disc'. It is the link between bone position and nerve channels that is its vital element. Activities of the tissues, organs and limbs are coordinated and regulated by nerve response. Mechanical pressure or irritation of a nerve causes inflammation and, say chiropractors, causes waste and disease of tissues served by that nerve.

It takes only a minor spinal displacement – or subluxation as it is called – to irritate a nerve. Pressure can be caused not only by bone but by muscular contractions and toxins which aggravate sensory nerves.

Chiropractic was founded by Daniel David Palmer in North America at the end of the last century. It was an accidental discovery. He had heard his janitor explaining how he had lost his hearing many years previously after bending over and feeling something 'go' in his back. On examination, Palmer found a vertebra out of place. He adjusted it gradually by manipulation and the janitor recovered his hearing. This remarkable recovery was dismissed as a scientific impossibility, but Palmer decided to pursue the principle behind it. He experimented and developed the technique he named Chiropractic.

Neither drugs nor surgery are used. X-rays are closely studied to find out the extent of the deviations of bone structure. A physical examination of great precision is given to locate lesions. To help endorse findings, chiropractors often use a machine which detects small differences of temperature along the spinal column – on the assumption that it is the inflammation set up by the lesions that registers temperatures.

Practitioners are the first to acknowledge that the success of their treatment often depends on rapport with the patient, and they achieve the best results when their hands take over, and the 'feel' of the patient unconsciously directs manipulation.

There is no fundamental difference between chiropractic and osteopathy. Chiropractors follow Palmer's rule that it is the obstruction of nerve forces that causes illness, while osteopaths assert it is a blocking in the artery that is the contributory factor. Nerves and blood are interlinked and both can be freed to heal through spinal manipulation. The chiropractor uses thrusts or direct techniques that demand precision, high speed and minimum force.

Chiropractors believe that disease is essentially functional – it becomes organic only if the life force is not put back into healing action in time. Apart from headaches, back complaints, disc syndromes and postural defects, chiropractic also helps acne, arthritic complaints, bursitis, mysitis, neuralgia, hypertension, constipation and conditions of the urinary tract. The idea of having spinal manipulation for such diverse ailments may seem odd, but if it is a free flow of nerve power from the spine which enables organs to function it becomes comprehensible and logical.

HERBALISM

Herbalism is believed to have originated about 5,000 years ago in the Far East. It was the mainstay of Roman medicine until the Middle Ages when it lost its original nature-cure character by an infiltration of astrology and magic, though the monks continued to cultivate gardens for the benefit of the sick. The use of herbs continued, too, as the basis of country cures and recipes were handed down from generation to generation. An invaluable guide – still on sale today – was Culpeper's *Complete Herbal*, a translation from the Latin of the herbalists' pharmacopoeia.

Herbalists have never claimed that herbs cure in the same sense as antibiotic treatments. All that the herb or its distilled essence can do is assist the body, stimulate its reactions and strengthen the life force so it may heal itself.

There are about 400 herbs classified into groups which singly or jointly bring about body fortification. A herbalist diagnoses symptoms and uses botanicals directly to influence the function of a particular ailing organ or of organs in need of attention. There are herbs to help every area of the body and they need not necessarily be distilled into medicine to be healing. They can be eaten raw as in the case of vegetables and cooking herbs; they can be applied externally as poultices or emollients to help inflammations and eruptions.

Herbs embrace all botanical matters that can be used for therapeutic purposes – plants, vegetables, fruits and flowers. Herbalists often treat patients whom orthodox doctors have dismissed and many of their cases centre around arthritic and rheumatic conditions, heart ailments, skin complaints, headaches and digestive troubles (see 'Natural Aids', page 281).

HOMOEOPATHY

Homoeopathy is a combination of natural healing and medical science. It embraces the knowledge of orthodoxy but rejects its method of drug prescription. There are three basic elements: the belief that like cures like, the high potency of a microdose and the treatment of the patient rather than the disease. It considers disease as the outward manifestation of the body's struggle to overcome antagonistic forces. Consequently rather than attempting to reduce the disease, it encourages it. The theory is that if you put into the body more of the disease it is exhibiting, then you are encouraging the body's healing mechanism and the natural defences are fortified and supported. What something can cause, it can cure, say homoeopaths, in much the same way that vaccines immunize by stimulating natural resistance to a particular disease.

Great emphasis is placed on diagnosis and history. The physician tries to build up a multi-dimensional picture, based on personality and emotions as well as the medical history of the patient and his or her family.

Remedies are prepared from pure animal, vegetable or mineral sources. They are given in highly diluted doses, easily absorbed by the sick body. What is often deadly in large quantities can be valuable in small. Iodine, for example, added in minute amounts to a diet lacking the essential minimum, is most beneficial – though clearly marked poison.

The system is to put one drop of the actual substance in 99 drops of spirit or water. This is mechanically and violently shaken to produce a distribution of properties. Then one drop is taken from this, further diluted and shaken. The process is repeated many times until the actual amount in solution is infinitesimal. It is claimed that the more diluted the material becomes in the ultimate dose, the greater its effect on the vital force.

Homoeopaths use herbs and botanical medicines. They also use drugs like morphine, cocaine and arsenic – again in highly diluted form so they are no longer poisonous, but beneficially effective. Other curative poisons are: snake venom for blood poisoning, spider poison for angina pectoris, belladonna for scarlet fever.

Homoeopathy was established just over 150 years ago by Samuel Hahnemann, from Saxony. He had trained as an orthodox doctor and had done considerable research in pharmacology. The cruelty and ineffectiveness of medicine at that time forced him to look for another way to help the sick. He believed the patient's life force was usually sufficient to cope with illness, if the doctor could give it some help. He also reasoned that as the patient's life force mattered most, any treatment had to consider the nature of the patient as well as the disease.

He came to the conclusion that illness was a process of purification, a form of cure in itself. His theory of 'like cures like' was revealed to him while testing the effect of quinine on a healthy person – himself. Quinine was used to cure the ague, and to Hahnemann's surprise he discovered that it produced in a healthy body the same kind of feverish symptoms.

He reasoned that it was only by their power to make sick that drugs cured sickness, and that a medicine could only cure such conditions as it produced when tested on a healthy body. If the ague were the body's way of fighting malaria, not malaria's way of fighting the body, a drug which produced the same kind of feverish symptoms could serve as an ally – as did quinine.

It was a whole new approach to disease and he set out to demonstrate the principle, subjecting all drugs he used to intensive 'provings' on healthy people before they were tried out on the sick. His remedies were all single compound substances and most of them have remained in the homoeopathic *materia medica* that is used today. Hahnemann also found that by decreasing the amount used in a dose its effect was not decreased – in fact quite the opposite, even when diluted almost to vanishing point.

Compared with allopathic treatments, homoeopathy does not give a speedy cure. It often seems slow, but the microdoses put the patient on a gradual road to recovery. It is an alternative and complementary method to the orthodox one. Usually homoeopaths are trained first in the traditional way, including surgery; they are not against orthodox treatments but object to the belief in a different drug for every disease.

NATUROPATHY

This is the branch of alternative medicine that is most understood. Awareness of the dangers of body pollution has turned an increasing number of people to naturopathy as an antidote. It is an age-old philosophy which teaches the principles of healthy living and is now part of what is called natural therapeutics. It encompasses many of the marginal theories of medicine, for anything that encourages the natural life force to heal the body comes under the regime of the naturopath. Thus many practitioners are also osteopaths or chiropractors while some hold qualifications in herbal medicine and homoeopathy. The entry of unnatural elements is considered the cause of disease; these could be toxins that upset body chemistry, structural faults or pyschological factors due to stress.

Some of the earliest naturopathic principles are to be found in Hatha Yoga which teaches simple diet, breathing, exercise, mental, emotional and spiritual tranquillity. The main basis for the modern revival was made by Dr Henry Lindhar. He believed that disease is a healing effort of nature and that the suppression of acute illness by drugs, serums or surgery could be the cause of chronic disease in later life.

Naturopathy has two aims: it treats disease and builds up health. It is a practical system of health restoration without the possibility of dangerous side effects – but it is also a way of living which ensures the optimum level of physical, mental and spiritual well-being.

Naturopaths diagnose by methods similar to orthodox ones but include a thorough spinal investigation and a more intensive appraisal of psychological aspects. They classify causes into three groups: chemical – due to faulty eating, drinking, elimination and breathing; structural – misplacements in the spinal column, muscular lesions, incorrect posture, stiff joints; psychological – hampered reactions because of emotion, fear, tension and frustration.

The way to restore the balance of the body through self-healing consists mainly of dietetics, fasting, hydrotherapy and structural adjustment. Structural adjustments can take the form of postural re-education, remedial exercise, osteopathic, chiropractic or neuro-muscular techniques. Rest and tranquillity are very important, so is the therapeutic use of water as in Sitz baths, sprays, massage.

A fundamental naturopathic argument is that for the body to be nourished only with the ingredients it needs, is its best defence mechanism. The first necessity, therefore, is to eat foods which are natural and whole, grown without fertilizers, unrefined and uncontaminated. Pre-cooked foods should be avoided, and all foods should be cooked for as little time as possible. It is not necessary to be on a vegetarian diet, though sometimes flesh-free diets are indicated.

Restoration of health depends to a large extent on a build-up of energy. Far from eating more, this may necessitate eating less, even fasting, to give the body a rest and the opportunity to devote all its energies to the elimination of toxins.

OSTEOPATHY

Osteopaths believe that disease arises from interference with the circulatory system stemming primarily from blockage in the spinal area. The method was founded in the U.S.A. by Dr S. R. Still around 1870. Osteopaths state that wherever blood is circulating normally disease cannot develop – because blood is capable of manufacturing all matter necessary for disease immunity. If blood becomes static it toxifies and illness follows. Osteopathy is the study and practice of certain principles applied to functional and organic disease – those not generally recognized by orthodox practitioners. The basis is that any deviation from normal in structure of bones, joints or soft tissues is capable of affecting the natural organic functions of the body.

These abnormalities are referred to as lesions and are centred on the spinal column. Their detection and removal is said to counteract both physical disability and organic ill health. It may not necessarily be an out-of-line bone that causes trouble; tension and contraction in muscles, overstretching or contracting of ligaments, tightened bands of connective tissue – all can obstruct normal blood flow. Of equal importance is the smooth functioning of the lymphatic system, which Dr Still coupled with blood as comprising the fluids of life.

Osteopathy demonstrates that many illnesses have a relationship to disorders of the spine and can be reversed by manipulating joints back into correct alignment. All Still's original researches emphasize that illness is due to the condition of the whole body and not an isolated outbreak in one part of it. He looked at the symptoms, but did not treat them directly. He traced them back to structural disturbances – the malposition of bones, strains and dislocations which he adjusted by manipulation and allowed the life force to do the rest.

The same method applies today. The theory is that a body cannot function properly unless it is structurally sound, and if the structure is sound then the vital force will take over to help restore health, whatever the disorder. Osteopathy involves the normalizing and adjustment of spinal lesions, the massage of soft tissue, muscles and ligaments. Modern osteopaths work with X-rays to examine the position of the joints, paying special attention to spinal lesions. Past medical history is studied. A method of diagnosing the condition of the blood in certain areas was established by Still and is an important part of the osteopathic assessment: areas of the body are touched to judge the speed, heat and quality of blood palpitating beneath them. It is similar to the pulse diagnosis of the acupuncturist.

Once the cause is removed the conditions set up are said to disappear. Osteopaths know of deficiencies which often cause the loss of muscular tone – bad diet, lack of essential vitamins and minerals – and the consequent falling out of alignment of bones. If such deficiencies are not compensated the body will revert to misalignment. Lesions can be caused by accidents, falls, twists, blows, bad posture, bad diet, prolonged tension.

If an illness has reached the organic stage it may be too late for manipulation to work satisfactorily. Certain arthritic conditions, slipped discs, asthmatic-bronchitic ailments, muscular atrophy, the Parkinson syndrome, pneumonia and some skin diseases can be helped – apart from every form of dislocation.

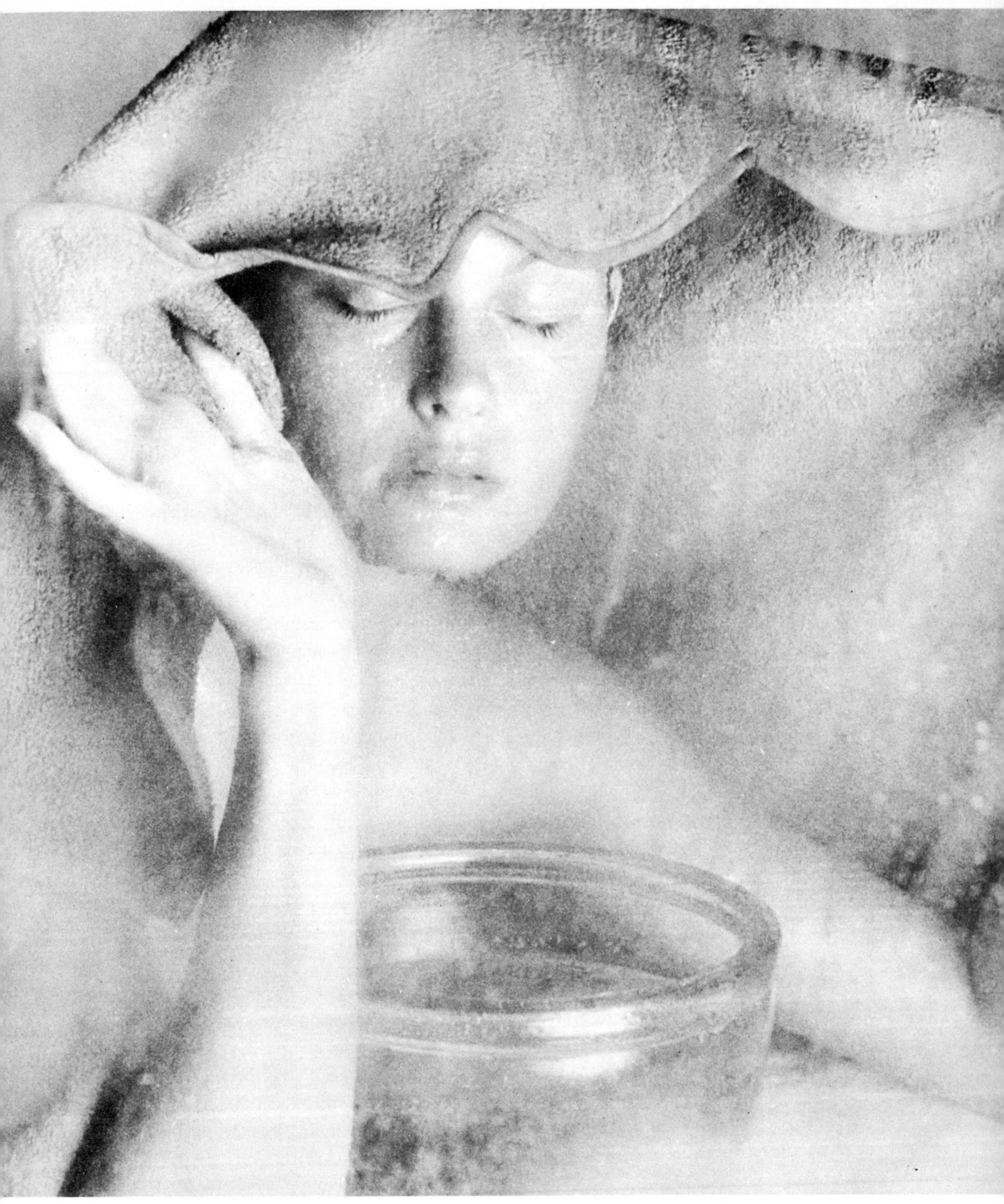

PENATI

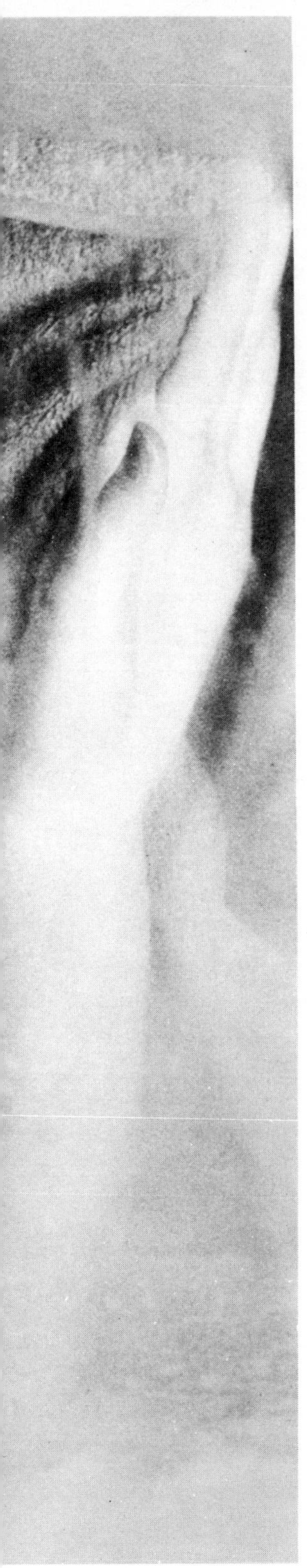

3

COMMON AILMENTS

Good health depends on many things – establishing regular physical and emotional patterns, coming to terms with hereditary inclinations, being conscious of the 'feel' of your body and being able to detect anything out of order. Most of us are midway between being sick and truly healthy. We are subject to many ailments which have become so common that they are often accepted as inevitable. Most of these common disorders – colds, headaches, backaches, asthma, constipation, high blood pressure, rheumatism – invariably have no one known cause, nor any definite cure. Treatment often falls back on rest, relaxation, warmth and positive thinking.

Listed here are some common complaints, their possible causes, symptoms and treatment.

ABDOMINAL PAIN: The stomach is in the upper left part of the abdominal cavity; the liver is above and to the right, the pancreas, spleen, bladder and intestines are below the stomach, and lower still, tucked away behind the pelvis, are the ovaries, womb and Fallopian tubes; the kidneys are towards the back of the stomach and protected by the last two ribs. Unless you know your body well, it is difficult to locate the pain exactly, though many aches are often caused by indigestion, wind and bowel upsets. If ordinary remedies fail, and if the pain continues for more than twenty-four hours, see a doctor.

ALCOHOLISM: A few years ago only one alcoholic in nine was a woman, now the ratio is one in four in Western countries. They are younger, the majority being under forty. Women are becoming problem drinkers because of boredom, frustration, the social acceptance of women drinking like men, the availability of alcohol. A drinker can be classified as medically alcoholic if she drinks the equivalent of two pints (1 l.) of whisky a day, has amnesia, and loses weight. A warning sign is the feeling that you must have a drink, not just at the end of the day, but early in the morning. Usually alcoholics can drink beyond the limit of others without appearing drunk. Heredity may play a part in problem drinking according to some experts. Others say that a biochemical factor is the influence, while others emphasize that stress and strain drive a person to drink. Whatever the cause, alcoholism is a real illness; it is a progressive disease which, unless arrested by total abstinence, inevitably leads to the deterioration of body and mind.

It takes time and patience to deal with alcoholism and an enormous amount of self discipline and control. One drink is like dynamite, and to abstain from that one drink is not easy. Group therapy seems to work better than any other treatment, and there are Alcoholics Anonymous branches all over the world. Here the drinker finds an atmosphere where there is no criticism, no hostility, only sympathy and understanding. Long-term plans are not even thought of; one day at a time without drinking is the aim.

Drugs can be used which, if followed by drinking within three or four days, make the patient feel extremely ill, with symptoms resembling heart-attack warnings. There is also aversion therapy, where injected emetic drugs make the alcoholic feel sick and vomit at the sight, taste or smell of alcohol. Neither treatment is pleasant, nor always successful.

Abstinence is the only cure. After a drinking bout an alcoholic can feel dreadfully ill for about a week, and it needs maximum courage and encouragement not to take the first few drinks that seem to cure the extended hangover. Unfortunately the compulsion to continue is usually too strong to resist.

ALLERGIES: Allergens or antigens are the medical names for the substances that cause allergic reactions, and they fall into four main groups: inhalants – pollens, grasses, plants, perfumes; ingestants – food and drink; contactants – dust, fabrics, cosmetics; injectants – insect stings and bites, injected medicines. Their effect is inconsistent: you can get a severe reaction to something you have eaten or inhaled for years without any problem. Sometimes the combination of allergens causes the reaction, and it is believed that several of the so-called allergy illnesses – asthma, migraine and eczema – could have emotional associations. In

Opposite and overleaf: Barry Lategan, 1975

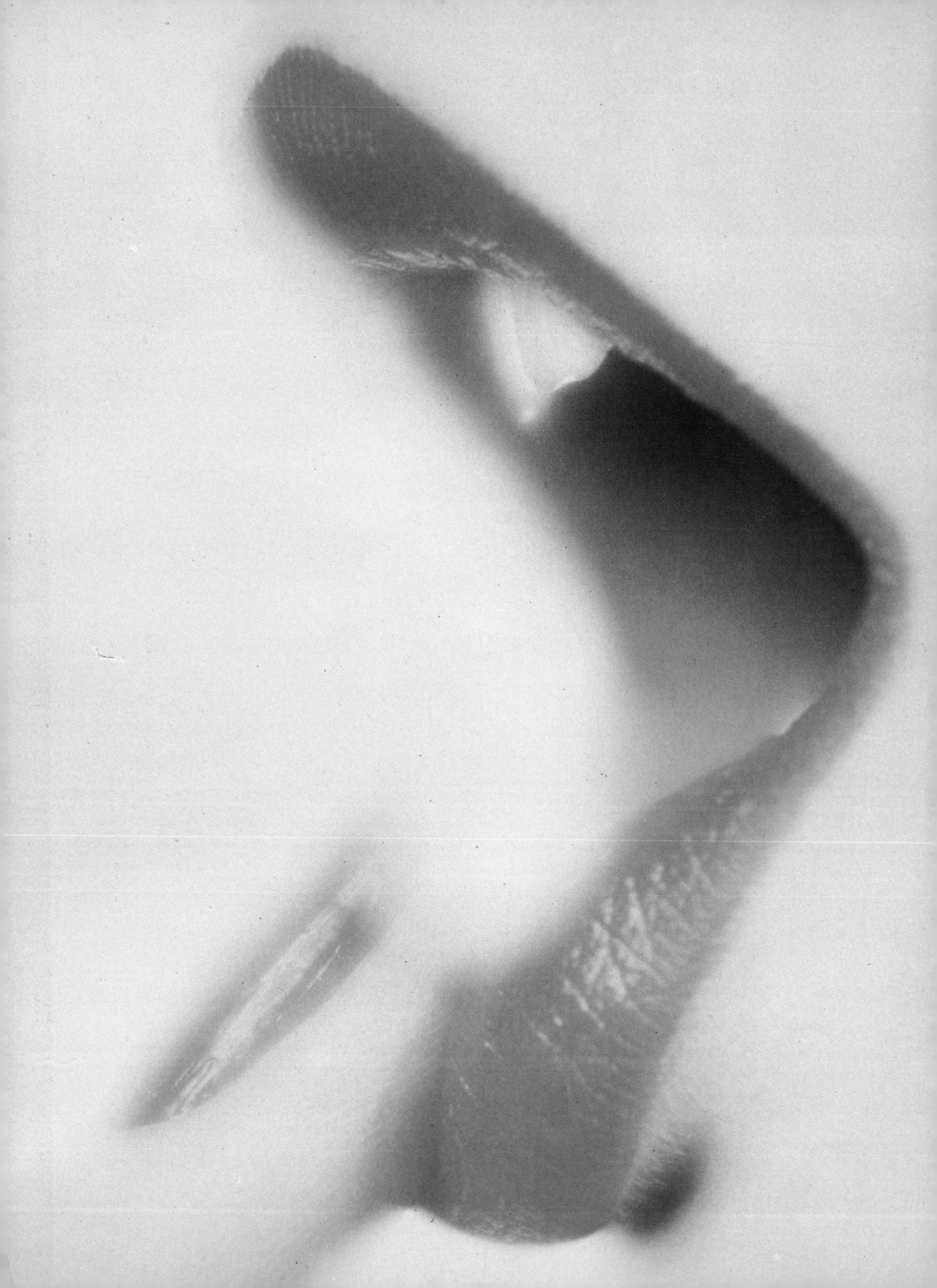

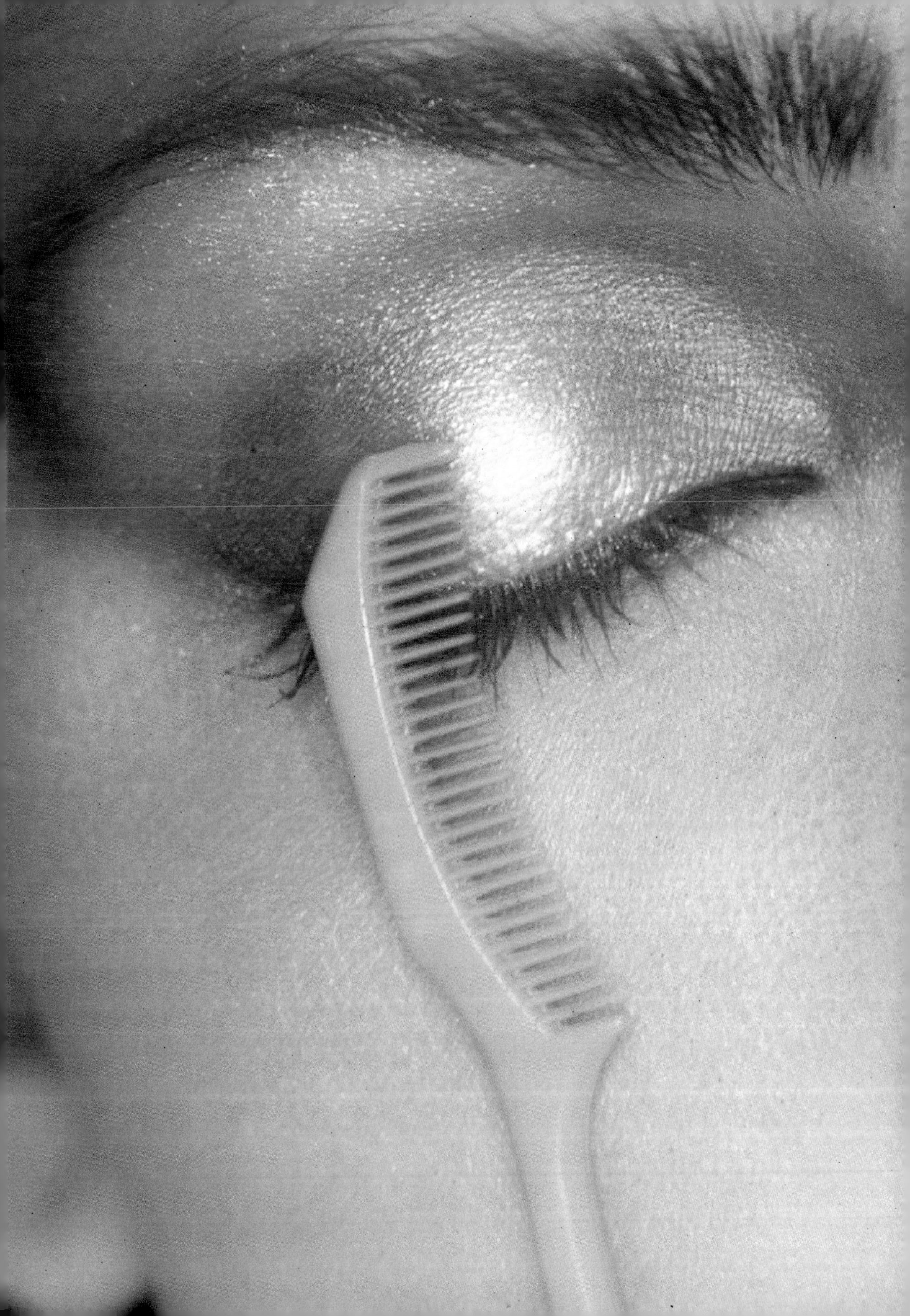

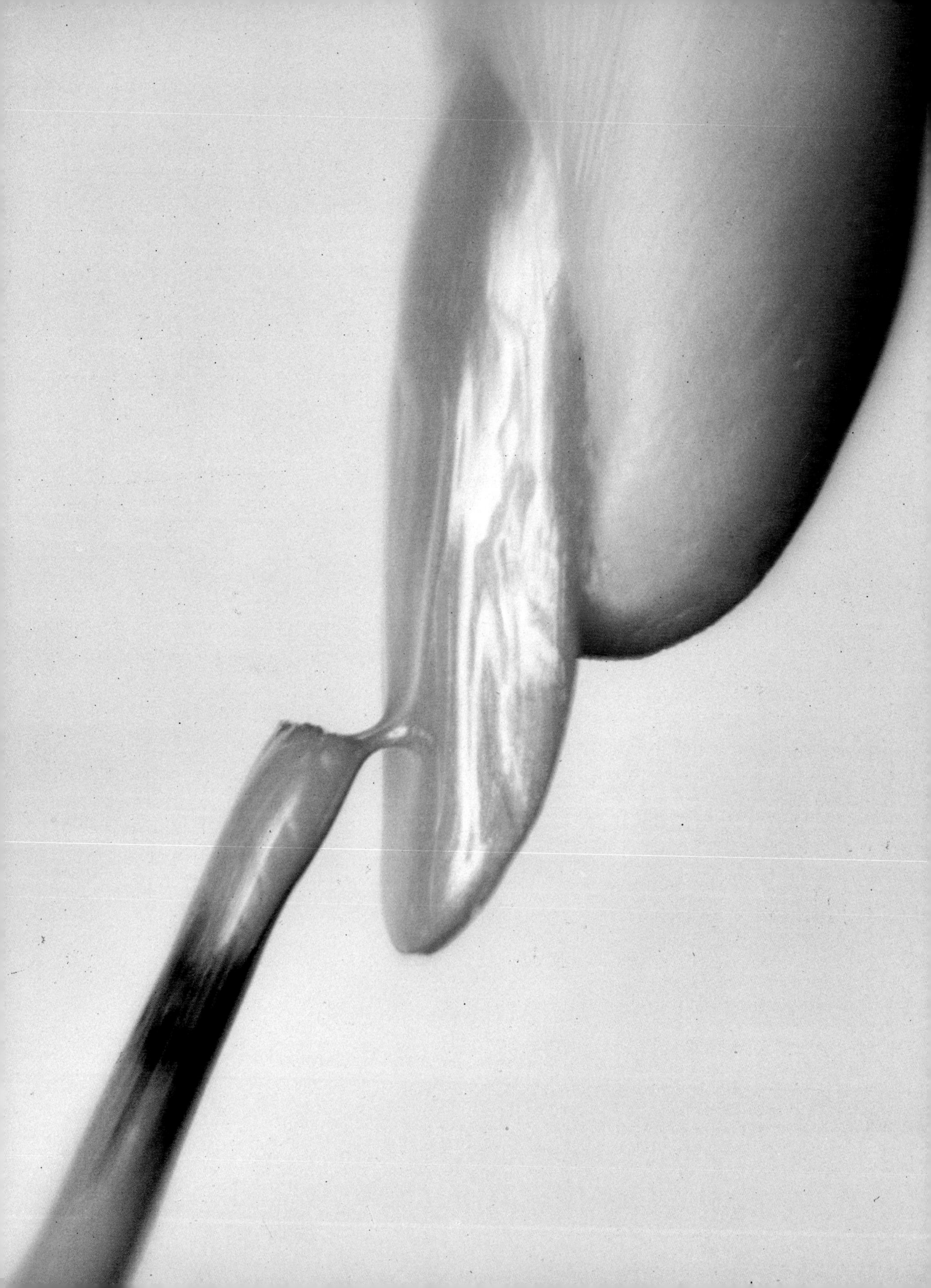

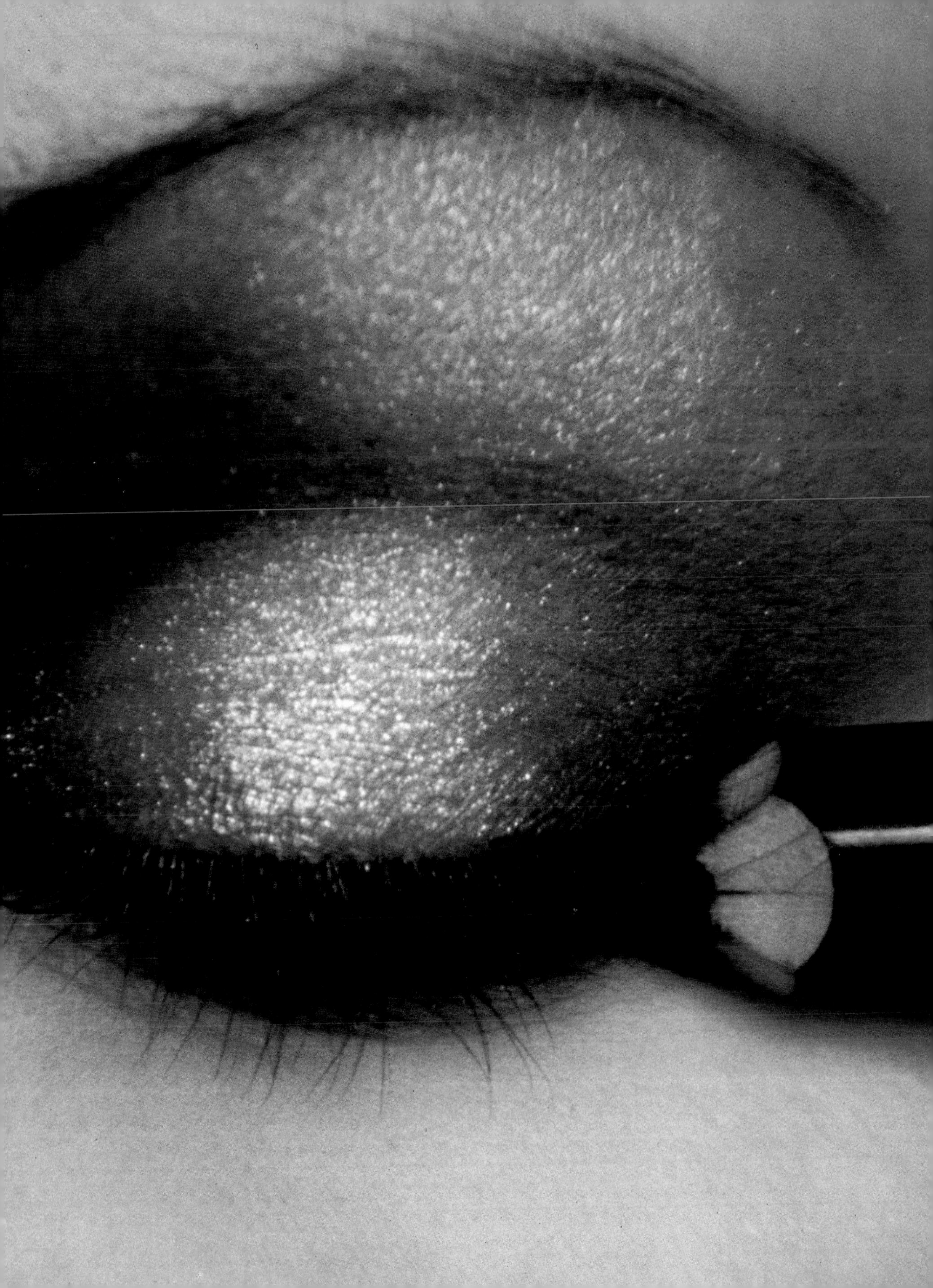

serious conditions, exhaustive tests are often necessary to trace the source.

The most common reaction is hay fever caused by pollen. Small amounts of pollen carried by the wind enter the nose and cause sensitization. Chemical substances in the body react with the pollen to produce the allergic reaction: blood vessels dilate causing red eyes, mucous glands secrete causing a running nose and muscles of the bronchial tubes contract causing wheezing.

During this allergic reaction, histamine is released into the tissues: this is a defence substance against the pollen but also responsible for the distressing outward symptoms. Many hay fever sufferers are put on medication known as antihistamine which stops the symptoms but there is a risk of a degree of sedation.

About one person in six reacts badly to stings from bees and wasps. If you are stung, apply ice to reduce the absorption of poison, removing the sting as carefully as possible. If swelling continues or is severe, check with a doctor or chemist.

Moulds are a common allergy producer. If damp, musty places make you sneeze, it is probably due to mould. Also be wary of aged cheese, wines and beers.

ANAEMIA: This covers a wide range of blood disorders, and is not always indicated by a pale skin. If you get tired easily it may be due to anaemia, so go to your doctor who will probably take blood tests and check the colour of the interior of your eyelids and gums. The most common version is a low haemoglobin count due to lack of iron. It can be caused also by an excessive loss of blood because of a heavy period, after childbirth or an accident. A diet of iron-rich foods is essential; and all the B vitamins should be supplemented, particularly B-12.

ASTHMA: It can begin in childhood and the sufferer may grow out of it, or it can appear in middle age. Its cause is not always known and it may be induced by an emotional upset or by an allergy to pollen, dust or animal fur. It affects the respiratory system: the bronchial tubes narrow due to muscle contraction and the linings of the tubes swell. Attacks cause wheezing and gasping for breath. Medication can reduce the swelling so that breathing becomes easier; in mild cases antihistamines are used, in severe cases drugs of the cortisone family.

BACKACHE: Almost everybody has backache at some time or another. In the majority of cases it is caused by lack of exercise resulting in

Opposite: Barry Lategan, 1975

muscular weakness, stress and strain. The wrong kind of exercise or spurts of excessive exercise often result in a bad back. Overweight, pregnancy, emotional tension and even sexual frustration are other causes. Real diseases are comparatively rare, though biological causes can be malfunctioning kidneys, arthritis, neurological damage or intestinal ailments; inflammation in the uterus and the ligament connecting it with the spine can also cause pain.

A 'slipped disc' is a misnomer as it is not so much a case of slipping as leaking. The rubbery disc covering herniates and some of the jelly-like substance escapes and presses on a sensitive nerve ending. It is the inflammation of the nerve that causes the severe pain. Many so-called slipped discs are often muscular problems. Disc trouble can also develop in the neck resulting in acute pain, stiffness and a frozen shoulder. Neck pain is frequently caused by anxiety and tension.

The causes of backaches are often complex and many people suffer from depression even if the pain is not of psychosomatic origin. It is a vicious circle: backache makes one depressed, one moves and sits in a slumped position, walks slower, aggravating backache and depression.

For all conditions, rest is essential. For low back pain and sciatica, rest in bed is advisable, always on a firm bed or a bedboard, while for the back pain, often called lumbago, heat is a help – preferably from an infra-red lamp or short-wave diathermy at a clinic. In severe cases, traction is helpful and this means hospitalization: the patient is anchored at the hips on a sloping bed so that the spine is stretched and the discs given a chance to readjust themselves. Or a surgical corset can give support to the lower back, a medical collar to the neck. The risk is that if these are worn too long or too often, muscles become even weaker through lack of use.

Treatment by an osteopath or chiropractor can be rewarding as spinal manipulation is the basis of their science. Massage and readjustment of vertebrae and lesions have been known to bring immediate relief.

Surgery for bad backs is very rarely performed and only when all other treatments have failed. One should never have back surgery without very careful consultation, probably with several physicians. Not all operations are entirely successful.

Prevention is the best solution. This includes keeping weight down, sleeping on a hard mattress, exercising smoothly and regularly. Be particularly conscious of posture and never bend forwards so the spine is used as a crane. When picking up something bend the knees to save the back. When sitting, sit well back in the chair so that the small of the back is supported.

To ease back muscles and aches, try these exercises:

1. Stand in a relaxed position, feet slightly apart; tense the buttocks, drawing them inwards and holding tightly for as long as possible; release slowly; tense again.

2. Lie face down with torso on a flat, firm support – a table or desk top; with hipline on the rim of the support, raise legs with knees straight to horizontal position; hold for a few seconds; drop feet to floor. Repeat many times. Turn over, repeat exercise, lying on back.

3. Sexual activity is good exercise and relaxing.

BLOOD PRESSURE: The concern is with high blood pressure, known as hypertension. Low blood pressure with no other abnormal clinical findings is less serious. Hypertension does not hurt and in the early stages produces no symptoms. Most hypertensive people feel fine, relaxed, energetic and generally cheerful. This means that high blood pressure can go undetected for decades, yet if left untreated can damage blood vessels all over the body and be a major cause of heart attacks.

High blood pressure is widespread and only a small number of people are aware they suffer from it. The method of taking blood pressure could be taught in about ten minutes and after practice you can become competent at reading the pressures. Two pressures are recorded, the upper (systolic) and the lower (diastolic) – the latter being the more important as this denotes the pressure in the circulation and strain on the heart muscle. Around 80 is normal, anything over 100 is abnormal. Blood pressure tends to increase with age and there may be occasional rises to abnormal levels which if transient are not significant.

Women tend to suffer more from hypertension than men but they tolerate it better. This means that women with high blood pressure probably can live longer without severe medical complications. There are times when it is important to check blood pressure regularly. First, when you go on the Pill. Second, during pregnancy: if it rises too drastically it can harm both mother and child. Third, at the onset of menopause: women tend to become hypertensive then and researchers believe that the physical and emotional stresses may be the reason, also the reduction of the oestrogen level.

Among the suspected causes are genetic factors, food habits, constant emotional strain. Although tension and anxiety may increase blood pressure temporarily most doctors feel the disease is not primarily psychosomatic. A few patients suffer from some specific disease – such as malfunction of the kidneys – which may be cured by surgery.

In treating hypertension, the aim is gradually to lower the blood pressure to near normal without producing distressing side effects. It is not always possible to do this as sometimes the circulation becomes geared to operating at a higher level and cannot function efficiently at a lower one. Moderate hypertension is treated easily. Keeping weight down is important; smoking is usually forbidden since this puts strain on the heart and alcohol allowed in moderation as this releases nervous tension. A low sodium diet is often prescribed and salt cut to an absolute minimum. Potassium supplements are sometimes necessary. If hypertension is very mild, diet alone may control it, with the possible addition of a diuretic to stimulate the kidneys to eliminate excess fluid.

There are drugs that depress the activities of the sympathetic nervous system but they may have uncomfortable side effects such as temporary fatigue, dizziness, weakness, depression or diarrhoea. These can often be eliminated, as at first it is difficult to judge the correct balance of drugs and dosage to control the disease while minimizing the side effects.

BLOOD SUGAR DISORDERS: There are two irregular conditions to do with blood sugar; one when it is too high (diabetes) and the other when it is too low (hypoglycaemia). They are often interrelated. Anyone who has consistently low blood sugar and no obvious biological problem should watch out for symptoms of diabetes. The diabetic is warned of the effects of hypoglycaemia – an overdose of insulin or an inadequate supply of food after an insulin injection may incite an acute attack of hypoglycaemia that can lead to mental disorientation, coma and even death.

Blood sugar disorders originate in the pancreas where either an over supply of insulin (meaning low blood sugar level) or an under supply of it (diabetes) can prevent the body from using glucose properly. Either condition has side effects – in the kidneys, arteries and, most significantly, the brain. This accounts for the mood swings, anxiety, depression and emotional outbursts that invariably go along with blood sugar disorders.

Tests easily reveal these conditions, which often can be treated by diet alone if detected early. The cause of blood sugar dysfunction is not clear. Heredity may be a factor and in the case of diabetes an overweight person seems more likely to become a victim. Diets too rich in carbohydrates and fats are said to bring on both conditions; also those too rich in sugar. Hypoglycaemia often comes from constantly mistreating the pancreas by skipping meals, excessive smoking, drinking instead of eating and by eating high-carbohydrate snacks in place of nutritious protein meals. Sometimes a weight-reduction regime does not provide adequate nutrition and an irresistible craving for something sweet precipitates a blood disorder. Hypoglycaemia can be cured by diet unless over production of insulin results from a tumour in the pancreas (which would demand surgery) or a liver disease. A diabetic needs to find the correct balance of insulin to be injected, and can then lead a normal and healthy life.

BRONCHITIS: Usually found only in cold, damp climates, very prevalent in industrial areas. It is an inflammation of the mucous membrane of the bronchial tubes and all too often called a chest cold: yet many people die from it every year. In the beginning there is a fever, dry cough and raw feeling behind the breastbone. As the cough progresses, mucus is produced, and if it becomes chronic, shortness of breath occurs. It is not hard to treat, but should not be neglected as there is always the possibility that it will develop into bronchial pneumonia. Also if the cough persists and is more or less permanent, it could be the symptom of a more serious condition such as TB or cancer.

Treatment consists of staying in bed and keeping warm; any vaporization system is recommended. Breathing in the fumes from Friar's Balsam (benzoin) freed in boiling water gives relief. Coughing and spitting up the mucus has to be encouraged, as this is the body's way of getting rid of the infection. Some cough mixtures and homoeopathic remedies help. The old-fashioned remedy of honey and lemon juice not only relieves the bronchial tubes but provides useful vitamins and minerals. Vitamin A is also of value.

COLDS AND 'FLU: A cold involves the upper respiratory tract and may be caused by any one of twenty viruses. A sore throat, running nose and a cough are the usual symptoms, while some viruses produce fever and weakness to become influenza. Vaccines have been developed for some strains of 'flu, particularly the epidemic kind that sweep through whole continents from time to time.

Colds are common and contagious. Why some people catch them and others not is unclear but it is thought to be a combination of biological weakness and psychological receptiveness. You invite colds by behaviour patterns; for instance resistance may have been lowered by poor eating, lack of rest, adverse weather conditions. There is said to be a connection between colds and depression, and although most people say they are depressed because they have colds, it may be vice versa. But catching a 'chill' is only too real and can give way to a more severe cold or 'flu. If the body is not adequately clothed or kept warm, the fighting force is fully occupied, leaving little power to fend off the cold germ.

There is no known cure for colds. Countless commercial remedies relieve the symptoms but do not keep you from catching cold again.

The best way to treat a cold is to let it run its course, making yourself as comfortable as possible. Stay in bed and keep warm; if there is a fever starve it and try not to take fever-suppressing drugs. Encourage perspiration by drinking warm drinks – citrus juices sweetened with honey are the best. Take large doses of vitamin C, 500–1,000 mg every hour. Vitamin C does not suppress a fever but it helps the body to win its own battle over the virus. Even large doses are non-toxic and harmless.

CONSTIPATION: Although it is ideal for the bowels to move smoothly and regularly each day, this is by no means essential to good health. A day or two can be missed without worry and without taking drastic measures. Artificial means of emptying the bowel disturb body chemistry and most doctors feel that a change of diet is better than medicine. A small dose of health salts is considered harmless, but a strong weekly dose is quite wrong; so is the use of mineral oil; either can result in colic, diarrhoea and dehydration. Medical opinion has come around to the old belief that constipation is largely due to a lack of 'roughage', so a diet of high fibre content is advisable – salads, leaves, stalks and skins of vegetables, fruit, wholewheat flours and breads.

CRAMP: Almost everyone gets this at some time – usually at night. It is frequently in the calf muscle and the pain can be extremely severe though often only lasting a few minutes. It is due to the shortening of the muscle fibres at a much higher rate than is usual. It can be caused by loss of salt through sweating, a calcium deficiency or sluggish kidneys. It often occurs during pregnancy. The pain can be relieved by forcibly stretching and massaging the affected muscles. It can sometimes be prevented by taking quinine sulphate tablets or building up calcium levels.

CYSTITIS: This is an inflammation of the bladder from which four out of five women suffer at least once in their lives. Symptoms include low backache, pain when passing water and an increased need to do so, occasionally some blood loss. It is caused primarily by an infection which lives naturally and harmlessly in the bowel but produces cystitis when it gets into the vagina and travels upwards to the bladder. Doctors usually prescribe antibiotics which may clear up the symptoms but attacks may re-occur. Keeping warm and resting in bed will aid a mild attack.

DRUG ADDICTION: A drug can be classified as any substance that has the capacity to produce measurable changes in mental and biochemical processes. There are many – botanical and chemical: some are valuable as medical therapeutics, others merely stimulate the brain and nervous system. The precise reaction within the body remains obscure, but whether beneficial or purely exhilarating most drugs can become addictive. This is a serious matter, for withdrawal symptoms are almost always fearful and can be severe enough to induce fits and finally kill. Even seemingly useful drugs such as barbiturates are able to produce different electrical brain patterns in different people. Many anti-depressant drugs interfere with hormonal metabolism; there is a group of prescriptive drugs that reduce depression, but change the amino-acid metabolism to a point where they may induce fatal results if eaten with cheese.

Addiction means you reach a point when you cannot do without a certain drug – you crave it, you do anything to get it. The mind directs the body to get what it wants and if this means giving up food for a drink, or walking across town to get a drug in the middle of the night, then you are addicted.

It is not advisable to self prescribe any drug. Once in the stomach anything we ingest must pass through the liver which attempts to render it harmless before it can pass into the blood stream. Because it has this capacity, many drug addicts prefer to use veins to get a quicker reaction.

Listed below are some of the more important drugs, their effect, use and addictive possibilities:

Amphetamines: Speed, meth, crystal, crank, dexies, ups, black beauties, 'pep' pills, Christmas trees. Chemical compounds that stimulate the nervous system. In medicine they are used mostly for depression and as an appetite suppressant. Their addictive power is moderate but an overdose can be fatal. They can produce high blood pressure and psychosis.

Barbiturates: Goofers, goof balls, downers, red devils, yellow jackets, yellow birds. Chemical compounds used as a depressant for the central nervous system, therefore given as a treatment for insomnia and as a sedative. Moderate to severe addictive possibilities, and an overdose can result in death. Especially dangerous in conjunction with alcohol.

Cocaine: Coke or snow. Increasing in popularity, for at first it gives quite pleasant perceptive side effects. When natural, it comes from the leaves of the coca bush found in Peru and Bolivia but can be synthetically produced. Stimulates the nervous system and can be used as a local anaesthetic. Addiction danger, plus a tendency to violence.

Hashish: Hash. The resin from the flower of the hemp plant and a more concentrated form of marijuana's active ingredient. Powers of perception are affected.

Heroin: H, horse, junk, skag. A derivative of the opium poppy. Acts as a depressant to the central nervous system and as a respiratory sedative. Opiates of the same botanical gender, such as morphine, are used as pain killers. Great danger of addiction.

LSD: Acid. Its compound has the complicated name of lysergic acid diethylamide. It produces intense hallucinations, changes perception of environment to a degree where faulty judgement of habitual surroundings can cause death. No known medical use. Dangers are psychosis and bad trips, suspected genetic damage.

Marijuana: Pot, weed, broccoli, grass, hemp tea, boo, mary jane. Comes from the female leaves of the hemp plant and alters perception of reality. Considered reasonably mild with possible dangers of psychological habituation, but rare psychosis.

Tranquillizers: Influence the emotional brain by calming it but do not affect the cortex where thinking, judgement and preservation instincts reside. Used medically to relieve emotional upsets and help insomnia by removing anxiety. Addiction to tranquillizers is rare, but the danger is combining them with alcohol; this can prove fatal, particularly in the case of excess of either.

DYSMENORRHOEA: The medical term for painful periods (see page 104).

FLUID RETENTION: This can cause bloating of the tissues, which is not only responsible for a degree of overweight but is the main reason for the formation of cellulite. It can be due to excessive salt in the diet, an underactive kidney or to a congenital defect. It can be helped biologically. First, keep salt to a minimum. Second, drink at least four glasses of water a day: this helps the elimination of salt and other minerals that require water in order to leave the body; a diuretic mineral water is of additional value. Anyone who drinks a fair amount of liquid other than water – even tea – is subject to fluid retention. It is more obvious in heavy drinkers.

HAEMORRHOIDS: Known as piles they can be agonizing, and are varicose veins of the anus – and like varicose veins are often hereditary. As soon as it becomes painful to evacuate or you notice blood, get medical advice: they sometimes occur as a secondary symptom of another disorder – such as a growth or liver disease – and should never be self-analysed and thought of as 'just piles'. The earlier they are treated, the better. In the initial stages, it may only be necessary to use ointments, suppositories or injections. If they continue to develop, surgery usually has to be used. This is not as painful as some people believe, though the first few bowel actions after the operation may be difficult. The veins that are clotting and bleeding are tied off or cut away. There is an alternative, a technique called cryosurgery – here piles are removed by freezing and this does not necessitate hospitalization. Another method which some doctors claim is as effective as surgery is this: the anus is dilated and the patient shown how to repeat the stretching process at regular intervals over a period of six weeks together with the use of a special laxative.

HEADACHE: Probably the most common type of pain in the body with causes ranging from a hangover to eye strain, from tension or too much sun to a brain tumour. Headaches can be divided into three types: vascular – includes migraine and cluster headaches; organical – from infections, tumours, eye and ear problems, nose and focal disorders; psychogenic – caused by tension, anxiety and depression. The clinical explanation is this: blood vessels in the head increase in size, and as these arteries are usually accompanied by nerves, when enlarged they press on the nerves and cause pain. Migraine starts this way and the warning signs of worse to come are visual disturbances and a general feeling of perception weakness. The blood vessels not only increase in size, but thicken and possibly release a fluid. At this stage, the pain is steady and agonizing and in extreme cases can continue for days.

What starts this activity is unclear. Heredity plays a part particularly in the case of migraine. Emotional strain and stress are possibly contributory causes; also food and allergies. For example, a chemical called tyramine that is found in some foods and drinks has been known to start headaches. It occurs naturally in cheese, chocolate, chicken livers, brown vinegar, yoghurt and most fermented food. Drinks with tyramine are beer, red wine, whisky, gin and vodka which may explain the typical hangover headache. A fast way to reduce such a headache is to take teaspoons of honey, slowly, one after the other – and as many as you like.

Headaches can be caused by low blood sugar, which is nothing more serious than bad eating habits. Many a headache has been cured by a good meal – protein, green vegetables, olive oil and garlic are recommended. Tension headaches are milder forms of the psychogenic variety and usually caused by fatigue and temporary stress. The more severe psychogenic ones usually require thorough tests and life-history research.

Cluster headaches are a form of migraine, but instead of being long and sustained, they manifest themselves in short violent attacks. They are considered the same as migraine when being treated. The migraine-prone person is usually highly intelligent, ambitious, creative and with a strong drive for perfection. Often the headache arrives after completion of an arduous task – musicians, writers, actors, may find themselves stricken once their creative work has been accomplished.

A change of weather is said to induce headaches – before a thunder-storm or a particularly strong wind the barometer drops sharply and weather-sensitive people develop severe headaches. This is because the atmosphere is positively charged. When the storm is over the air molecules become negatively charged and bring relief to the sufferer.

Most people rely on aspirins and their like to relieve headaches. Migraines respond unpredictably to treatment. Most relief drugs are based on ergot but they can have side effects. The heavier, habit-forming painkillers such as morphine should be avoided. A redirection of blood often helps; moving hands to make them warmer can lessen dilation of cranial blood vessels. Try lying on your side with the weight of your head resting on a thumb placed at the centre base of the skull (between the two muscle tendons); just a few seconds of pressure on each side can relax and relieve the headache. Acupuncture and spinal manipulation are considered helpful.

HEPATITIS: From time to time this disease can reach epidemic proportions. It is extremely contagious and also carried by persons who have no sign of it. Initially the virus is picked up in food, such as shell fish, that has become contaminated. There are two types of hepatitis – infectious and serum. Though caused by different viruses, they are both called viral hepatitis. One significant difference is the period of incubation. Infectious hepatitis (once known as epidemic jaundice) takes between 15–40 days to appear and serum hepatitis between 60–100 days.

Infectious hepatitis is easily transmitted by the faecal-oral route. Therefore it can spread quite rapidly within a family, school or an office. Isolated cases can appear. Children frequently get the disease but so mildly that it is not diagnosed as such – but it is equally contagious.

Serum hepatitis can be carried in adults as well and herein lies its epidemic danger. Healthy carriers can be detected by certain tests, but few healthy people take them. In northern Europe and north America carriers compose about 1% of apparently healthy people, but the number is much higher in tropical, Eastern and some Mediterranean countries.

One of the early symptoms of hepatitis is depression. Often there is sweating for no apparent reason – of the palms, the face. Usually there is inflammation of the liver, and it is frequently possible to feel it, somewhat enlarged and tender. Loss of appetite and nausea are often signs. Not all patients go yellow. It is essential to have a blood test.

There is no effective treatment for hepatitis. It can cause a day or so of discomfort or necessitate months in hospital. Rest and relaxation in bed is essential. Alcohol is forbidden, not only during, but for a long time after, an attack. This is because the liver cannot break down alcohol with its usual efficiency. Rich and fatty foods should be avoided.

HERPES: There is one strain of herpes that is closely linked with chicken pox and shingles, but the other one is the common annoyance that frequently crops up in connection with colds – this is the Herpes Simplex. It begins as a small area of irritation around the mouth or just inside the nose and generally makes its appearance towards the end of an ordinary cold, sore throat or chest infection. It can become very painful and raised, then forms a blister. This can take from forty-eight to seventy-two hours. Frequently the blisters burst and a watery fluid is emitted. The affected area usually crusts over and heals within two weeks. Sometimes the sores become re-infected and need treatment with an antibiotic ointment. Once a person is subject to a herpes infection it is frequently re-activated when another cold virus enters the system.

HYPERIDROSIS: Excessive sweating which cannot be controlled by anti-perspirants. It can be helped by surgery.

In the case of the underarm area, two to three days are generally required in hospital. The area of trouble can be as large as 3 inches (75 mm.) by 2 inches (50 mm.); the skin is excised and stitched. There is a scar, but in such an area it is of little significance. The operation for treating the hands and feet is more complicated and could mean up to 10 days in hospital. It involves removing the part of the sympathetic nerve chain that supplies the affected area. For the hands, the procedure is either through an incision on the side of the chest underneath the arm, or above the collar bone. For the feet, an incision is made in the abdomen at the level of the navel.

INSOMNIA: The word really means total inability to sleep, but this is virtually non-existent as a medical condition. People who say they can't sleep at all, usually do to some degree, but believe they lay awake night after night without closing their eyes. There are two main causes – anxiety, depression and psychological disorders of all sorts, and pain or discomfort.

Doctors usually prescribe a sleeping pill, barbiturate or tranquillizer, which often only adds to the problem. Barbiturates may interfere with REM sleep (see page 329). They make you drowsy and usually help to get you to sleep but because they interfere with natural body rhythms, the sleep is very light, so you wake up easily and often in a state of anxiety. The next step is usually to take another pill, then another. Barbiturates are dangerous because not only are they addictive, but one can wake up suddenly and not be entirely rational or conscious. A small overdose, especially in combination with alcohol, can be fatal.

Loss of sleep undermines physical and mental health. Not everyone needs eight hours of sleep at night but if a person is constantly exhausted during the day – because of insufficient sleep – it has to be made up somehow. The insomniac is fully aware of this, and trying to force sleep is a prescription for sleeplessness. It is a vicious cycle. Lying in bed at night, rigid and tense, waiting for relaxation and drowsiness, can be psychologically painful and physically exhausting.

Most people should be able to put themselves to sleep by a form of self-hypnosis or auto-suggestion. Here is one method. Lie looking upwards at the ceiling, hard enough to put a slight strain on your eyeballs. Untense hands by clenching and stretching alternatively a few times. Next focus eyes inward as well as upward, as though looking down your nose. Close eyes slowly, counting backwards from ten to one in rhythm with breathing. On the last count, take a deep breath and let it out slowly. Relax the entire body and imagine yourself asleep in the most pleasant way. Open your eyes and think of relaxation only.

MONONUCLEOSIS: Also called glandular fever or the kissing disease. It is actually a non-malignant leukaemia, where the white blood cells increase over the red. It is self limiting although it can continue in a mild form for months, and sometimes recurs.

The cause is not known, though it is suspected to be a virus. It is often incorrectly diagnosed at first, as the symptoms are like those of scarlet fever, german measles or undulant fever. There is always a definite fever, high temperature, fatigue, aches and pains, sore throat and headache. A chemical analysis of the blood can accurately detect it. It is infectious.

There is not much to be done except to allow the illness to take its own course. Stay in bed while the fever continues, eat nourishing food and take vitamin B-complex supplements. Antibiotics are useless against viruses though the side effects can be relieved.

MOTION SICKNESS: Some stomachs react adversely to movement, giving a series of shocks to the nervous system resulting in nausea, giddiness and vomiting. Anti-travel pills are not always recommended. As a precaution don't begin a trip on an empty stomach – a bowl of warm soup into which has been stirred a quarter of a teaspoon of cayenne pepper is beneficial. Keep the bowels open.

RHEUMATISM: Arthritis and gout are all different manifestations of the same disease – inflammation of the connective tissue in the joints. While not fatal it can cause a great number of disabilities. As it progresses the involved joints are moved less and less because of the pain. In consequence, the surrounding muscles begin to atrophy, resulting in crippling.

There are several causes: heredity, an accident which can leave a joint vulnerable, an improper diet. Medicine is largely unable to cure rheumatism. Drugs can relieve the pain but not the condition. It is always worse when the weather is cold and damp. Warmth is one of the best remedies and a thermal cure can often considerably help a chronic condition. Spinal manipulation can give relief. Exercise, rest, relaxation, proper food, vitamin and mineral therapy, plus vitamin B-12 supplements will help reduce the pain and discomfort. Fruit and vegetable juices are good, particularly raw carrot juice. Celery, cabbage and parsley are also recommended. It has been found that many arthritics have oil deficiencies, so should add a good vegetable oil to their diet.

ULCERS: Affect 10% of the population mostly between the ages of forty-five and fifty-five, though symptoms may begin quite young. Women are more subject to them after the menopause. Ulcers occur because the lining in the stomach or duodenum in certain spots is unable to withstand the digestive action of acid and pepsin. A duodenal ulcer tends to afflict those who produce an excess of acid, while a gastric (stomach) ulcer is developed by those who produce less acid than normal. The main symptoms are upper abdominal pain and hunger feelings. Vomiting sometimes occurs and may be tinged with blood. The diagnosis is confirmed by barium meal X-ray or by passing a flexible telescope through the mouth into the stomach to look at the ulcer directly.

Stress and pressure are said to incite a duodenal ulcer, also smoking, alcohol and spasmodic eating; people of Blood Group O appear to develop it more frequently than those of other blood groups.

Treatment involves removal of stressful situations, often a change in diet, alkalis to relieve the pain and sometimes a liquorice derivative which is claimed to increase the rate of healing. Surgery is a last resort.

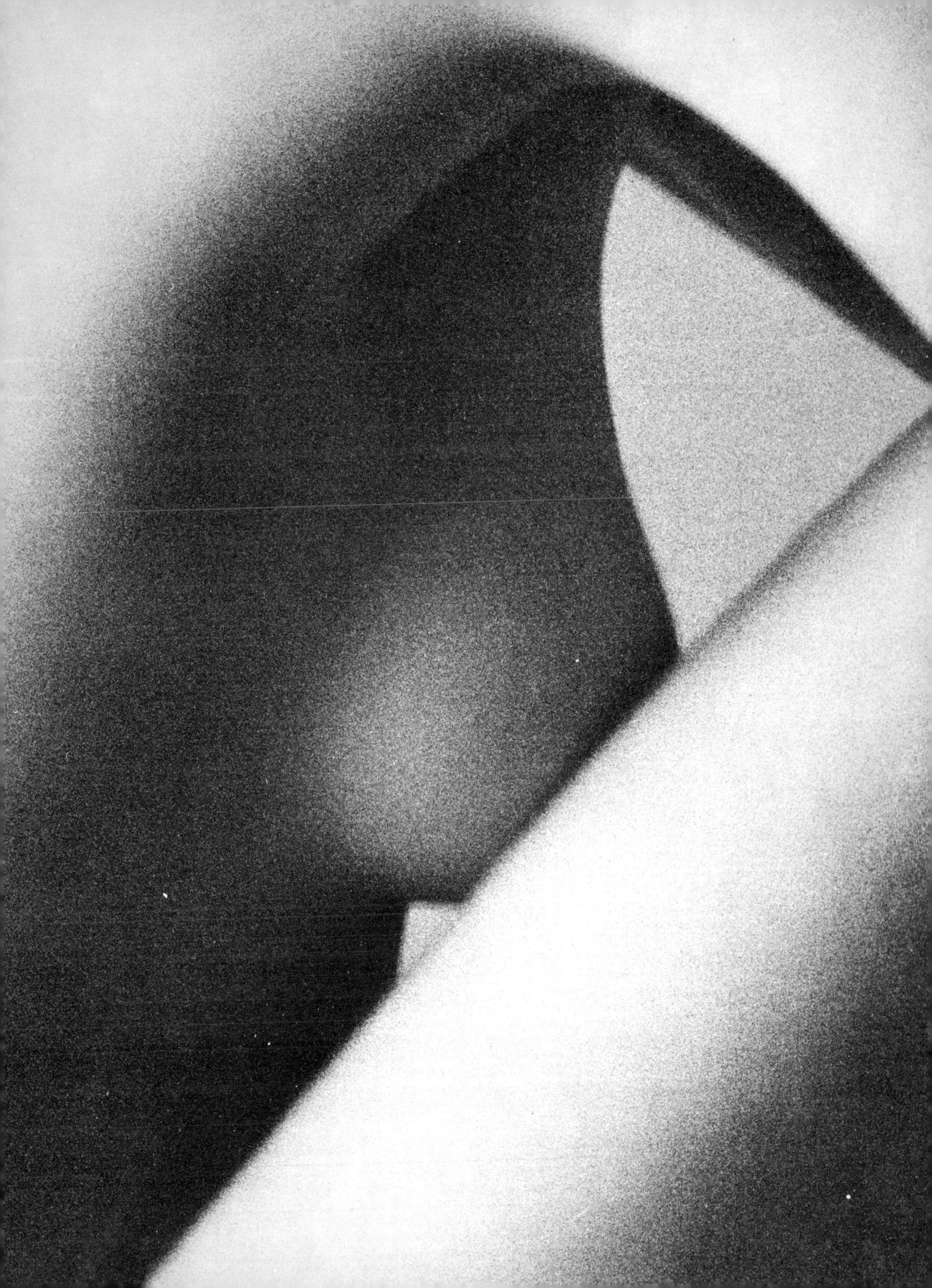

4

PLASTIC SURGERY

As a science and an art, plastic surgery has developed incredibly over the last twenty years or so. It can give young people more confidence, and for many adults it can provide a new lease of life. It is a natural follow-up after considerable weight loss. Although many improvements last a lifetime (nose structures, ear and chin corrections for example) even those that last a matter of years can be rewarding.

The modern plastic surgeon is one of the most interesting of medical specialists. In addition to being highly competent, he must have a certain amount of artistic ability if he is to perform his work with any degree of distinction. There is every reason to have confidence in him as the qualified plastic surgeon has had to go through a rigorous training.

Plastic surgery is basically either cutting away or adding – the former normally costs more than the latter. Surgeons, as might well be expected, are highly individual, sometimes using different methods or techniques. Bones, skin and fat can be reduced by simply taking part of them away. In lifting techniques (which also pull out wrinkles and lines) the skin is drawn into natural folds where it will be least conspicuous.

Inserted substances can build out an area. Human bones and cartilage are still widely used in corrective surgery, but in several cosmetic procedures, silicone prostheses (artificial implants) are popular and most effective, particularly the sponges which are constantly being improved, and for example too-small breasts can have implants of fluid silastic encased in a plastic bag (see details later). No more liquid injections are given as in earlier years when they were also used to fill out face and hand wrinkles as well as expand bosoms. Whereas the bulk silicone and the encased fluid can be safely secured and isolated, the liquid silicone was simply injected and did not always stay where it was put.

One of the most frequent questions asked is: how long will it last? It depends – on the person, the age, the metabolism, future care and stress. Some things once done are there for ever: those that have to do with bone structure or areas entirely uninfluenced by muscles or fatty deposits such as noses, chins, ears.

There is a new theory that a prevention-lift in the late thirties or early forties will keep a face in better, younger shape relatively longer: on the basis that the face can be re-arranged before muscles lose too much of their elasticity. However, not many people are so far-sighted. Nor can you have surgery and forget to care for the skin and body from that time on. One of the leading body-surgeons never ceases to emphasize that a sensible diet, exercise and skin care must be continued after surgery.

At an interview the surgeon will examine, advise and explain, and it is terribly important that you ask him about everything: what he will do in the operation, how long it will take, what about anaesthetic, how long is the hospital stay, when do the stitches come out, how soon can you use make-up, will any marks finally disappear – and the cost. It is impossible to give an estimate on fees for operations as they fluctuate not only from country to country, but also from doctor to doctor.

Here are the main corrective possibilities, which give a general idea:

EYES

Operating time: 1½ hours
Hospital time: 1 to 3 nights
Recuperation: 7 to 10 days
After-care: moderate
Benefit duration: 5 to 10 years

Eyes are a fair barometer of health, age and how a person feels. They are also possibly the most important focus of beauty and personality. This together with the fact that an eye job is one of the simplest, cheapest and most successful in the plastic surgeon's repertoire, accounts for the fact that this operation is one of the most popular.

Often facial ageing or disfigurement is nothing more than problems centred around the eyes. As one surgeon says: 'I'd have anyone who is considering a face-lift come first for the eyes. Having these done alone can make an enormous difference and it is frequently unnecessary to consider a total lift for many years.'

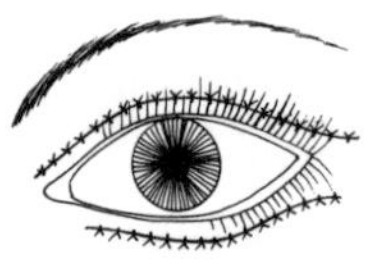

Under-eye bulges or crêpy, puffy skin on the upper eyelids can be removed. It is not only women in their middle years who are candidates, but quite young women too. This is because the so-called bags under the eyes may be an inherited family feature and nothing to do with age, late nights or a dissipated life. No amount of sleep or healthy living will rectify them. In this case, it is little hernias (ruptures) that are causing the swellings – pads of fat which escape the control of muscle surrounding the eye. These fatty ruptures can also appear above the eye, creating puffiness, but are not likely to be as noticeable as the underlid bags. In later years, it's another matter. Skin loosens whether there are hernias or not, while the upper eyelid can become as much of a problem as the lower; to such an extent that vision may be affected.

For either above or below the eye, the operation is relatively brief – about an hour and a half under local or general anaesthetic depending on the doctor. The surgeon makes a fine incision just below the lower lashes and/or in the hollow where the eyeball curves inward to meet the arch of the bone. In the case of the younger patient with smooth skin, he removes the fat and sews up. With an older patient whose skin is sagging and lined, he removes a section of the skin – so the puffiness, looseness and wrinkles are eliminated at the same time.

The healing of the tissues around the eye area is so accommodating that scars almost never occur, and if they do are no more than lines so fine as to escape the naked eye. Healing depends on the individual, but in general the patient can be out and about in three to four days (with dark glasses). Stitches can be taken out after five days. Bruising and discoloration usually remain for three to four weeks. Eyes are inclined to swell as they heal, though this is purely temporary and can be helped with ice application. Discoloration progressively becomes paler and make-up can usually be used after ten days to camouflage.

FACE

Operating time: 3 to 4 hours
Hospital time: 3 to 5 nights
Recuperation: 2 to 3 weeks
After-care: moderate
Benefit duration: 5 to 10 years

The face ages progressively. As a rule, at thirty, personality lines usually appear; around thirty-five or forty, muscle lines show up near the eyes, and from then on skin lines, wrinkles, neck marks, folds and pouches appear due to the general progressive degeneration of tissues.

The aim of the face-lift is to achieve exactly what its name implies: to pull up anything that is sagging and at the same time pull out the lines that invariably are concentrated around the eyes, mouth and on the forehead. In an older skin, the loss of supporting fat pads contributes to the increase in wrinkles, even over the cheeks, and also accounts for much of the folding. In a complete lift, the skin of the throat is smoothed if necessary, and the tightening of a double chin may also be included.

Originally a face-lift consisted of simply making an incision in the skin diagonally above the temple in the hairline. The skin was pulled, the

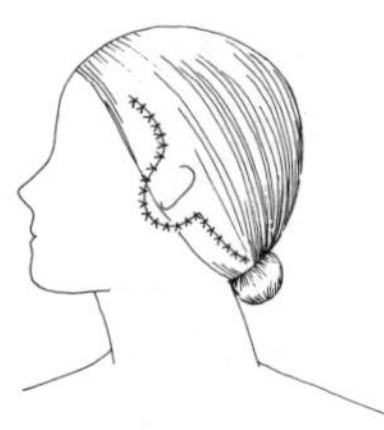

excess cut off, and all sewn together again. However, the pull of the facial muscles on the stretched skin soon caused the face to relapse. This is why the so-called mini-lift is a waste of time and money.

To do a good face-lift, it is essential to work also on the underlying muscular bed. Involved in this is considerable undercutting of the skin, and facial muscles are re-attached to minimize their pull. The secret is to decide which muscle action to eliminate or reduce. Unfortunately, although this greatly extends the life of the lift, it can cause a loss of expression. So it is possible to end up looking very much younger, but also with a rather blank face.

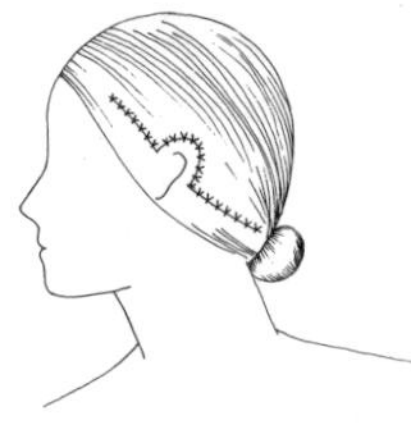

An incision is usually made in the natural fold in front of the ear, running under the lobe, up behind the ear and then diagonally into the scalp, though some surgeons prefer to make all incisions inside the hair-line or behind the ear. In these ways a really good lift can be made. Some surgeons don't even shave the hair, but simply divide it. The only scar that shows, even in the early stages of healing, is the one in front of the hair, but this should fade completely within a couple of months. The others are hidden by hair right from the start. A local anaesthetic is often used even though the operation is a long one, three to four hours, but this is the joint decision of the doctor and patient. Some surgeons also prefer to divide the face, and work on a section at a time.

The stitches are removed after five to seven days, then there's another five days for full healing. There may be some swelling at first, but you are usually quite presentable after a week or two to go out with make-up. Sometimes puffiness and bruising can be prolonged; this depends on skin chemistry.

NECK

Operating time: 1½ to 2 hours
Hospital time: 2 to 3 nights
Recuperation: 2 to 3 weeks
After-care: moderate
Benefit duration: 5 to 10 years

This is really a partial face-lift and involves smoothing out the neck and getting rid of a double chin. The skin is taken upwards and the incision is made behind the ears in the shape of a long inverted hairpin. It is not often that this operation is considered alone, as most faces in need of such treatment usually require other improvements. However, there are women who don't mind facial lines, but have a complex about a double chin. Also many young women are affected this way.

NOSE

Depending on skin texture and on thickness, the nose can be straightened, shortened, softened, narrowed and built-up. The operation is performed

Operating time: 1 hour
Hospital time: 3 nights
Recuperation: 2 weeks to 1 month
After-care: moderate
Benefit duration: for ever

from the inside, so there is absolutely no scarring. For reduction, the surgeon chisels away to remove excess bone, cartilage and superfluous tissue. Cartilage and silicone implants are used for enlarging. Afterwards there's a little discomfort as a plaster cast is put on the nose and you have to breathe through the mouth, but it is no worse than having a heavy cold. The cast is removed after 7 to 10 days. There will be sensitivity, pinkness and swelling, as well as bruising around the eyes. This discoloration lasts for a few weeks, but it is usually possible for a patient to go back to everyday life after 2 weeks. It may take a month for all swelling and sensitivity to disappear.

This is one cosmetic operation that may be desirable for the adolescent. If a young person clearly has a nose of such shape or proportion that it is bound to have deep psychological effects, it is well worth while getting it corrected as early as possible.

BOSOM (*Lifting or enlarging*)

Operating time: $1\frac{1}{2}$ hours each breast
Hospital time: 3 to 4 nights
Recuperation: 3 weeks
After-care: moderate
Benefit duration: up to 10 years

Breasts that droop are rarely corrected by simply taking a tuck in tired muscles. After excess skin is removed, the breasts would probably be small. So they are enlarged and filled out where necessary to achieve an even, rounded bosom. The same technique is used as that for providing a reasonable bosom for the flat-chested. In this instance, the stretching property of skin is for once an advantage, as the skin expands smoothly to cover any additional matter that is put in. The usual method is to insert prostheses (implants) made of gel or saline-filled sacs that sometimes have mesh backs; these come in many sizes and feel, and look, completely natural. They are firmly stitched to the chest wall. Incisions are usually made in a half-moon curve under each bosom; sometimes sacs are inserted through incisions in the armpits. In the case of flat-chested patients, some surgeons prefer to secure an empty sac, then inject saline afterwards. This method is particularly advantageous when the operation is for breasts of unequal size. Small breasts should not be tampered with until after childbirth.

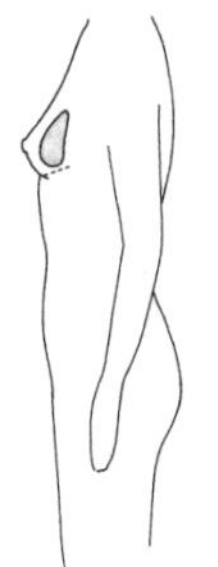

BOSOM (*Reduction*)

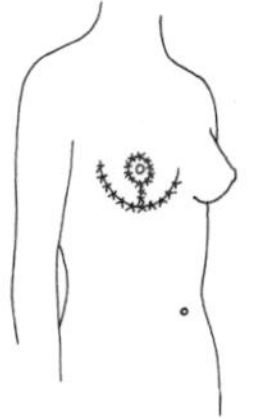

Besides being the cause of much embarrassment, the large bosom can be a health hazard, not to mention the strain on the spine. Many doctors consider it more susceptible to malignancies.

Reduction is a complicated and delicate operation and can take up to two hours for each breast. It is done under a general anaesthetic and the

Operating time: $1\frac{1}{2}$ to 2 hours each breast
Hospital time: 4 to 5 nights
Recuperation: 3 to 5 weeks
After-care: considerable
Benefit duration: up to 10 years or longer

surgeon's task is to remove excess fat and skin, and to replace the nipple if necessary – and it usually is. There are several methods of incision, but generally it involves a vertical cut from the nipple down, another that curves under the breast's fold, and a third around the nipple. Scars come close to disappearing in a few months but rarely go completely. The operation sometimes involves the risk of hampering the nipple's normal function, such as lactation, but surgeons are terribly careful to control this whenever possible. Depending on each case, the doctor will always give implicit instructions for post-operative care. After three to five weeks the bosom should be in shape and the scars reasonably faint. However, the nipples take some adjusting and will settle into their final, natural position about ten to twelve months after the operation.

CHIN *(Receding, prominent or double)*

Operating time: 1 to 2 hours
Hospital time: 2 to 3 nights
Recuperation: 2 weeks for minor surgery, up to 12 weeks for major surgery
After-care: moderate
Benefit duration: for ever

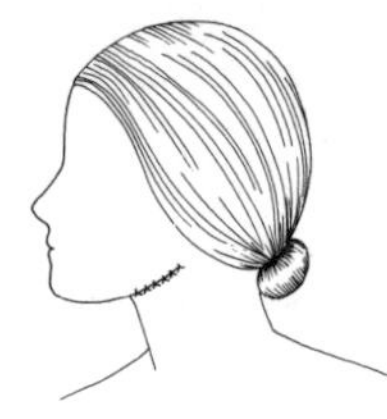

A receding chin can be built up by adding bone and cartilage or inserting a shaped silicone implant. An incision is made inside the mouth in front of the teeth. Often a nose irregularity and a receding chin go together, but an operation to bring the chin forward may balance the profile to such a degree that a nose correction is unnecessary.

A double chin is usually corrected as part of a face-lift or a neck operation, but if the trouble is just a pad of fat under the chin, flabbiness or loose 'turkey' skin, there is a simple operation that is done under local anaesthetic and takes about an hour. A Z-shaped incision is made directly under the chin, excess tissue removed, excess skin is cut away. Stitches come out after a few days.

EARS

Operating time: 3 to 4 hours each ear
Hospital time: 2 nights
Recuperation: 2 weeks
After-care: moderate
Benefit duration: for ever

Fly-away or 'bat' ears can be easily repositioned to the head, leaving behind each ear an almost invisible fine-line scar. A tiny incision is made behind each ear, the excess cartilage is removed and the skin correspondingly tightened. All is then stitched up. The ear is bandaged flat against the head. Healing takes about two weeks and the bandages must remain in place during this time. Children can suffer undue teasing over this defect, and because this operation is one that can be successfully performed at an early age – from the age of four on – the sooner it is done the better. For adults, the technique and result of the operation are exactly the same.

BUTTOCKS AND THIGHS

Operating time: 2 to 3 hours
Hospital time: 7 to 10 nights
Recuperation: 3 to 4 weeks
After-care: considerable
Benefit duration: 5 to 10 years

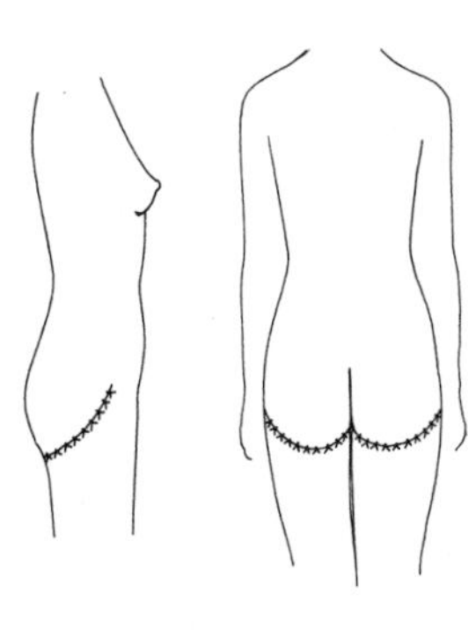

Buttocks and thighs can be operated on together under general anaesthesia, to remedy what is known as the 'riding breeches' problem. It is a long and complex operation, for the young and middle-aged only, and not all surgeons will do it. It is recommended to try to lose some weight first, though usually this is the area where fat refuses to budge and is in the form of cellulite. The first step is to calculate the quantity of tissue to be cut away; this is done standing, for maximum accuracy and better aesthetic assessment. Two lines are drawn on the buttocks – one above and one below the original gluteal folds – to indicate the section to be taken away. The upper line establishes the new level of the fold and is the first line of incision. The lower one is the second incision and the adipose tissue is removed from under this crescent-shaped flap. The skin line is pulled upward and backward towards the inner side of the upper thighs, excess cut off, then sutured to the upper skin line. This means that the flabbiness of the inner thigh is corrected along with the outside figure line. The final stitching line is tucked neatly within the buttock fold, but extends to the outer thighs curving around a little in front to almost reach the hip-bone. After the operation, it is usually possible to walk without too much discomfort within two days but to sit down normally takes about two to three weeks. The scars do pale, but very slowly.

STOMACH

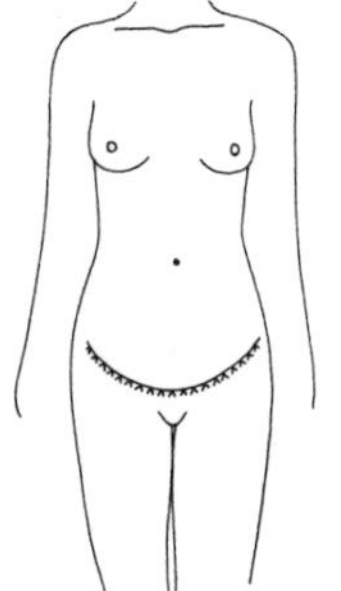

Operating time: 2 to 3 hours
Hospital time: 5 nights for stretch marks, 8 nights for more extensive surgery
Recuperation: 3 to 4 weeks
After-care: moderate
Benefit duration: 5 to 10 years

Fat can be removed from the stomach, though not every surgeon will perform the surgery. It is a most delicate procedure and can also include the reconstruction of an ugly, malformed navel. To a much lesser degree, the concern of many women lies in stretch marks that come from pregnancy or drastic loss of weight. These can be smoothed out by basically the same procedure – at considerably less time and cost. Stomach reduction works on the same principle as a face-lift, except that it goes in the reverse direction. It is a matter of taking away excess fat and skin and controlling the muscles. The incision is low on the belly and is carried in an upward curve over the hips. The scar coincides with the pubic hairline so it is virtually invisible. In time the scar on the hips will pale but it rarely completely disappears. Sometimes the navel has to be repositioned.

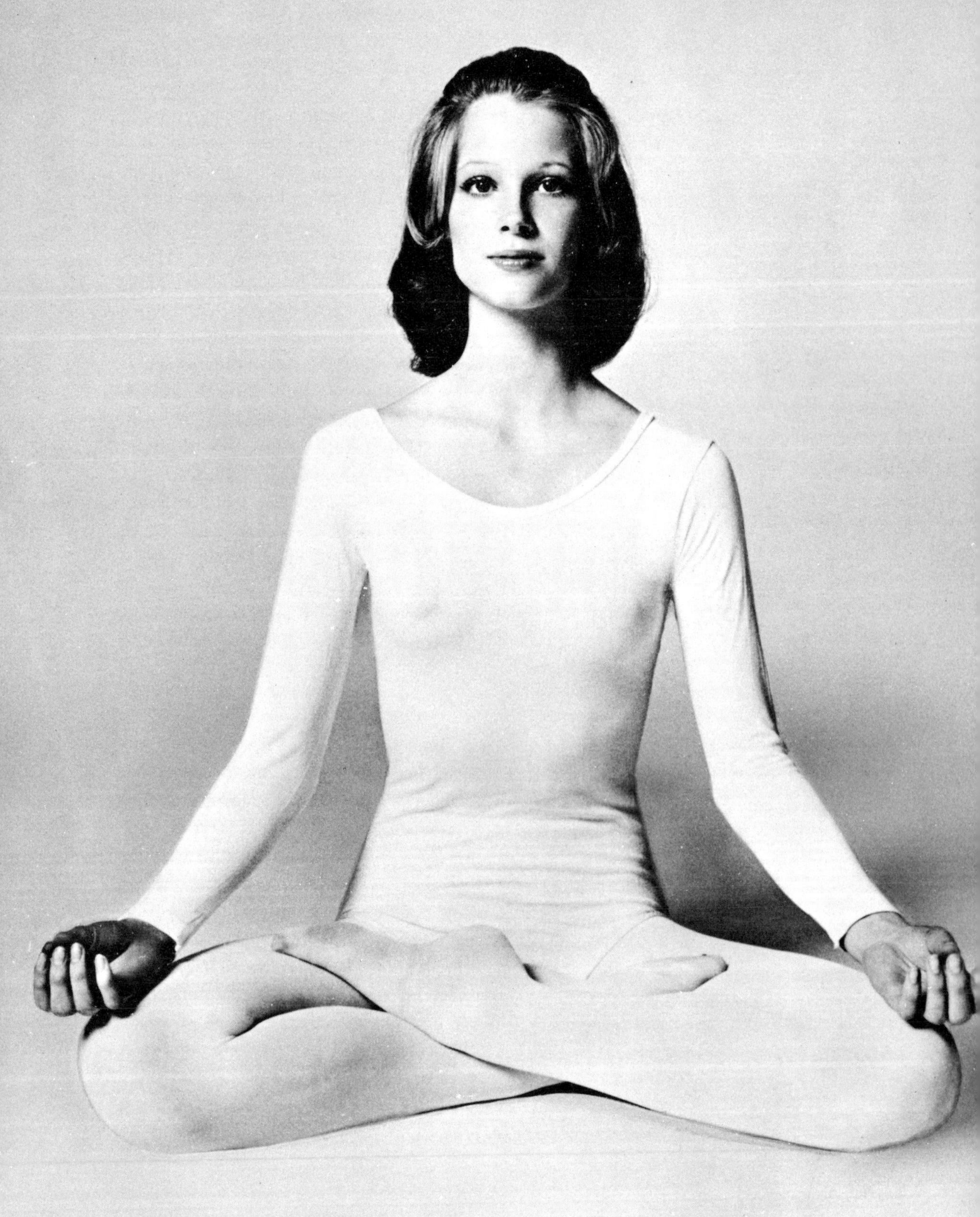

5

NERVES AND TENSION

Tension is not an illness; it is a symptom, a reaction to stress. It can, however, trigger off a real illness, finding its outlet in physical, nervous and mental disturbances.

How does it start? Tension is primarily the result of unresolved inner conflict. It indicates a clash between impulses that demand action and a counterforce that stops it. Whether this involves a physical or mental process is of little importance as nerve reactions are basically the same.

Whenever stress signals go out to the brain, the nervous system prepares the body to react on a fight-or-flight basis. Adrenalin is poured into the bloodstream, the muscles flex, blood pressure rises and the body is equipped for attacking or retreating. Then comes the counter signal of civilized training and reason: stop, it's wrong, a bad decision, too emotional, too aggressive, risky, selfish. The result is no action and no outlet for accumulated energy; tension follows.

Many people can be unaware that they are in a state of neuromuscular tension though congested nerve channels can cause headaches, backaches, fatigue, insomnia, dizziness and general inertia. Do you find your hands are clenched, palms sweating, your feet tapping? Such nervous reactions in themselves can create further anxiety by altering the chemistry of the blood. It is a vicious circle.

Stress levels are individual. Each of us has a limit as to how much stress we can stand before the brain is alerted and changes take place in

FRANCES MCLAUGHLIN-GILL

the hormone system. Our stress quotient is the barometer of our reaction to environment. Stress always has to have a stimulus. Some people find ordinary everyday life so full of stimuli that their over-reaction to living is a permanent trial and even seemingly harmless stimuli can cause stress and become 'the last straw'. Morbid depression and mental illness lie at the end of this path; both are essentially an alienation from society and environment. Indecisive or negative reaction can cause stress. This is where inner conflict is at its zenith and can become paralysing. When there is no positive action, physical or mental, tension remains and builds up. Indecision is fed by anxiety, guilt and fear. Negativeness is expressed in self doubt about emotions, ability and judgements. To help yourself means slowly to accept everything for what it is, your limitations and those of others too. With positive actions you can ease the stress gradually and alleviate the tension; sometimes medical help is necessary through psychotherapy and drug relief.

Anxiety is extremely common, particularly in women. It is different from fear, which is a normal emotional reaction to a definite real danger. Anxiety is a neurotic response, for it anticipates a catastrophe that is invariably imagined. Most women who suffer from anxiety are never quite sure exactly what it is they are so anxious about, although they will list generalities such as money, the future, security, losing a job, husband, the home, growing old. All nebulous, but such is the power of the imagination that it can direct the brain into action as though real ordeals were imminent, and a stress and tension pattern follows.

The hypothalamus reacts immediately to anxiety and drugs that depress this can help but do so only by suppressing the symptoms, not eliminating the cause. Diet is thought to play a role in anxiety: anyone deficient in any of the vitamin B complex shows signs of nervousness. Even missing a meal can put some people in a stressful state.

To help control anxiety, try rationing yourself. List the most important things to worry about and concentrate on those. Live from day to day; don't look back, don't peer into the future. Balance your anxiety with physical and mental recreations that leave little time and thought for fretting. Women with time on their hands worry more, and the more you worry the less inclined you are to go out and take action. Try to make one positive decision a day, starting with little things such as choosing a new lipstick. It is surprising how quickly confidence can build up to enable you to face a major decision without the nagging anxiety that you have made the wrong move.

Unbalanced emotions can cause considerable stress. You have to know when to let go and when to restrain. Bottling up some things is a sure way to build up tension. The problem is often fear – fear of showing emotions beyond the bounds of what you consider to be proper; or more correctly, beyond the bounds of what you think others consider proper. Fear of letting go sexually runs under the surface of most psyches. Fear of aggression follows closely and is related. Both often simply represent the wish to admit to an inner need for some form of self-expression.

People are afraid to cry, to unleash their feelings of loneliness and loss in case they get carried away in a flood of emotion. A good weep has its limits, and whether you are crying for someone, something or just out of self pity, it can ease stress and tension. By the same token, if anger has no outlet, you can look and feel washed out from inner exhaustion.

Jealousy is one of the most stressful and destructive emotions; it can maim the spirit and almost paralyse the will. You can be jealous of a person, a thing, a situation. At its most intense it cannot be sustained without nerves going to pieces. The cure for jealousy is to see it exactly for what it is: a dissatisfaction with oneself, a complex of inadequacy and insecurity. Your energy is better directed into doing something constructive and positive. Another emotion, frustration, stems from envy. It thrives on unhappy compromise and can turn into habitual resentment. Again action is the answer.

Guilt is closely akin to anxiety as it is a clash between an inner urge and a fear of its consequences. It is particularly insidious because it is unconscious with quick automatic response. On an emotional level it appears as anxiety, confusion or depression. On a physical level it is manifested in aches, pains, fatigue, digestive and circulatory disorders.

Its roots lie in right-and-wrong guidance during childhood. It is like a computer in the super-ego ruling actions with all that has been fed into it, and handing out punishments. It judges the conscious rational self, the ego, and the deeper intuitive raw self, the id. There is no choice but to come to terms with guilt, putting it in perspective. Whatever the specific situation – an action, a misdeed, a break-up of a marriage, ending of an affair or friendship – to live healthily means to learn to accept reality and to make peace between an inbred sense of morality and immediate needs for survival. It is not selfish, it is practical.

Depression is a morbid sadness accompanied by a sense of futility. All these stress factors can lead to depression, but it doesn't mean necessarily you are going to get depressed if you suffer from any of them.

Psychiatrists say it is unconsciously motivated by a loss of some kind – a person, a thing, a possession, a job, security, confidence, looks, money.

The loss can be spontaneous or anticipated, but the depression is an inner reaction to the events that led up to it. It is quite different from grief, which is a realistic and appropriate reaction to a loss. Once in a state of depression every move seems to take you down further. It needs the most determined will and constructive methods to get out of it.

Women are more prone to depression than men. Many feel frustrated, bored and trapped in house-bound monotony. Boredom is the surface state; underneath is conflict supported by thoughts of repression, rebellion and dreams. A woman may feel she is lacking something important if she is satisfied with the traditional female role – and this depresses her. Or she may expect more out of her life – but what is not altogether clear. She feels inadequate, ineffectual and frustrated. Women are more prone to depression after childbirth, in the mid-thirties and at the menopause when hormone disturbances are significant. Failure in sexual relations is often a cause for depression, so is criticism or rejection.

The signs of depression are only too apparent. Sleep is often affected – sometimes there is difficulty in getting to sleep and early waking; sometimes sleep is an escape and you simply can't get enough of it. Psychosomatic illnesses are often a cover-up for depression. Intellectual lucidity diminishes, concentration is low, conversation dull and listless, reflected in passive facial expressions and a general air of boredom and indifference.

A depression can be stemmed if you recognize the symptoms and tackle them early enough. It means making a tremendous effort to meet people, to go out, to get involved. Psychic fatigue is part of depression. Loss of interest and apathy makes you too exhausted to do anything. It is necessary to force yourself to do something stimulating: specific exercise or sport is good; energy creates energy.

All causes of stress are connected with nervous response. Excessive control of stress builds up tension, and if you live under conditions of great strain, you have to find a way of relaxing. The best way to discharge neuro-muscular tension is through pleasure. The more absorbing and more physical the better.

RELAXATION

Just learning to relax and let go is the basic way to combat tension. Try some or all of these methods, but always one a day:

Breathing: Nature's way of releasing tension is to bring oxygen to all parts of the body. More important than breathing in is learning to breathe out so that the lungs are completely emptied of stale air. Breathe out longer and harder than you breathe in. Standing or sitting cross-legged on the floor, inhale to the count of four, breathe out to the count of eight. Breathe in through the nose and out through the mouth, which should be partially opened with jaw relaxed.

Lying at a slant: This is a Yoga position of relaxation, where the head is down and the feet raised twelve inches above the floor, so the body goes in a smooth backward slope. Use a firm board – a plank covered with a towel is perfect – propped or secured at the correct angle. Relax for fifteen minutes every day, eyes closed, hands by your sides. At this angle the spine straightens out and muscles, ordinarily tensed while standing, sitting or walking, are relaxed. A good time to relax like this is after a day's work, before a bath or an evening out.

Head rolling: With arms behind your back, breathe in deeply, then slowly rotate head from left to right making a complete circle. Be conscious of muscles in neck and shoulders. Do very slowly, twice in each direction.

Dangling: With legs wide apart, allow the body to fall over from the waist, so the head becomes a weight at the end of the spine. Hang and sway from side to side for about half a minute. Slowly lift up, using stomach muscles to raise the back, one vertebra at a time.

Slapping: Throw your arms alternately across your body, over the shoulder to give yourself a good slap on the back in the area of the shoulder blades. 10 slaps with each hand.

MEDITATION

This is the next step after relaxation because it releases from tension the mind as well as the body. While the body is at rest, the mind empties itself and you emerge from meditation physically revived and more mentally alert. It can also serve as a self analysis session, for when you meditate, you are forced to observe your thoughts. The process can be difficult. At the beginning it is a great strain to sit still for fifteen or twenty minutes and to clear the mind of all trivia. After practice it can be achieved. During meditation there is a drop in the rate of breathing and heart activity, brain patterns change to a more relaxed form. Experienced meditators say that you can begin to see problems objectively and dependence on forms of relief such as drugs, alcohol or cigarettes, is considerably lessened. The two most prevalent forms of meditation are Raja Yoga and Transcendental, both of which use a 'mantra' (a sound to be spoken aloud or in the head) to clear the mind. It is advisable to go for initial instruction as this gives you a better understanding of the philosophy behind meditation plus practical help on technique.

The rules are simple:

Choose a comfortable position. It is not necessary to sit cross-legged, but once accustomed to it, it helps achieve regular relaxed breathing.

Breathe slowly and rhythmically, taking twice as long to breathe out as to breathe in.

Now determine which 'mantra' you will use. The traditional ones are like our vowel sounds of ah-eh-ih-oh-uh. Repeat them all and decide which one suits you best. It is said that ah relieves anxiety, eh tension, ih aggression, oh pain and uh sexual excitement.

Introduce the chosen sound into your mind, saying it aloud at first if it helps you to concentrate. Repeat it over and over again in your head, pushing out every other thought – not with force, but with detached observation of the mind's wanderings. At first the mind runs wild and other thoughts refuse to go; both practice and patience are needed. If you find it difficult to meditate with eyes closed, focus on some object, a picture or a sculpture. This sometimes increases concentration.

Make yourself sit and learn the technique for a minimum of fifteen minutes a day. Make it a regular habit. In time you will begin to look forward to it, and find it absolutely necessary.

SLEEP

Sleep is imperative for mental and physical health. Deprived of it, we can become tense and nervous. It has always been a physiological necessity but only recently has the significance of various aspects of sleep come to light. The repose of sleep and lowered metabolism may rest and revive the body, but dreams restore the mind and discharge tension.

When we fall asleep, the eyelids close and the pupils become small. Breathing is diminished, blood pressure falls, the heart slows down, the temperature drops and the digestive juices and saliva decrease. Consciousness is lost, but only temporarily; a noise, a light, a jab can cause wakefulness. There are several stages from drowsiness to oblivious sleep where all muscles are relaxed and it is difficult to be woken. The brain still receives every sound and touch, but though it responds, it does not express messages in actions – unless you are prone to sleepwalking. Sleep is not a tranquil posture; a normal person may change position from twenty to sixty times a night.

There are two kinds of sleep – slow-wave sleep, which is dreamless and usually starts the sleeping sequence, and dreaming sleep, known as REM sleep, as it is characterized by Rapid Eye Movements. The two types alternate during the night.

REM sleep is the deepest and most refreshing, for it is both a physiological and psychological process. Dreams are said to restore the central nervous system but how is still not quite clear. They may help in the working out of emotional problems, and are necessary for psychic survival. Research has shown that if one is deprived of slow-wave sleep, it does little physical damage, but if REM sleep is interrupted it can be more serious, resulting in increased tension and nervous reactions. The natural recuperative reaction is to dream more during the next sleeping period – making up for lost dreams and lost tension relief. Dream activity therefore is good for mental health which is why you often wake up depressed after taking alcohol, barbiturates or tranquillizers – because all these decrease the amount of REM sleep.

Eight hours sleep a night is considered average and necessary to restore normal body functions and alertness. It is possible to get sufficient sleep in short spurts, provided all the benefits from the full slow-wave and REM sleep cycle are obtained. Some people claim they need more sleep than others and studies have been done on the personality types: short sleepers are usually active and outgoing, flexible, sociable and relatively high on social conformity. Long sleepers tend to be more introverted and creative but are successful at sustained work.

It doesn't matter when you sleep provided it is daily, regular and within a twenty-four hour cycle. It is the rhythm that is important, and each body has its own inner clock known as circadian rhythm – a cycle in which a 90 to 120 minute period of sleep – or wakefulness – alternates with a 5 to 10 minute dream period. It goes on unceasingly twenty-four hours a day like breathing. It is combined with an almost clocklike regularity in the rise and fall of the body's temperature. The highest points are when you feel most alive and alert, the lowest when you are daydreaming or sleep-dreaming. It is much easier to get to sleep during one of the low points in temperature, and many sleeping difficulties could be circumvented if we kept track of them. Try this, and relaxation exercises, and check other remedies detailed under 'Insomnia' (page 311).

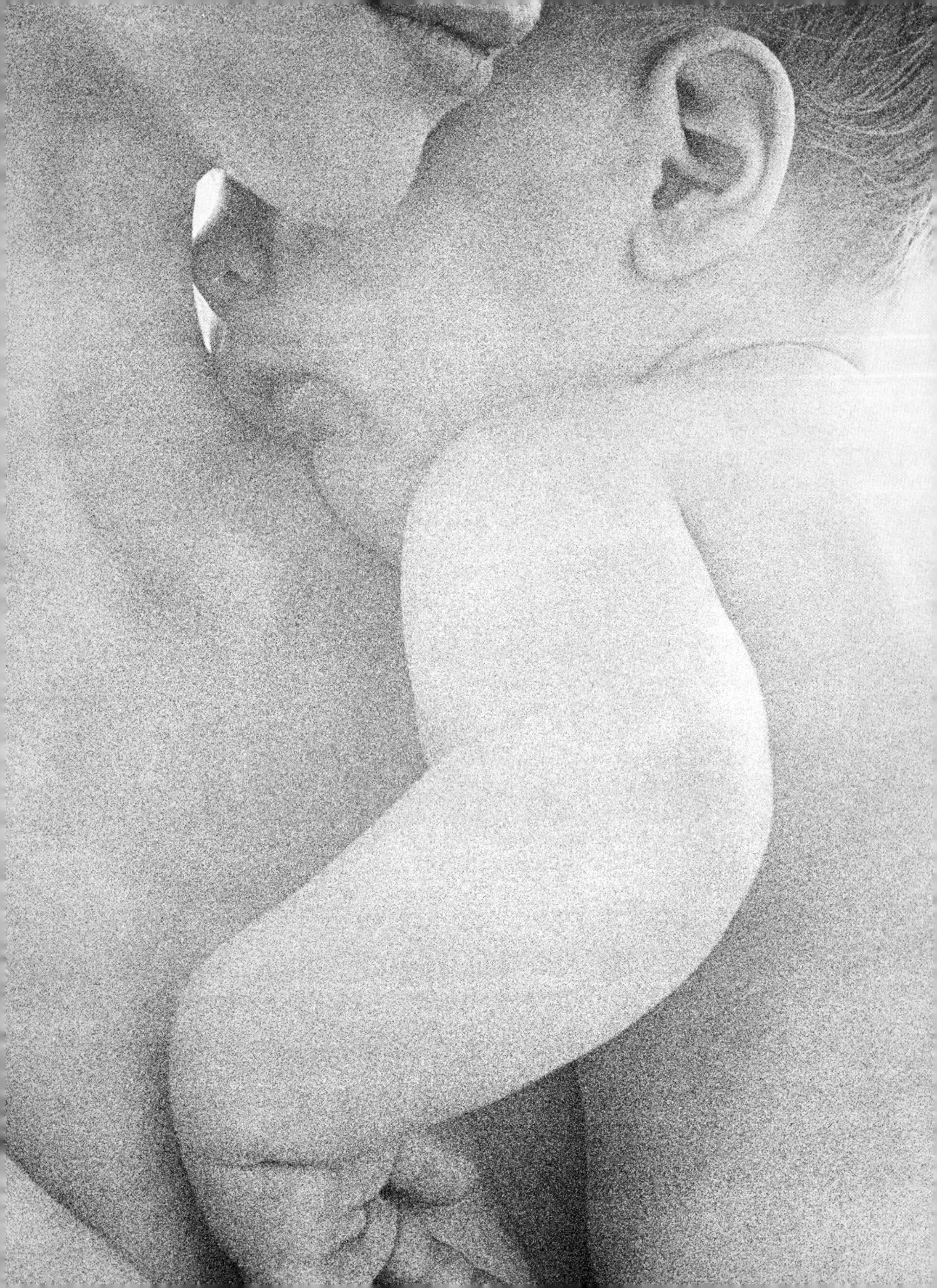

6

AGEING

Fifty years ago a woman of forty was finished. Now the boundaries are extended, but although the surrender to ageing no longer has a deadline, the ageing crisis starts earlier and lasts longer due to the emphasis on extreme youth. There is a survival instinct that pushes women through each decade with determination to keep things at a status quo; this plus a supply of survival equipment enables women to look younger, longer. What we call ageing is not the same for everyone; one woman's forty is another's sixty. Doctors cannot determine with any assurance whether a person is thirty, forty or fifty; they may misjudge by as many as fifteen years. Biological age is what matters and this can be self-determined and adjusted.

There is no mysterious fountain of youth but there is a great deal that can be done to make you look and feel younger at any age. Rejuvenation therapies are going on in many different fields – cosmetics, nutrition, psychology, surgery, endocrinology and chemistry, but the most remarkable have been in the hormone and chemical fields. The aim is not so much to prolong life as to make it more vital and rewarding though added years are often a bonus. Various elixirs of youth have claimed unbelievable things, now the approach is more realistic.

Visible ageing varies and there is no way of estimating when it will start. As we get older, the cells' capacity to reproduce, grow and renew themselves decreases – clearly seen in the way our bodies cannot heal a wound as quickly as they used to. This happens at different rates throughout the body but it is a progressive reduction which means a decline in the regulation and intensity of the vital processes. There comes a point when cells not merely fail to reproduce but actively destroy themselves. No two people age at the same rate and different cells have different life

LATEGAN

spans. A cell forming part of the tissue that lines the alimentary canal lives only thirty-six hours, while nerve cells may live until you die. Blood cells show early changes, cartilage cells change little in form during life and may even survive death by several hours.

There are many theories as to why cells become disorganized but the precise reason is by no means established. It is possibly a combination of several factors:

We age because we wear out and cells produced later in life are inferior to those produced earlier.

We are programmed to age. This is determined by heredity; we have an inbuilt mechanism scheduling cells to divide a certain number of times, after that the body reaches its limit of renewal.

A mistake in biochemistry causes dysfunction. This is connected with the theory that metabolism is maintained and directed by catalysts such as minerals, vitamins, enzymes, micro-elements and amino acids. If we succeeded in substituting the catalysts, then the cells would begin to reactivate normally and youthfully.

The accumulation of harmful hinderants blocks the tissues to such an extent that the cells are unable to perform efficiently.

The connective tissue deteriorates – the colloid theory. Many of the symptoms typical to ageing such as wrinkling and flabbiness of the skin, hardening of the arteries are related to the properties of the colloid molecules in the connective tissue.

The body loses its ability to differentiate between its own proteins and foreign ones and begins to reject its own new ones.

Whatever the reason, cell growth slows down because of the decreasing ability of the organism to renovate itself. If the laws governing activations were known, nature could be forced into regeneration. Only the control and regulation of human chemistry can lead to the final conquest of age.

PREVENTION: SELF-CARE

Growing older and staying younger is not entirely dependent on chemical control. There is a whole range of aesthetic and skin aids ranging from plastic surgery and dermabrasion to the reviving effects of fragrances but all these depend on the skill of others. Heredity, habits and environment all play a part in the way we age. The best way to look young and feel good for decades is to start early building health and care habits to last a lifetime. But it is never too late to improve – start with diet, exercise and attitude:

Diet

Keep your weight down; you will not only look younger but will have a good chance of by-passing such ageing maladies as diabetes, high blood pressure and hardening of the arteries. If blood pressure and cholesterol levels are too high you may be biologically ten years older. Not all people who are overweight die young, just as not all people who smoke get lung cancer, but statistics show that excessive weight anticipates an earlier death.

You need less food as you get older, usually no more than 1,800 Calories a day. You need the right food – vegetables, fruit, lean meat, milk, cheese, fish, little or no animal fat. You need to weigh yourself daily, even if you've never been in the habit of doing so before, as the secret is never to put on more than a few pounds above your norm. These can be taken off without too much effort or sacrifice. Starvation and crash diets are not a good idea, as these tax temper and nerves, shrivel the body and collapse the face, because the skin is no longer capable of re-adjusting its elasticity and coverage.

Be sure you are getting an adequate supply of vitamins and minerals. Supplement your diet with brewers' yeast, kelp, rose hips, yoghourt and honey. Use garlic and onions a lot; include ginseng tea in your beverages; make apricots, fresh or dried, one of your most important fruits. Vitamin E is thought to be particularly good as a regenerator, and one of its best natural sources is wheatgerm. Vitamin C is recommended to help regulate hormones and keep the collagens of connective tissue healthy.

If you have a sweet tooth, substitute these honey balls for commercial confectionery.

1 cup sesame seeds
1–2 tablespoons solid honey

Grind sesame seeds, pour into honey and knead until a firm dough; make into balls, sprinkle with coconut if you like.

Pollen tablets as a diet supplement are considered by many to help build up stamina and body resistance. They are made from pollen, which is the male sex cells of flowers and contains a concentration of essential food elements. Pollen, together with unstrained honey, is an integral part of the diet of the longest-living peoples such as the Hunzas and the Caucasians.

Exercise

Life-long exercise is ideal not only in the interests of a young figure, but for keeping circulation at its peak and thus maintaining the overall health of the body. Anyone who wants a thirty-year-old figure at sixty had better start early. Don't take up exercise suddenly, it can do more harm than good. If you've never exercised much, start gradually and with the more gentle regimes. The Mensendiek routines aren't strenuous, nor are those done in the bath or in water. Massage and electrical stimulation are relaxing. Active sports are the most enjoyable way to exercise and usually the most consistent. And walk – with a spring and with good posture; don't get into the habit of dragging yourself along – it looks and is ageing.

Attitude

Boredom and lethargy will age a person almost as quickly as poor diet or lack of exercise. Keep optimistic and interested. Never retire from living, even if you have to retire from a job, but progress from one stage to another. Remaining sexually active is an important youth preserver. It is a myth that sexual desire and ability decline in the course of ageing.

Research reveals that those who live longest do not appear to be endowed with much competitive spirit and have a pragmatic fatalism about life. This does not mean sitting back and letting things happen, but an absence of exhausting aggressive characteristics. The body needs a certain amount of stress but the amount must be controlled.

Puritans claim a relationship between a short life and a merry one. They couldn't be more wrong. Happiness and gaiety are interwoven with health and vitality.

Appearance

Looking younger doesn't mean clinging to an image of earlier days. It means accepting your age without giving in to it. Uniformity is essential: body, attitude, camouflage. It is pointless to have a young face on an old body, or bright hair over wrinkles, or to act like a young girl when you look more like her mother.

Your personality shows when you are older. What you have been thinking for years is revealed in facial expressions, gestures and sounds. Your faults can become exaggerated and permanent.

The attention a mature woman gives to her appearance must be specialized and consistent. Looks are not luck but a daily responsibility.

You need not spend a great deal of time each day, but it must be every day. The good-looking vital woman with the young figure, the smooth skin, the shining hair is a study in discipline.

THE MENOPAUSE

Women are the only animals who outlive their capacity to reproduce. Throughout adolescence and maturity, female hormones affect a woman's sexuality, appearance and temperament. There are two hormones involved – oestrogen and progesterone – and for the duration of a woman's productive life they appear in a cyclical pattern. Oestrogen is more plentiful in the first half of the cycle and progesterone during the second. Primarily they cause the lining of the womb to thicken each month in preparation for a possible pregnancy and lead to menstruation if conception does not occur.

When most women reach their middle or late forties, the supply of oestrogen in the body is greatly reduced and finally stops altogether. This is known as the menopause and has far-reaching effects. No more than 20% of normal women are fortunate enough to undergo a menopause free of symptoms.

Strictly speaking, the menopause is the date of the last menstrual period, and the climacteric is the transition phase of ovarian function which can extend for some two years before or some two years after. The average age is 48, with a normal range from 45 to 52. No two women have the same experience. The more rapidly the ovaries fail, the greater the likelihood of severe symptoms. A few women menstruate as usual and then suddenly never have another period. Often periods gradually become scanty and irregular, sometimes disappearing only to return before ending completely. Signs and symptoms can begin before any alteration in the menstrual pattern; sometimes they come at the same time as cessation or may not occur until years afterwards. One symptom usually appears first, to be joined by others:

Hot flushes and sweating – probably the most distressing of the early symptoms; a feeling of heat rises from the chest to the head and the face becomes red; it may be accompanied by excessive perspiration; in many women, stress or excitement tends to bring on these symptoms.

Emotional changes – include feelings of nervousness, irritability, depression, weepiness, difficulty in concentrating, loss of memory and confidence, apprehension.

Sexual implications – loss of vaginal tissue and less plentiful secretions can cause dryness to a degree of atrophy so severe that intercourse is often impossible; in addition there is often a decrease in sexual responsiveness.

Bone alterations – changes often take place in the skeleton; bones may lose some of their protein, slowly becoming more brittle with a tendency towards osteoporosis (weakened bones). This is why women often break their hips or wrists even in minor accidents. The spine often becomes weak and curved, a condition known as dowager's hump. Bone aches and associated muscle pain are common.

Body and skin changes – skin as a whole becomes thinner, less firm and loses its elasticity; breasts shrink and lose their contour as muscle and skin tone diminishes; hair becomes brittle and thinner.

Until recently women have had to put up with the menopause with little help except aspirins, tranquillizers and reassurance that it was 'normal'. It is now becoming accepted in medical circles that hormonal supplements are of enormous value in counteracting all the effects of the menopause.

HORMONE REPLACEMENT THERAPY (HRT)

In recent years, oestrogen has had considerable publicity as a factor in controlling the adverse effects of ageing, particularly the menopause. It has been a controversial issue, but now doctors are more convinced that this is a correct and indicated treatment.

Replacement oestrogen does not make a woman fertile again but it does continue its protective and constructive jobs. It keeps bones strong and prevents osteoporosis, it helps to keep tissues healthy and preserves muscle tone, it keeps the vagina in shape and lubricated, it cures the hot flushes and the sweating, and by raising the level of tryptophan (an amino acid) in the blood, emotions are once more better balanced, most notably depressions are lifted. It is also believed to help prevent heart disease to which women are as prone as men after feminine hormones begin to decrease. In fact, replacement of oestrogen reverses the effects of the menopause.

For some women, the glandular imbalance may appear to make little or no difference for some years because oestrogen continues to be produced by other glands. But it is estimated that up to 50 per cent of women do need HRT and another 25 per cent would look better and feel happier with it. Specialists, however, stress that it should only be used under medical control, and that each patient must be individually assessed for treatment and dosage. A simple test establishes oestrogen level. There is sometimes a little weight gain at first, and the breasts can become larger and more active. Usually both return to normal in time.

The correct administration is extremely important. Oestrogen should be prescribed on a cyclic basis of three weeks out of every four and preferably with the addition of progestagen. The doctors who pioneered HRT advocate the combined therapy. It works this way: replacement oestrogen not only restores normality to many body functions, but builds up the lining of the womb. Although impregnation is impossible, it is not a sound idea to thicken the walls of the womb for a long period. Abnormal thickening can lead to a condition called hyperplasia, which has been known to precede or coexist with early cancer. The answer is to stop oestrogen for one week in four, thus allowing the level to drop and usually permitting any build-up to shed – more or less in the old menstrual pattern. To be sure of this the second female hormone of progestagen should be used for five days at the end of each cycle. However, many women are reluctant to accept obligatory withdrawal and subsequent bleeding. It is a rather short-sighted attitude. An additional point for the case of progestagen is that regulated bleeding prevents a possible break-through of blood and any subsequent examinations and tests to find out why it happened.

There is no evidence that HRT increases the risk of cancer in the breast or uterus or elsewhere. At first this was a fear, together with apprehension about it being a contributory factor in thrombosis. These doubts have no clinical support. These hormones have been submitted to many tests and questions – and survived. Some are manufactured from extracts in the urine of pregnant mares, others are chemical compounds.

CELLULAR THERAPY

This treatment is reactivation for the whole body. Organs are stimulated into renewed action and thus motivate metabolism back to its earlier more vigorous state of activity, avoiding the necessity of medical supplements or substitutions.

It began with Professor Paul Niehans in the early 1930s, and despite constant and current scepticism on the part of orthodox medicine, it still ranks high among rejuvenation methods. Niehans died (in his eighties) in 1971 but his exclusive La Prairie Clinic in Vevey, Switzerland continues treatment. There are other centres scattered over Europe, and in Germany alone there are 500 doctors registered as cell therapists, though not necessarily devoting their entire time to it.

Early in his career, Niehans was regarded as an outstanding expert in endocrinology. By chance he stumbled on a way for the body to accept organ replacements. A patient arrived in a parathyroid condition with no time left to be helped by surgery. On impulse Niehans chopped up the parathyroid gland of an ox, put it in a saline solution and injected it. The patient tolerated the intrusion, recovered and lived on for a quarter of a century.

From this example of human tolerance and acceptance of an animal organ (hitherto denounced as impossible and unsafe), Niehans reasoned that the body might be able to accept, or at least in some way exploit, animal cells. He decided to use embryonic cells where regeneration power and possibilities were strongest. He worked on the old medical principle of like heals like, and injected the identical cell to that in the human body in need of revitalization. For example, if the patient has a liver condition, fresh liver cells are used to stimulate the patient's own liver; heart cells combat heart disease; placenta cells alleviate angina and after-birth exhaustion. The fresh embryonic cells come from the foetus of a lamb, and Niehans preferred to use them as fresh as possible, literally minutes after extraction. Whether they are assimilated or whether they act as a catalyst is not understood, but they do help to begin a reactivation process, and it has been photographically shown that injected cells do migrate to the corresponding organ in the body. The recharging only works so long as organs have not deteriorated beyond a certain point.

The case for cellular therapy is still based on empirical evidence. Positive subjective reports or analysis of individual case histories showing before and after findings, are not sufficient for orthodox acceptance. Patients are first examined and a thorough diagnosis is made of what organs are ailing, confirmed by special analytical tests. The appropriate extracts are prepared and injected into the patient's buttocks. Treatment lasts 3–5 days usually. A diet is given, some restrictions imposed, such as no alcohol for several months, no sun, no saunas. Patients often claim to feel better at once but this improvement is usually temporary and frequently in the mind. The real benefits are not experienced for about three months, when visible and physical improvements appear.

Not all cellular therapists inject fresh cellular matter; some use dried cells in solution, others extracts of cells comprising the essential ribonucleic acids which contain the blueprints for renewal. Treatment can be used as a preventive measure, to ward off the effects of oncoming age rather than help counteract them. Treatment is not a once-in-a-lifetime project. A repeat is recommended every five years or so depending on how early you received the first treatment and how old you are. Niehans never claimed that his therapy could help keep anyone alive and younger indefinitely, but stressed that a better, more youthful life was possible throughout the natural span.

Organically the system can be improved; digestive disturbances respond well, so do conditions involving the heart and the arteries. Liver and kidney ailments are frequently treated. It is possible to treat any part of the body where malfunction or slow metabolism is the problem. The best results are seen in glandular disturbances, degenerative and stress disorders. The most frequent demands are for help with impotence and frigidity, menopausal and menstruation difficulties. In the case of the menopause, improvement is claimed in all the usual resulting disorders.

Despite the resistance of medical authorities to these ideas and claims, many women continue to seek out cellular therapists. One thing is a fact: the records of cellular therapy since Niehans began in 1931 have shown that it is certainly safe. Whether effective or not is a personal judgement.

PROCAINE THERAPY

Another approach to age retardation is a drug called Gerovital (also known as GH-3) which has the reputation of diminishing almost all the inflictions of ageing. The discoverer of Gerovital is Professor Ana Aslan of Romania, who over the years has treated more than 100,000 patients in her clinic in Bucharest. Gerovital is a white soluble crystalline substance known as procaine hydrochloride, commonly familiar as novocain and used as a local anaesthetic in dentistry and minor surgery.

Like other revitalizing agents, it was not the result of planned research at all. Professor Aslan was treating elderly patients suffering from rheumatism with procaine injections to alleviate pain and discomfort. She found and observed over a period of seven years that it also made them more active in mind and body, in addition cleared up many skin troubles. From these incidental findings developed Gerovital, which also contains other ingredients including benzoic acid and potassium salts which alter the action of procaine, expanding and prolonging its effect.

Professor Aslan was put at the head of a special geriatric clinic and large-scale experiments were initiated. She did not know exactly how and why it worked, but it did, and she was able to produce substantial clinical evidence to back her claim. The first change is normally in mental functions and physical changes occur shortly afterwards. One of the earliest visible signs is improvement in the skin – it softens, wrinkles smooth out, colour brightens and pigmentation improves. Hair has been known to grow more thickly again. Its effect on psycho-mental functions is particularly significant because the depression so often associated with ageing causes many other diseases. Once this is alleviated the related disorders are often removed. Professor Aslan and other protagonists of Gerovital say it is successful in stimulating cell renewal, in stimulating the circulatory system, in strengthening bones and joints, heightening the endocrine glands, and has a mobilizing effect on cholesterol.

Initially it was met with doubts by the medical hierarchy though the interest and support of the public were overwhelming. The Romanian government gives its complete approval to the treatment and dispenses the drug in 150 centres throughout the country. Patients at the Bucharest Clinic need a series of 12 injections over a period from 10 days to 2 weeks. Effects wear off, so it is advisable to repeat them before a year has passed. In some countries the drug is considered acceptable as an anti-depressant measure but discounted as an anti-ageing method.

The Germans recognized the potential of Gerovital and developed the drug in tablet form, quickly named 'The Youth Pill'. It is known as KH-3 and is a combination of procaine and haematoporphine which acts as a catalyst. It is readily available in European pharmacies, and the prescription is one capsule a day for five months. Its effectiveness has still to be substantially proved. It is not advisable for women under 30 or pregnant women; no side effects are known, but it is a cautionary measure. Generally speaking KH-3 is said to have the same effect as a super-vitamin, but it is also believed to have a direct catalytic effect on the chemistry of the cell itself. No one really knows.

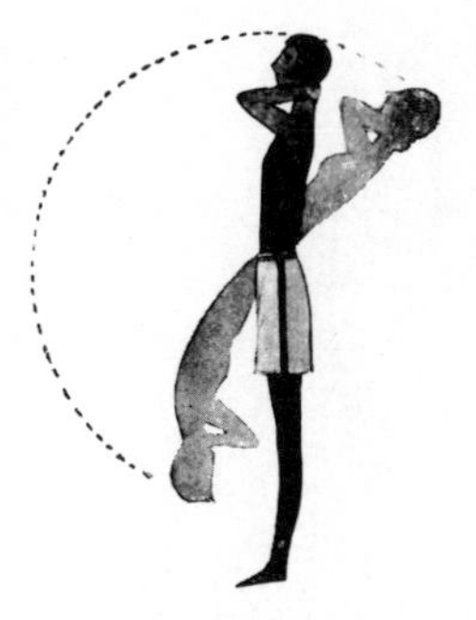

THE BODY

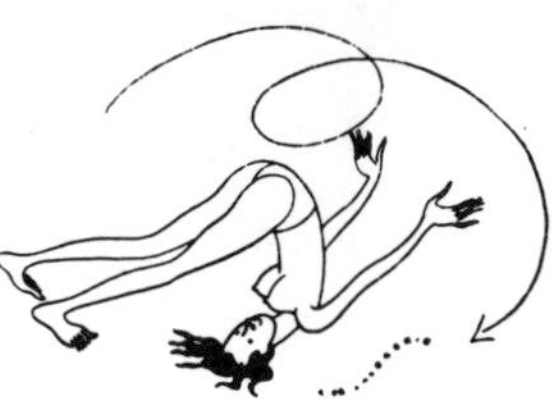

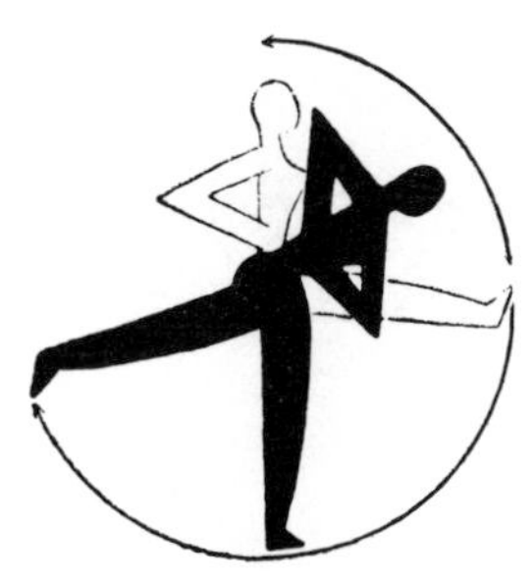

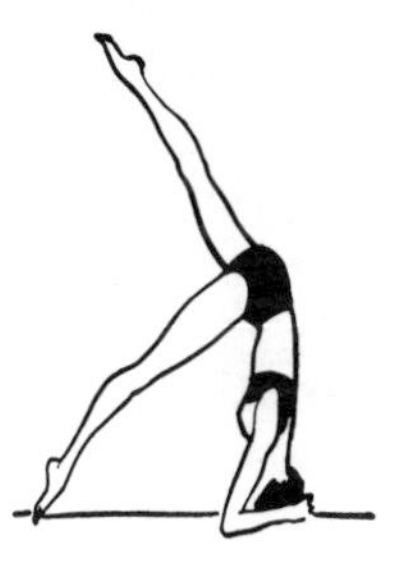

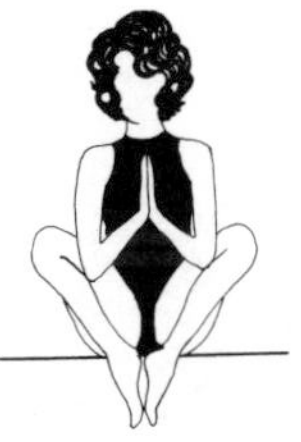

In the 1920s women sailed, swam, skied and played tennis – poker face Helen Wills and temperamental Suzanne Lenglen were the idols. It was chic to be thin – and for thinning legs, ankles and for tired feet 'Sculpto Crystals' were 'unsurpassed'. 'A new aid for those who are troubled by excess of avoirdupois is the Rub Away, an excellent massage roller composed of hollow cylinders of rubber.' 'Excessive underarm perspiration' was the 'menace to every woman's daintiness' and you could send for a sample of ODO-RO-NO for only 3d. With the 1930s came the great open-air cult. Sunbathing was the craze and stripped, oiled sun worshippers lay on roofs and beaches, toasting each side. Kensington's 'perfect spa' for the culture of health and beauty had 'every kind of bath ever invented – Vichy, Brine, Wax, Pine Needle, Foam, Aeration and Sulphur'. To the question, 'Please Vogue my brow is wet with honest sweat. And not only my brow. What can I do to keep fresh?' the reply was, 'We, personally, swear by Perstik and Perstop.' The 1940s was the age of health care and the 'diary of a bright young thing': feed the glands, the body reduces itself . . . and don't rely on the War to 'slim away' stoutness. Vogue *said: 'The new beauty has stiffened her spine and improved her figure.' The psychologists moved into the beauty field and recommended the overweight to think less about 'how delicious' and more about 'how many inches'. With the 1960s came the health food kick, growing your own vegetables and eating pure foods without preservatives or additives. More and more of the body was bared and by 1966: 'Bikinis have never been more minimal, nor the chance of a smooth tan from head to foot more possible.' Comfort was sacrificed to the youth cult and the ideal was to look like a thin coltish child in the early teens. What now, what next? People look less self-conscious, more natural, more relaxed. 'Today people are more than just aware of being overweight, they are doing something about it. To be obese is an offence – against society and yourself.'*

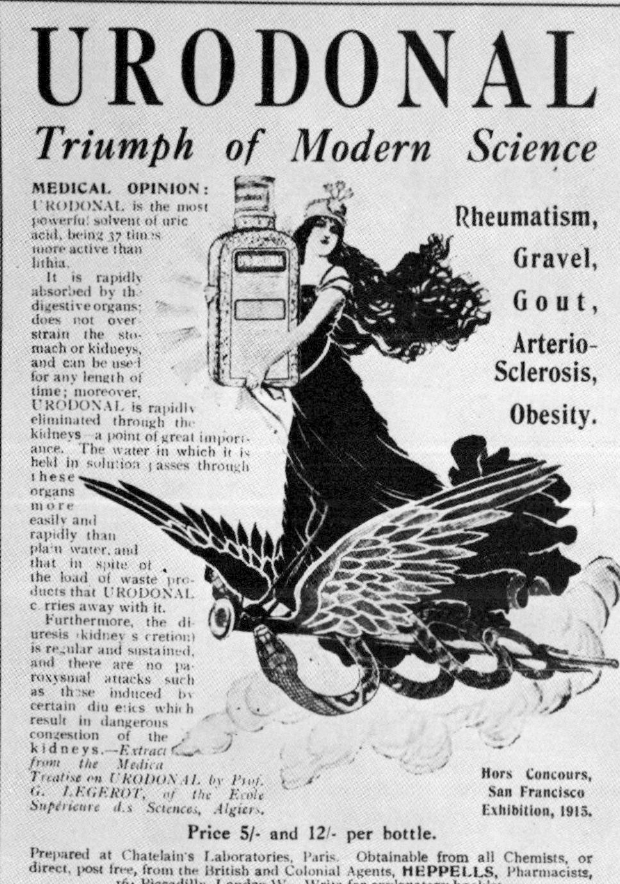

URODONAL
Triumph of Modern Science
MEDICAL OPINION: URODONAL is the most powerful solvent of uric acid, being 37 times more active than lithia.
It is rapidly absorbed by the digestive organs; does not overstrain the stomach or kidneys, and can be used for any length of time; moreover, URODONAL is rapidly eliminated through the kidneys—a point of great importance. The water in which it is held in solution passes through these organs more easily and rapidly than plain water, and that in spite of the load of waste products that URODONAL carries away with it.
Furthermore, the diuresis (kidney secretion) is regular and sustained, and there are no paroxysmal attacks such as those induced by certain diuretics which result in dangerous congestion of the kidneys.—Extract from the Medical Treatise on URODONAL by Prof. G. LEGEROT, of the Ecole Supérieure des Sciences, Algiers.
Rheumatism,
Gravel,
Gout,
Arterio-Sclerosis,
Obesity.
Hors Concours, San Francisco Exhibition, 1915.
Price 5/- and 12/- per bottle.
Prepared at Chatelain's Laboratories, Paris. Obtainable from all Chemists, or direct, post free, from the British and Colonial Agents, HEPPELLS, Pharmacists, 164 Piccadilly, London W. Write for explanatory booklet.

1917

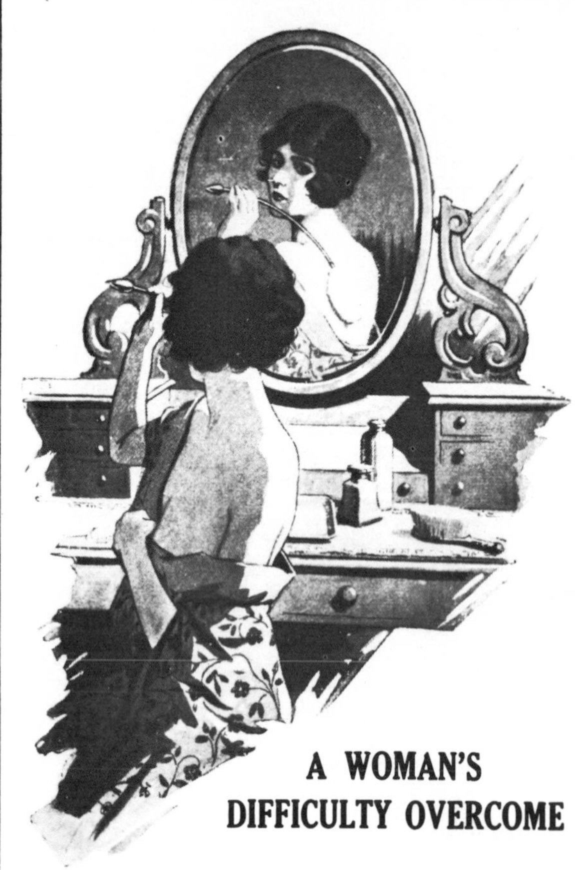

THE AMBEDIA BACK PUFF

(Patent No. 182060).

Price 15/- Complete.

Of all High-Class Chemists, Stores, and Ladies' Salons, or direct from—

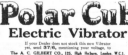

DEARBORN Ltd.,

(Dept. V.)

37, GRAY'S INN RD.,

LONDON, W.C.1

1922

'To achieve beauty without make-up
by means of electricity
and gentle massage is the secret
of a beauty specialist.'

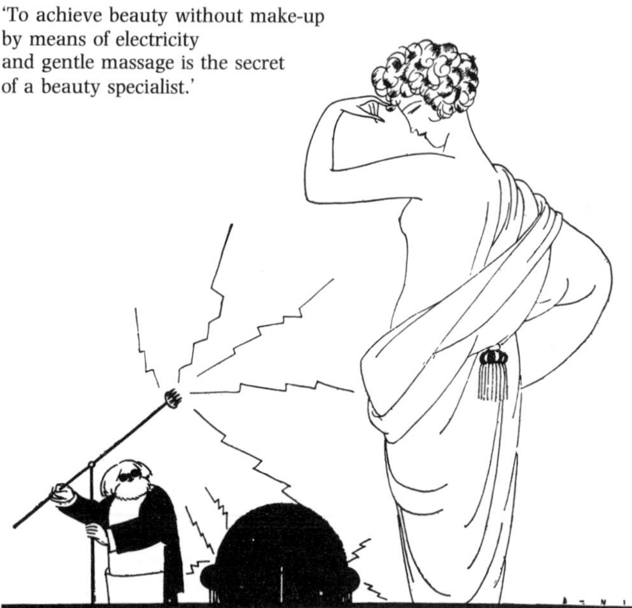

BENITO 1922

Be your own Beauty Specialist

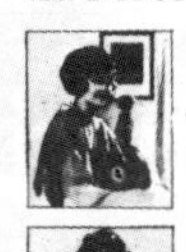

THE Polar Cub Electric Vibrator enables every woman who cares about her appearance, to gain in the privacy of her own home the full benefits of *electric massage*—the most successful and up-to-date treatment for preserving the beauty of the face and figure.

Polar Cub treatment really does remove wrinkles and hollows. Polar Cub Electric massage is splendid for your scalp. Polar Cub Electric massage is recommended for nervous disorders. It brings instant relief in cases of headache, fatigue and general "nerviness." Order a Polar Cub Vibrator to-day.

To use it is simplicity itself. Just remove the electric light bulb and attach the Vibrator. It is perfectly safe and perfectly harmless.

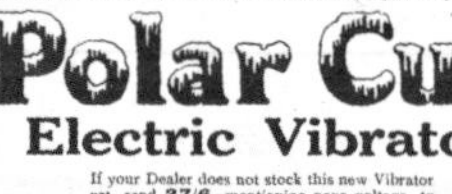

Electric Vibrator

If your Dealer does not stock this new Vibrator yet, send 37/6, mentioning your voltage, to
The A. C. GILBERT CO., 125, High Holborn, London, W.C.1.

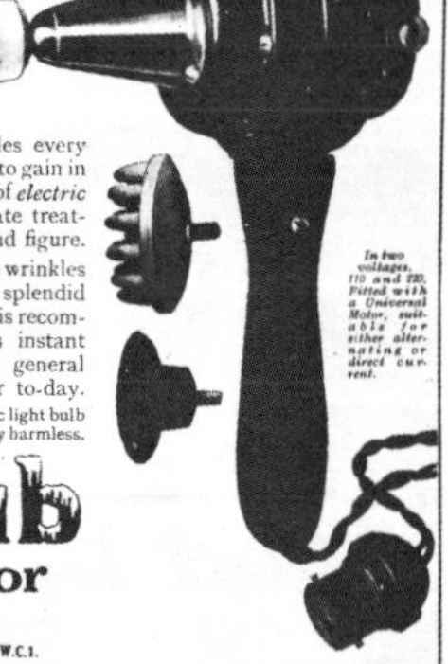

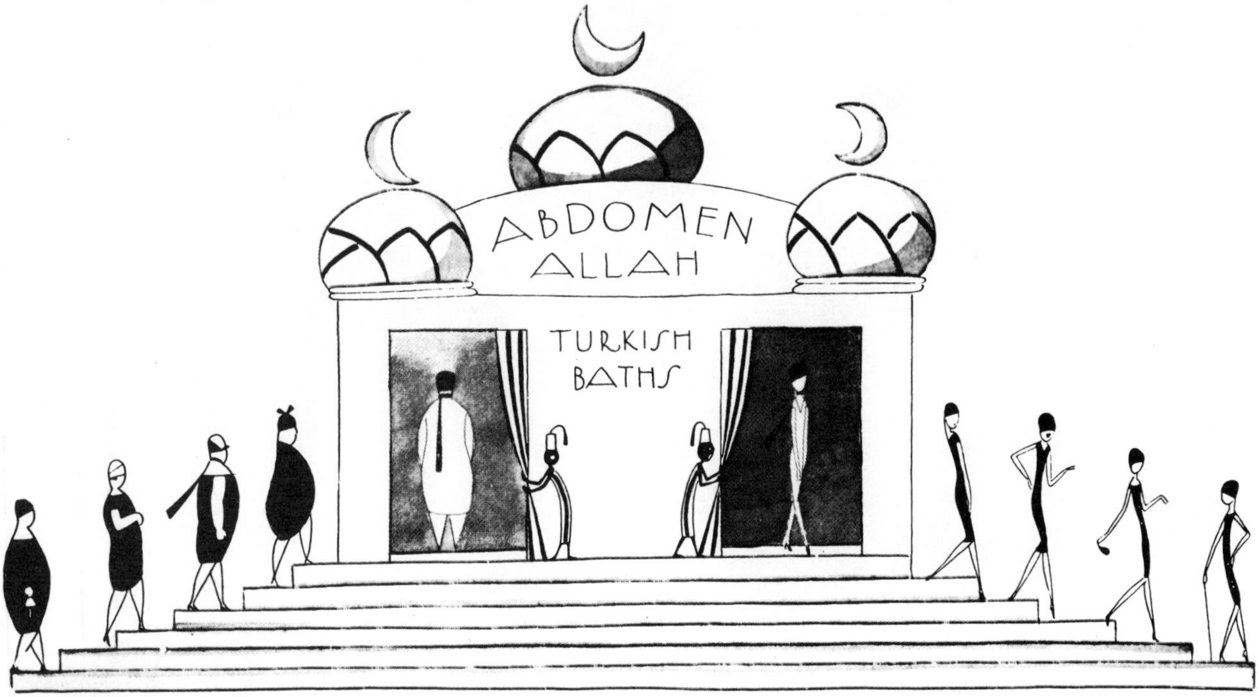

FISH 1925

'Entering the left hand portal of Abdomen Allah's fashionable aquarium, we see the portly female clientele on their way to take the waters, the steam bath, the hot room, the massage and other tortures prescribed by the terrible Turkish regime. Notice that the ladies resemble five of the most upholstered ottomans in the Ottoman Empire. But wait . . . Incredible as it may seem, the quintette of slim *Vogue* silhouettes, making their exit at the right, are the same monumental matrons who, at the left, occupied more than their full share of cubic space. The Turkish Bath has done it. Now they can face their modistes unashamed and slip into small size frocks without ignominy, shame, or rubber girdles.'

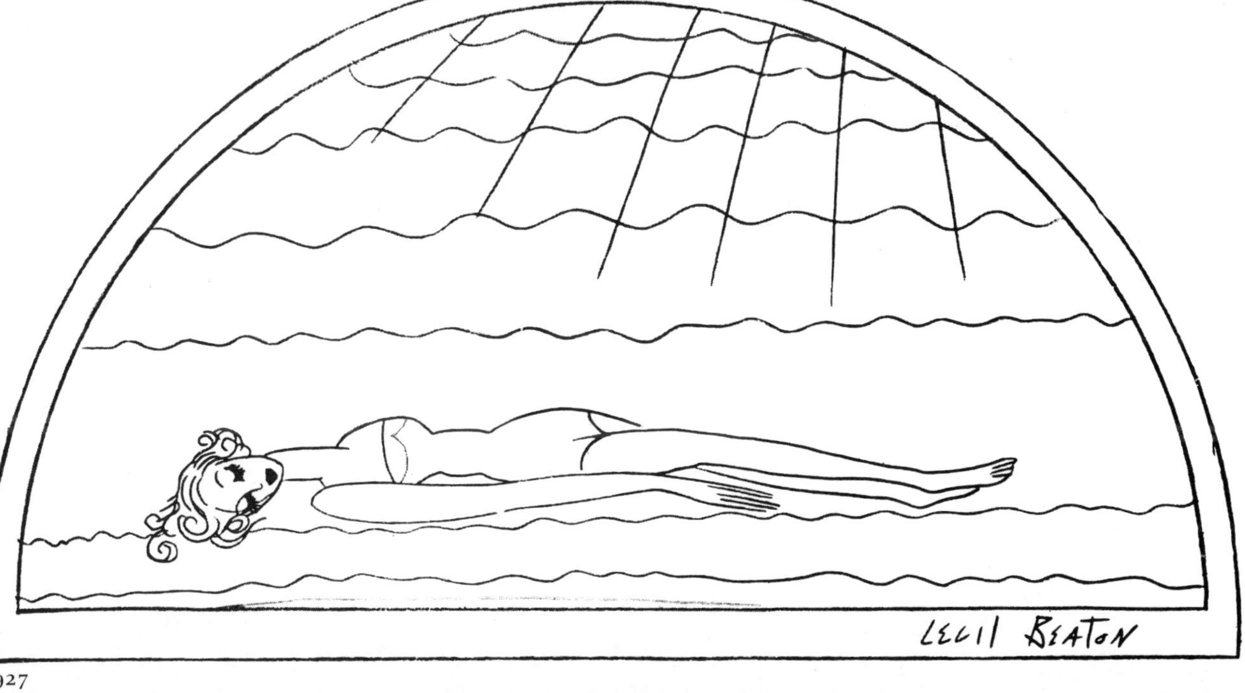

1927

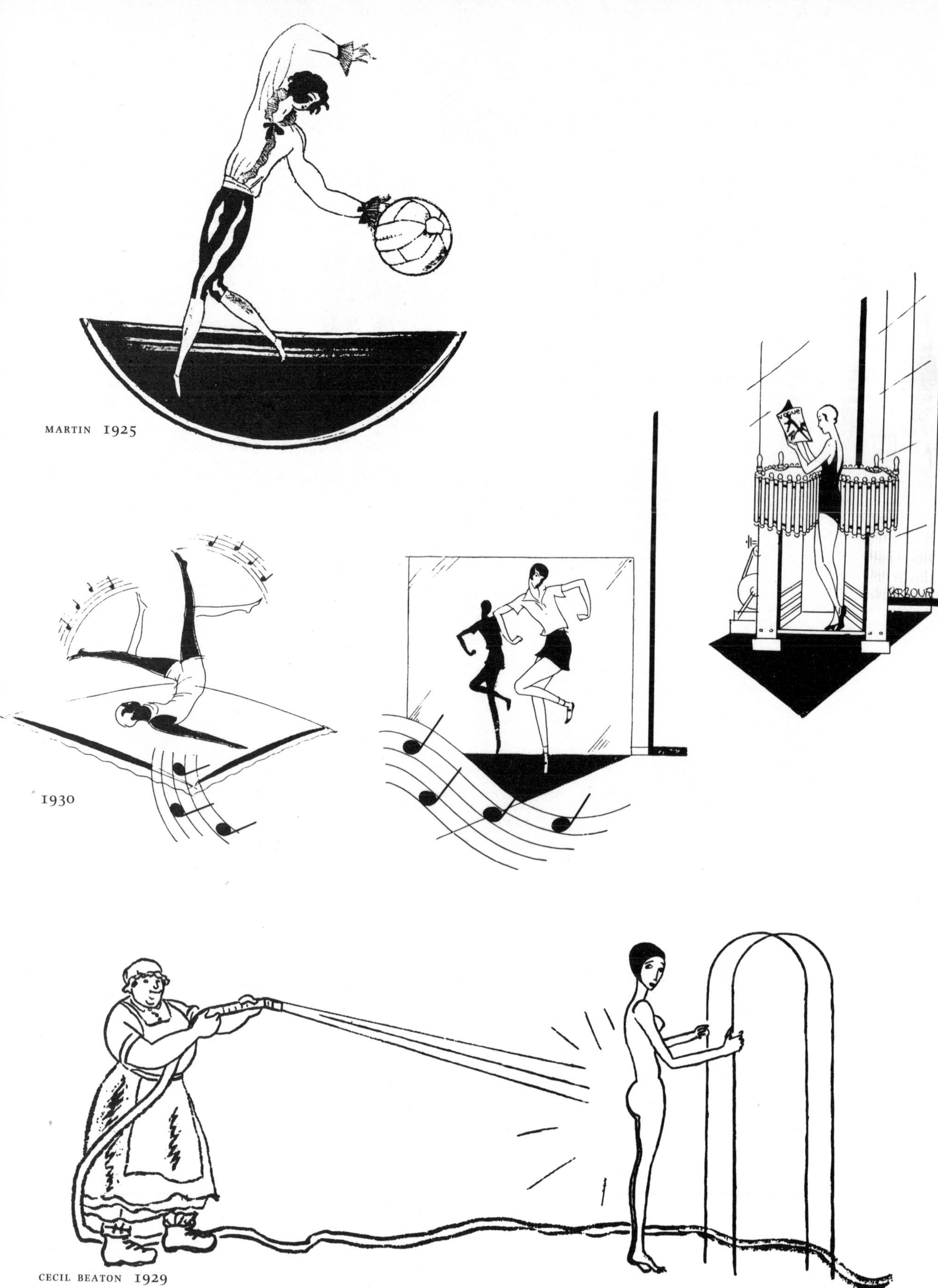

MARTIN 1925

1930

CECIL BEATON 1929

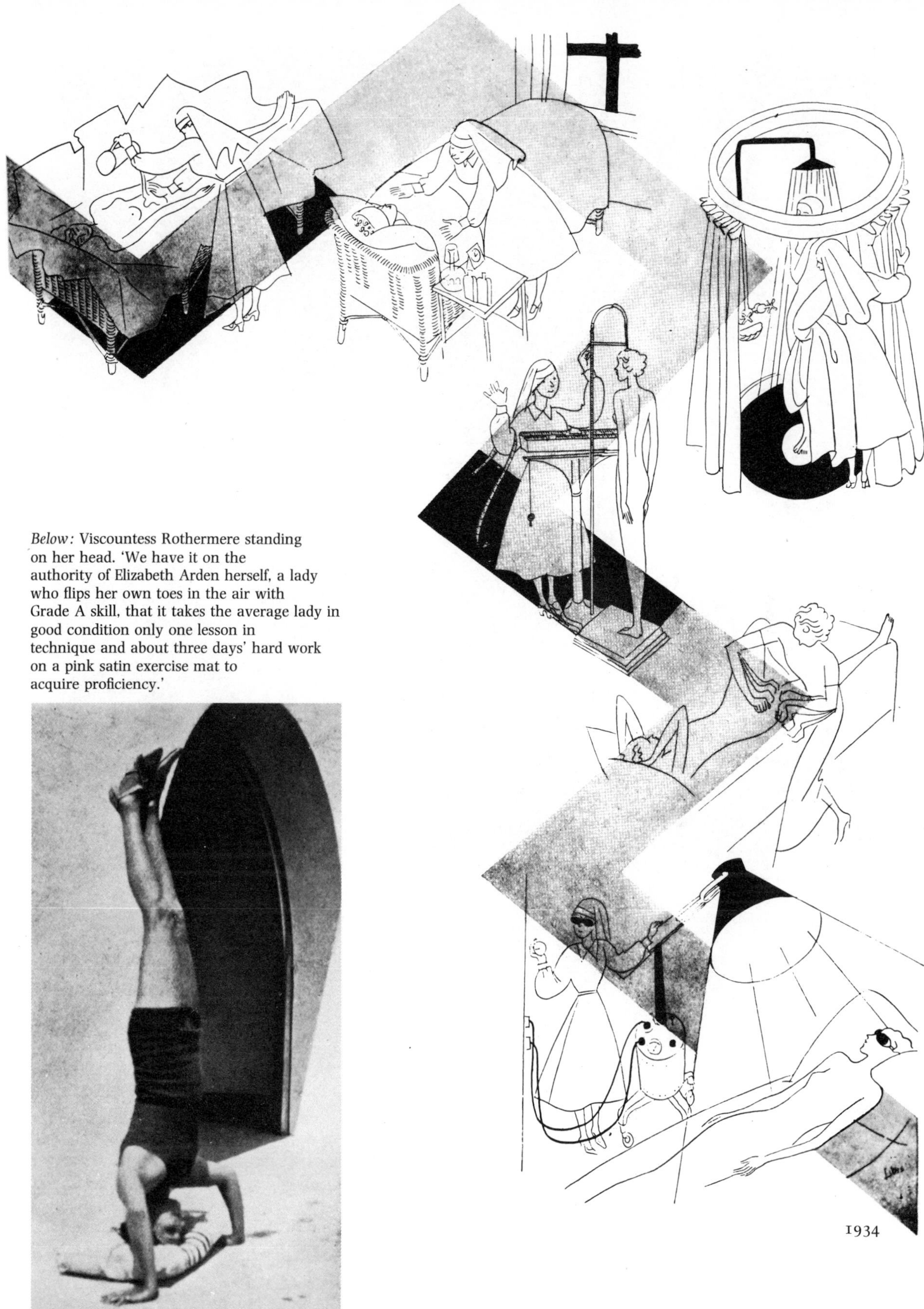

Below: Viscountess Rothermere standing on her head. 'We have it on the authority of Elizabeth Arden herself, a lady who flips her own toes in the air with Grade A skill, that it takes the average lady in good condition only one lesson in technique and about three days' hard work on a pink satin exercise mat to acquire proficiency.'

1934

1932

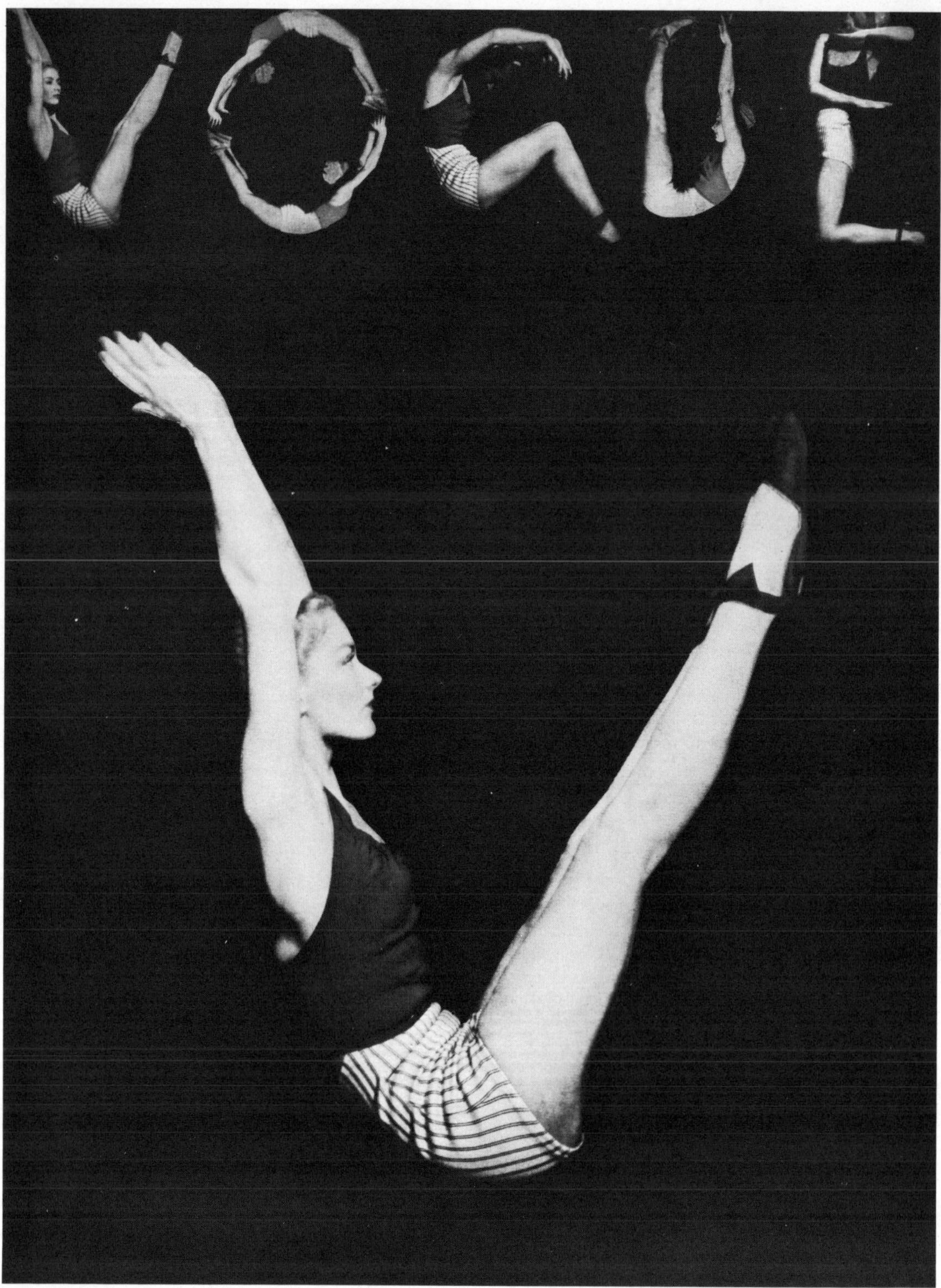

HORST 1940

GJON MILI 1943

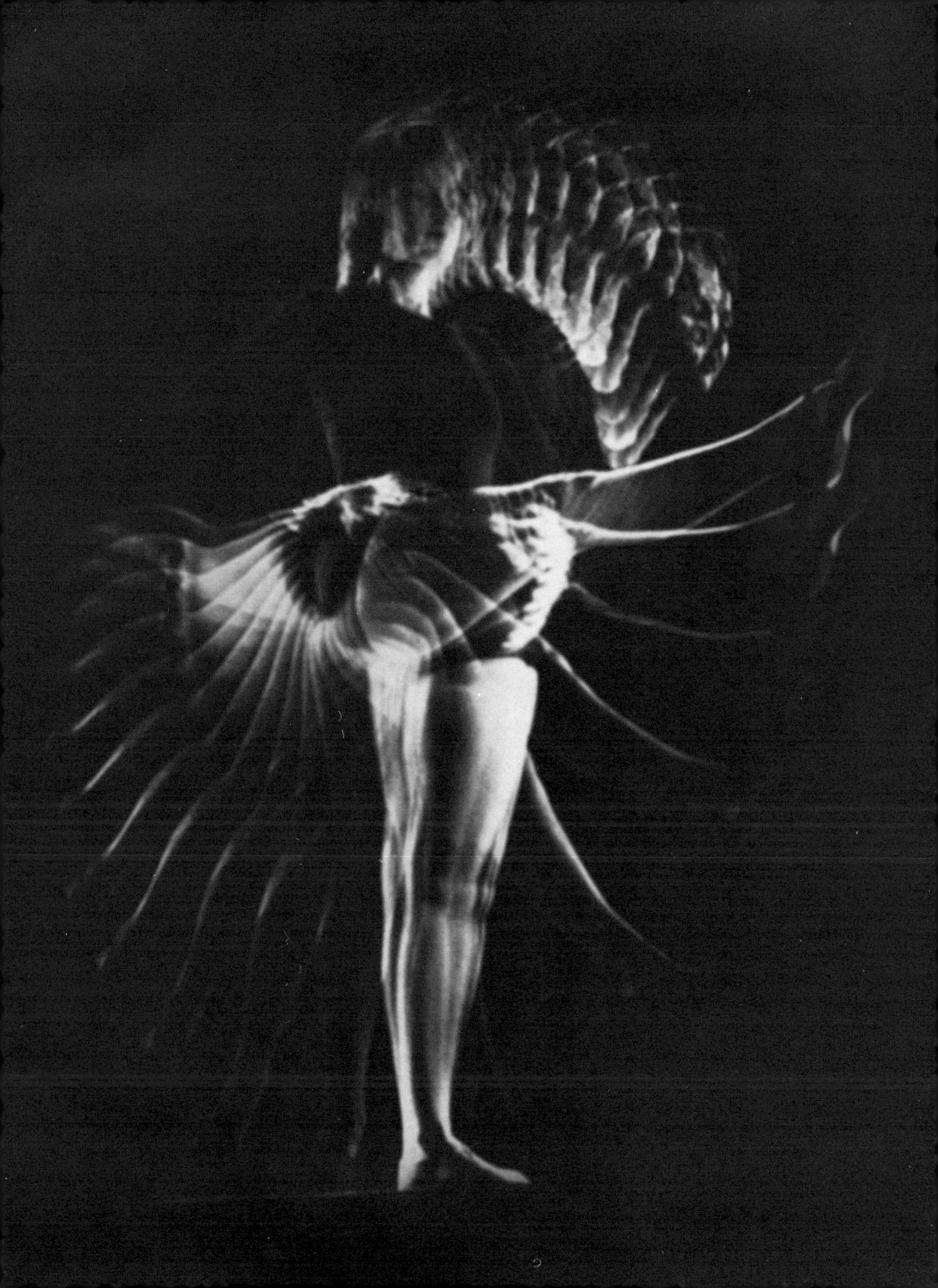

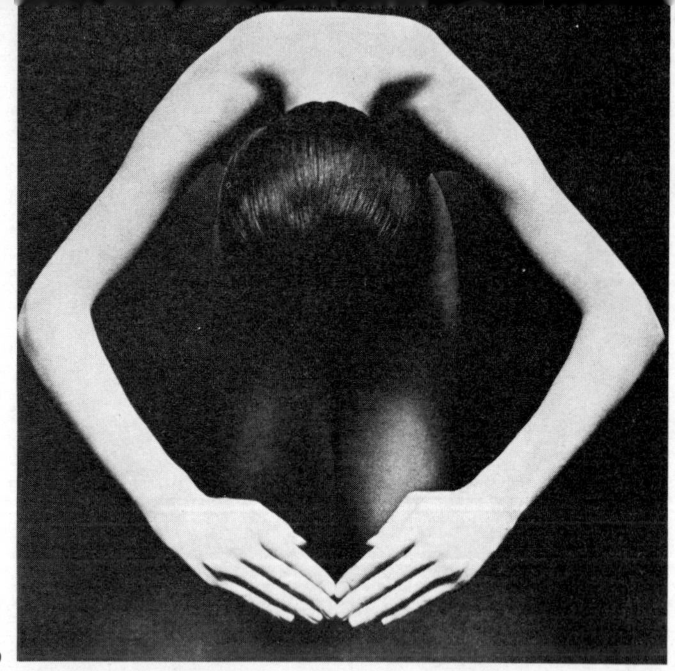

GUY BOURDIN 1969

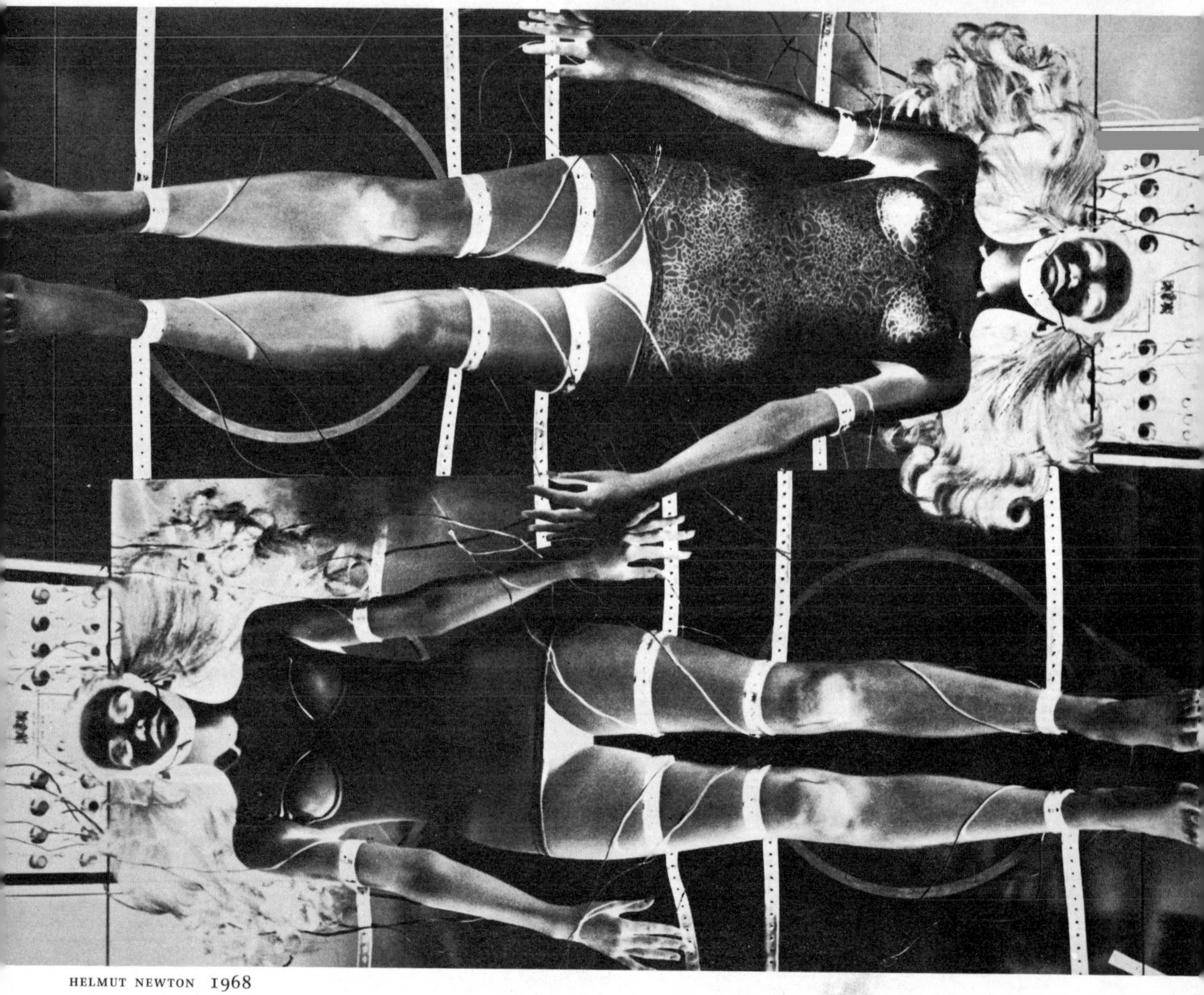

HELMUT NEWTON 1968

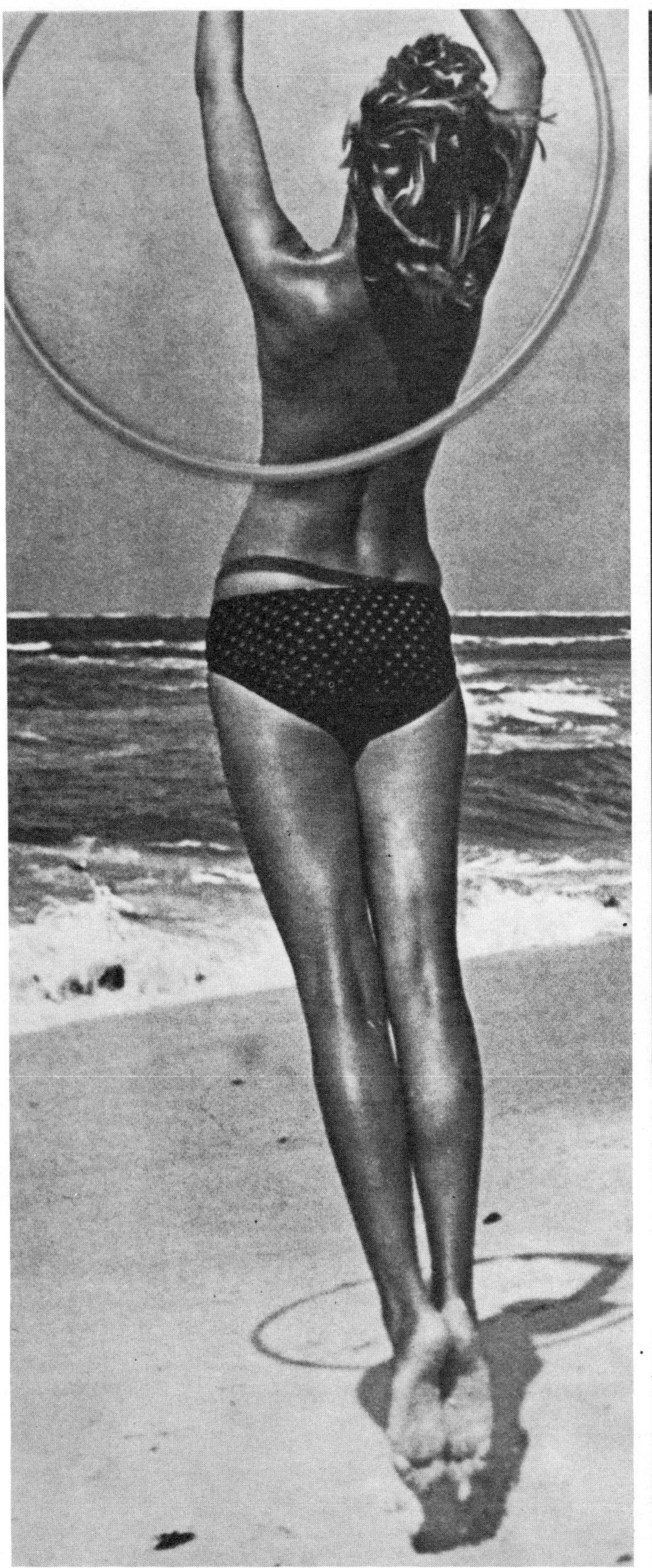

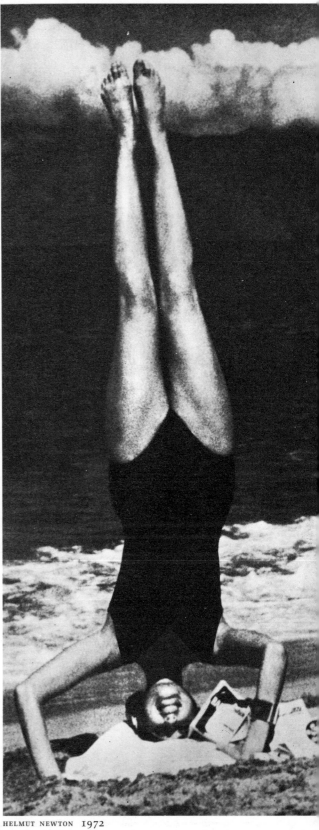

MIKE REINHARDT 1972

HELMUT NEWTON 1972

INDEX

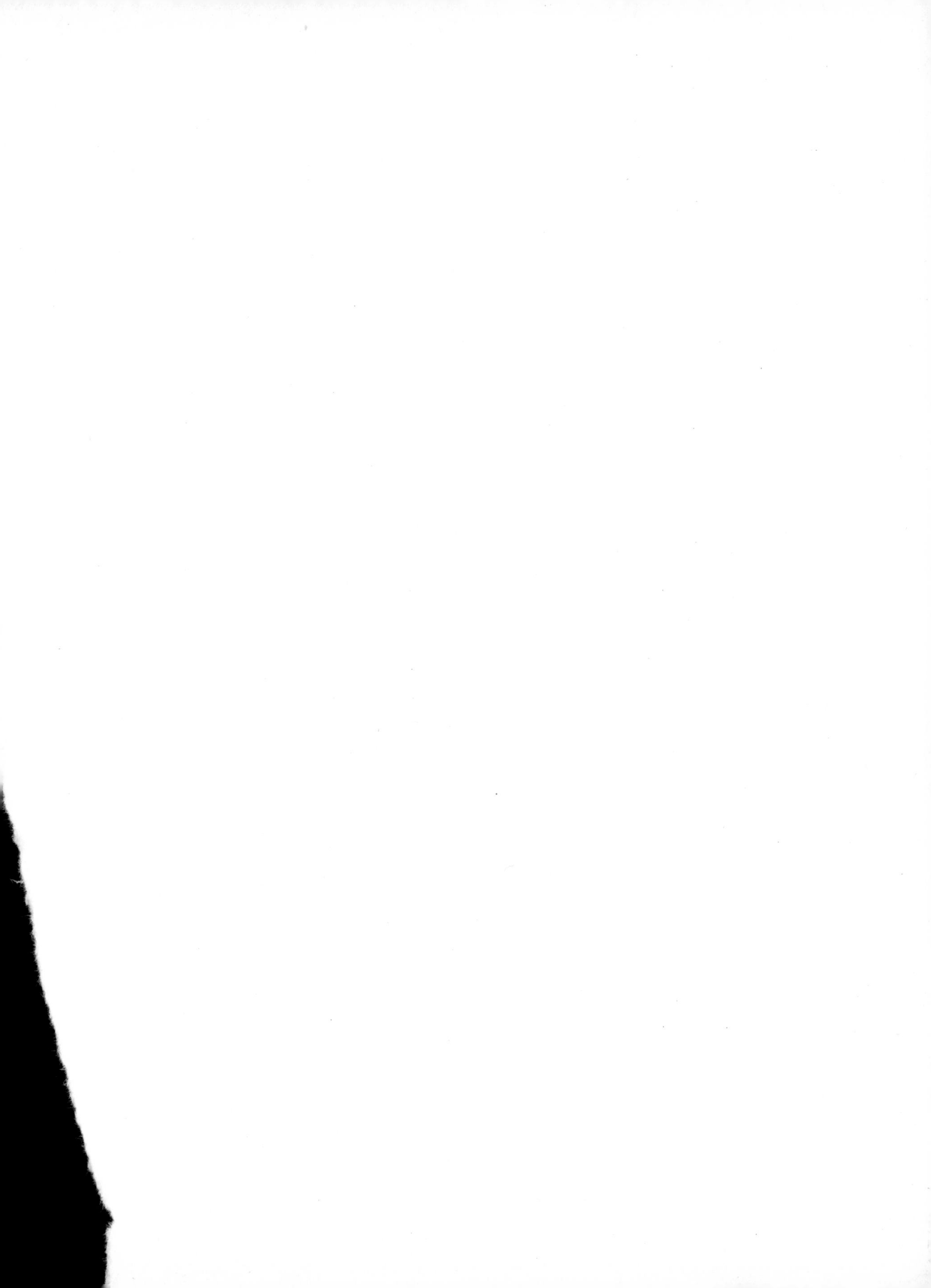

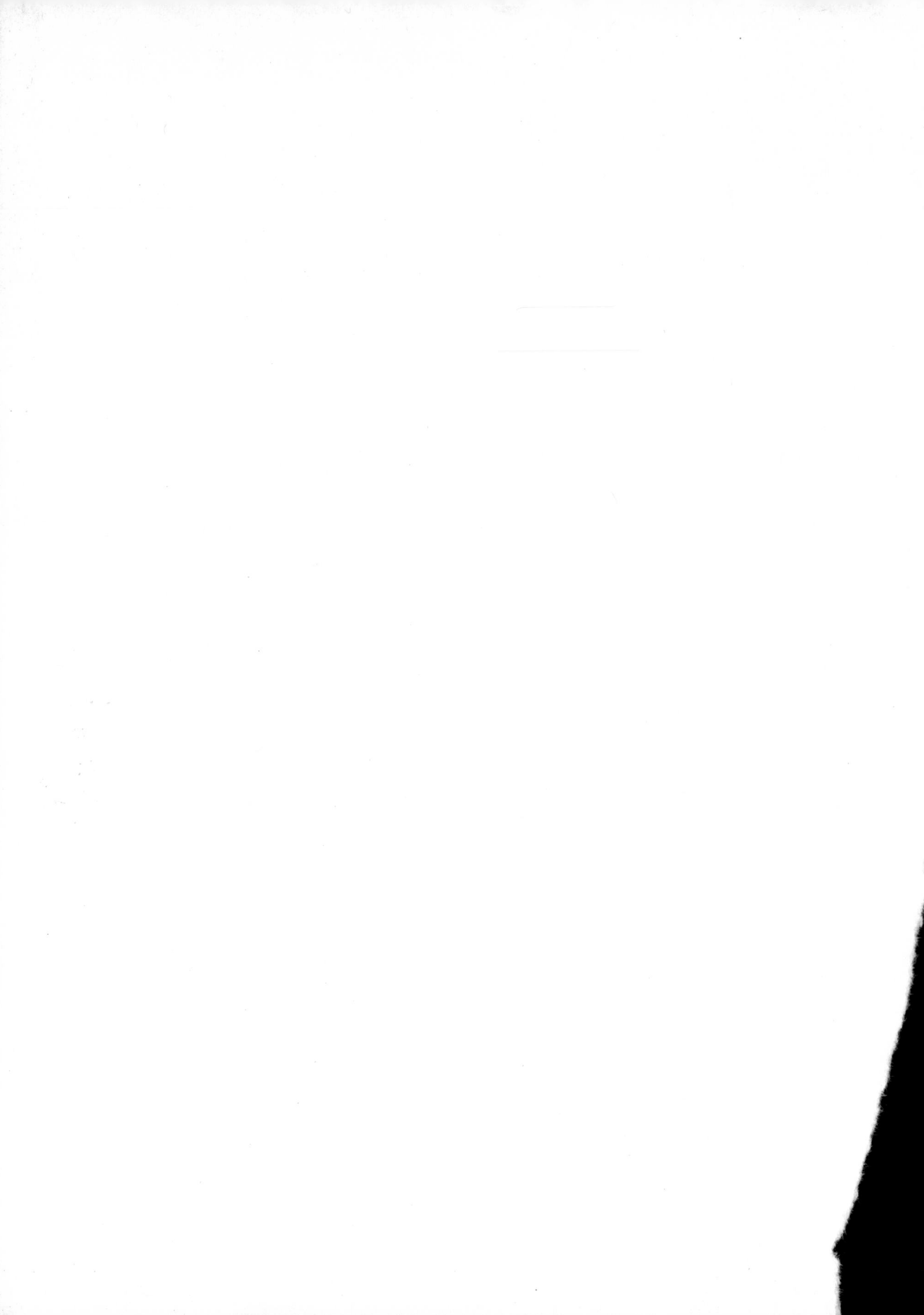